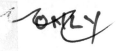
Handbook on
Animal Diseases in the Tropics

Handbook on Animal Diseases in the Tropics

Fourth Edition

editors:

M.M.H. Sewell
Centre for Tropical Veterinary Medicine, Easter Bush, Roslin, Midlothian, Scotland

D.W. Brocklesby
Professor and Director, Centre for Tropical Veterinary Medicine, Easter Bush, Roslin, Midlothian, Scotland

Baillière Tindall
London Philadelphia Toronto Sydney Tokyo

Baillière Tindall

WB Saunders

24–28 Oval Road
London NW1 7DX, England

The Curtis Centre, Independence Square West
Philadelphia, PA 19106–3399, USA

55 Horner Avenue, Toronto
Ontario M8Z 4X6, Canada

Harcourt Brace Jovanovich Group (Australia) Pty Ltd
30–52 Smidmore Street
Marrickville, NSW 2204, Australia

Harcourt Brace Jovanovich (Japan) Inc.
Ichibancho Central Building, 22-1 Ichibancho
Chiyoda-ku, Tokyo 102, Japan

This book is printed on acid-free paper

First published by The British Veterinary Association in 1962
Fourth Edition 1990

British Library Cataloguing in Publication Data is available

ISBN 0–7020–1502–4

Typeset by Colset Pte. Ltd. Singapore.
Printed in Great Britain by The University Press, Cambridge.

Contents

DISEASES CAUSED BY HELMINTHS *J.A. Hammond and M.M.H. Sewell*

DISEASES CAUSED BY VIRUSES   *G.R. Scott*

Preface

It is with great pleasure that this new edition of the *Handbook on Animal Diseases in the Tropics* is dedicated to Professor Sir Alexander Robertson, CBE, LLD, MA, BSc, PhD, DVSc, CChem, FRSc, FRCVS, FRSE.

It was Professor Robertson who inspired the production of the first edition of this Handbook in 1962 under the auspices of the British Veterinary Association and he was the editor for the first three editions. Sir Alexander was admirably suited to this task through his long held interest in tropical veterinary medicine, his experience of veterinary education in many countries, which included advising on the foundation of most of the now well established veterinary schools in the anglophone tropics, and as the first Director of the Centre for Tropical Veterinary Medicine near Edinburgh. The staff of this Centre have again undertaken the bulk of the revision and up-dating of the text of this edition.

The aims of this edition remain the same as those stated in Professor Robertson's preface to the second edition. These are "to provide a concise summary of the more important infections and conditions causing ill-health in domestic animals in tropical and sub-tropical countries, emphasising the special features applicable in these countries in the case of diseases of a wider distribution."

Despite the great increase in recent years in knowledge about diseases of animals in the tropics and sub-tropics, there has been a determined effort to prevent the Handbook growing into a tome. This has inevitably meant asking the authors to strictly limit the material they have presented. In making this selection, it has been the intention to concentrate on those practical aspects which will be of most assistance to the veterinarian in the field, possibly far from alternative sources of information. However, many of the chapters include recommendations as to further reading which will assist those who wish to obtain more detailed information on that particular topic.

M.M.H. Sewell
Centre for Tropical Veterinary Medicine,
Easter Bush, Roslin, Midlothian, EH25 9RG, Scotland

Note

The names of parasitic diseases in this Handbook are in general conformity with the *Standardized Nomenclature of Animal Parasitic Diseases (SNOAPAD)* drawn up by the World Association for the Advancement of Veterinary Parasitology (see *Veterinary Parasitology* (1988), **29** 299–326).

Diseases caused by arthropods

A.R. Walker

The ectoparasites of livestock are all of the phylum Arthropoda and within the order Acarina or the class Insecta. They include numerous biting flies that are often called micro-predators, rather than ectoparasites. Numerous groups of arthropods cause minor nuisance to livestock or transmit disease. Only those which cause economic losses to livestock producers in the tropics will be considered here.

The Acarina comprise the mites and the ticks, which have four pairs of legs as adults, and a body that is divided into a capitulum that bears the mouthparts and the opisthosoma. The Acarina never have wings and their ecology is influenced by their inability to move far except when they are on a host. Large infestations of ticks or mites may accumulate at the resting sites or pens of their hosts.

There are seven families of mites and two families of ticks. All ticks are ectoparasites, but most mites are free-living. The economic significance of ticks is due both to their parasitic activity and to their being vectors of numerous serious diseases to livestock. Although mites can produce serious infestations in livestock, they are not implicated in the serious transmission of diseases.

The Insecta, which are ectoparasites or micro-predators of livestock, comprise the lice, fleas and flies. As adults, all insects have only three pairs of legs and a body that is divided into segments, grouped into a head with mouthparts, thorax with legs and wings, and an abdomen.

The lice are primitive insects, the immature forms of which look like small adults, and they go through several moults before reaching adult size. Lice have no wings, but this is a modification for parasitic life. The fleas are advanced insects, the larvae of which look like maggots and which grow to the size of, and then transform into, adult fleas. This transformation is called complete metamorphosis – from larva to pupa to adult flea. As a parasitic modification, adult fleas do not have wings. The flies also experience a complete metamorphosis. Those flies that bite or cause nuisance to livestock have harmless larvae; however, a number of flies have larvae which are parasitic to livestock but the adult flies are harmless. This is known as myiasis. Most insects are of economic importance to livestock as direct parasites, but the tsetse flies are almost exclusively responsible for the transmission of trypanosomes.

ACARINES

Mites

Dermanyssidae

This family contains the gamasid mites of the genera *Dermanyssus* and *Ornithonyssus*, which are non-specialized micro-predators of birds. Their life-cycle is completed within 1–2 weeks and consists of a larva, two nymphal stages and an adult stage. The female lays repeated batches of small numbers of large eggs and takes repeated blood meals to support egg production. Poultry mites can accumulate in poultry houses and cause a very severe infestation. The stress and blood loss in the poultry leads to loss of weight gain and a fall in egg production. The mites infest the structure of the poultry houses and they feed on the poultry at night. There are others families related to the Dermanyssidae that contain the *Pneumonyssus* mites, which infest the lungs of their hosts, and the *Raillietia* mites, which feed on ear wax in cattle.

Demodicidae

This family consists of the highly specialized genus *Demodex*, all stages of which live only in the hair follicles of their hosts and which feed on sebaceous secretions. Many mammals have *Demodex* as a normal inhabitant of the skin, but in dogs, goats and cattle the infestation sometimes becomes severe and the mites penetrate the epidermis, causing loss of weight gain, a reduced value of hides and even death. Secondary bacterial infections often worsen the damage.

Psorogatidae

This family contains the genus *Psorogates*, the sheep itch mite. The life-cycle and effects of the Psorogatidae are similar to the Psoroptidae (see below).

Sarcoptidae

This family consists of the genera *Sarcoptes*, *Notoedres* and *Knemidocoptes*. These are the mange mites, highly specialized for life entirely within the skin, where all stages of their life-cycle are found in burrows between the *stratum corneum* and *stratum germanitivum*. Mating takes place on the surface of the epidermis and spread is by close contact between hosts. In the tropics, sarcoptic mange is a severe problem in camels, and it also affects young swine, sheep and goats. *Sarcoptes* also infests dogs, but mange in dogs and cats is more commonly caused by *Notoedres*. *Knemidocoptes* (*Cnemidocoptes*) *mutans* burrows into the skin of the legs of poultry causing scaly leg, crippling the birds. *K. gallinea* infests the base of feathers and causes depluming behaviour in poultry. Mange infestations cause loss of production due to hyperkeratinization of the skin and severe pruritus leading to anorexia. Severe infestations may occur in animals already in a poor condition, leading to death.

Psoroptidae

This family contains the genera *Psoroptes*, *Chorioptes* and *Otodectes*, the scab mites. Infestations by these mites are always superficial on the epidermis, but the piercing of the skin by the mites leads to exudation and exfoliation, causing scabs to form. The mites continue to feed at the edge of the scabs. Their entire life-cycle takes place on the host. Spread occurs by close contact with infected hosts and also by fomites and contaminated animal housing. *Psoroptes* scab is a severe problem in sheep, but it is also found in goats and cattle. Though less common, *Chorioptes* causes similar problems in cattle and horses as *Psoroptes*. Loss of production is due to pruritus leading to anorexia, and excessive grooming leading to wool loss. *Otodectes* infests the external ear canal of cats and dogs.

Control of mites

The intradermal mites Sarcoptidae and Demodicidae are susceptible to a wide variety of acaricides, but problems may be caused by the poor penetration of externally applied acaricides. Systemic treatments, such as ivermectin injectable or trichlorphon or phosmet pour-on, may thus be useful. For the control of sarcoptic mange in herds of camels or cattle, spraying with conventional acaricides such as lindane, diazinon, amitraz or permethrin is effective. The spraying usually needs to be repeated at least once, after a period of about 1–2 weeks. Benzylbenzoate is most useful for treating ear infestations.

The superficial mites of the Psoroptidae are often the subject of control by mandatory legislation, using conventional acaricides such as lindane, toxaphene, coumaphos, amitraz and carbaryl. Sheep are usually treated in dipping baths. Though repeated treatments are often not required, it is usually mandatory for the entire flock to be treated annually.

The control of Dermanyssidae mites is directed at poultry houses. The modern design of poultry houses reduces the number of resting and oviposition sites for mites, and good sanitation and cleaning assists this. Acaricides can be applied to the poultry houses, usually in a dust formulation of malathion, carbaryl, coumaphos or tetrachlorvinphos.

Ticks

Ixodidae

This major family consists of the hard ticks, so-called because they have a hard shiney scutum or dorsal shield.

Life-cycle and feeding

All ticks are obligate parasites of vertebrates. Their life-cycle consists of alternate feeding through the skin of their hosts and long periods spent on vegetation or in animal housing. This has led to their extreme physiological adaptation. During the questing stages, the ticks survive upon the food reserves built up during the previous stage spent on a host and by extracting atmospheric moisture. At the feeding stage, the ticks must ingest enough blood in a single meal to support their survival at the next stage or to enable them to produce thousands of eggs. To ingest such large quantities of blood, ticks change their physiology during the early stages of feeding so that they are capable of a final phase of rapid engorgement. For this reason, ticks attach to their hosts for days or weeks, using both cement secreted in their saliva and a feeding tube (hypostome) with barbed teeth. A lesion is created in the dermis of the host by an acute inflammatory reaction. The ticks then feed on the plasma and whole blood which enters this lesion. Immune reactions to the saliva cause pruritus, leading to anorexia in the host. The blood is concentrated during feeding, so that with heavy infestations of adult ticks blood loss accounts for a substantial proportion of loss of production. The sterile abscess that forms at the feeding site damages hides, and this is true even of the small *Boophilus* ticks which feed on sites of good hide potential. The large *Amblyomma* and *Hyalomma* ticks feed at vulnerable sites, including between the toes, and on the teats and genitalia, causing lameness and malfunction.

All of the hard ticks have only three stages in their life-cycles and each stage feeds only once. Most ticks are known as three-host ticks because, at the completion of feeding, the engorged tick detaches, moults and then waits for a host. When the female feeds, she produces a single batch of eggs numbering many thousands, and then dies. The males remain on the host where they attempt repeatedly to mate. With a few species of ticks, the engorged larvae remain on the host where they moult rapidly to nymphs and continue to feed. In one-host ticks (mostly *Boophilus*), the nymph also remains on the host, so that all three feeding stages take place on the same individual host. Engorged females drop to the ground to lay their eggs, and the larvae adhere to vegetation.

When poor management leads to a heavy infestation of pastures or livestock housing, or when breeds of livestock are introduced which cannot resist the feeding ticks, the parasitic activity causes direct economic losses. Through immunological and behavioural responses, livestock which are indigenous to tick-infected areas are able to demonstrate a resistance, thereby reducing the infestation of pastures. However, exotic stock are unable to do this.

A variety of poorly defined syndromes are caused by the feeding of ticks, including some soft tick species. During the final phase of engorgement, hard ticks excrete a lot of water from the blood meal so as to concentrate it. This is done via the saliva, at which time the host may suffer from a moist eczema (i.e. sweating sickness), generalized malaise or flaccid paralysis, which leads to death in extreme cases. Proteins of unknown function in the saliva have, in some cases, been isolated as the causative agent. There is no obvious advantage to the tick of such activity, and the toxins do not appear to have an adaptive function for the ticks.

Ixodes

Though widely distributed, *Ixodes* spp. are unimportant in the tropics, except for the paralytic species. *I. rubicundus*, which is found on sheep and goats in southern Africa, causes a paralysis that can kill lambs and kids. *I. holocyclus* occurs in eastern Australia where it normally infests bandicoots, but when it infests cattle, dogs or humans, paralysis often results. Commercial antidotes and experimental vaccines are available.

Amblyomma

Widespread throughout the tropics, *Amblyomma* spp. are often large three-host ticks, many of which infest reptiles. However, those that infest mammals feed on a very wide variety of hosts, particularly as larvae or nymphs, and the immature stages of some species infest birds, thereby further dispersing the ticks. If unsuccessful in finding a host, adult *Amblyomma* are able to survive on vegetation for several years without feeding.

The African species *A. variegatum* and *A. hebreum* are of the greatest economic significance, because they transmit the rickettsial pathogen *Cowdria ruminatium*, which causes heartwater in cattle and sheep. In addition, *A. variegatum* is associated with streptothricosis, the actinomycete infection of the skin of cattle, caused by *Dermatophilus congolensis*.

In the Americas, *A. americanum*, *A. cayannense* and *A. maculatum* are of economic significance to livestock, due to the damage caused by their feeding sites. In areas infested with myiasis flies, tick infestation sites are attractive to female flies for laying their eggs.

Boophilus

The genus *Boophilus* contains five species, all of which are one-host ticks, specially adapted to feed on cattle. Though *B. decoloratus* is restricted to Africa and *B. annulatus* to the Americas, *B. microplus* – which originated in South East Asia – has spread throughout the tropics, including Africa. Cattle are the preferred host of *Boophilus* spp., but small numbers do feed on sheep, goats, horses and wild ruminants.

Boophilus spp. are small ticks with short mouthparts that are unable to penetrate very deeply into the skin of their hosts. Nevertheless, they cause pruritus in cattle leading to anorexia, which increases the loss of gain in liveweight. Research has shown that this loss in gain in liveweight throughout the entire feeding cycle of one female plus her mate, is 0.6 g for each engorged female tick. The hides are also damaged. Because *Boophilus* ticks have all their feeding stages on a host compressed into about 3 weeks, and the egg-laying stage lasts about 1 month, it is possible for there to be up to six generations in a year, unlike most three-host ticks which usually only have one generation per year. Thus *Boophilus* ticks have a high intrinsic rate of reproduction, pastures may become very heavily infected with their larvae and severe infestations accumulate on cattle.

In contrast, ticks may not accumulate on cattle which are farmed on extensive range-land systems; however, the transmission of diseases then becomes more serious. *Boophilus* ticks are the main vectors of *Babesia bovis* and *Babesia bigemina* and an important vector of *Anaplasma*. *Babesia* spp. are highly adapted to transmission by *Boophilus* ticks, and they are able to invade the developing eggs and thus infect the larvae. This is transovarial transmission.

Dermacentor

Though widely spread throughout the world, *Dermacentor* spp. are only locally important in the tropics as a parasite of livestock. *D. andersoni* is notorious as a vector of the causative agent of Rocky Mountain spotted fever in humans, and as a cause of paralysis in cattle in Canada. *Dermacentor (Anocentor) nitens*, the tropical horse tick, stretches from the southern USA through Central America and into tropical South America. It is a one-host tick with a predilection for the ears of its host, and severe infestations lead to loss of condition and predispose the host to attack by myiasis flies. The tick transmits *Babesia caballi*, the causative agent of equine piroplasmosis.

Haemaphysalis

Though distributed worldwide, *Haemaphysalis* is only of importance to livestock in South East Asia, where *H. bispinosa* transmits *Theileria mutans* between cattle. However, in Africa, the yellow dog tick, *H. leachii*, transmits *Babesia canis*, the causative agent of canine biliary fever, and *Rickettsia conori* the causative agent of tick typhus or Boutonneuse fever in humans.

Hyalomma

Hyalomma spp. are widespread throughout the tropics from Africa to China and many species are adapted to desert conditions, including cold-winter conditions in the dry areas of the Middle East. Though most species are three-host ticks, they are also able to feed as one- and two-host ticks, depending on the host available, and they are able to feed on a wide variety of hosts. *Hyalomma* populations often concentrate around livestock housing, where successive generations find it easy to find a host. Adult *Hyalomma* ticks actively run out from their resting sites when a host approaches, unlike most other hard ticks which wait attached to vegetation until a host brushes past.

Hyalomma ticks have long mouthparts and cause large feeding lesions. *H. rufipes*, which feeds on the feet of sheep and goats, can cause lameness. Some species (e.g. *H. truncatum*) cause a toxic syndrome known as sweating sickness, the obvious clinical signs of which are a moist eczema around the head and shoulders, severe malaise and possible paralysis. The aetiology of sweating sickness appears to be the same as tick paralysis.

Numerous *Hyalomma* spp. transmit the causative pathogen of tropical theileriosis, *Theileria annulata*. The theilerias are highly adapted to their vectors, but not to the extent of transovarial transmission. Two separate transmission cycles occur: from infection of the larvae to transmission by the nymphs, and from infection of the nymphs to transmission by the adults. This is because the theilerial stages that take place within the tick are highly adapted to propagation in the salivary glands of the feeding tick. When the tick completes feeding and moults to the next stage, the salivary glands regress to primordial glands that are unable to support the *Theileria*. Infection can persist in adult ticks for up to a year while it waits for an available host. *Hyalomma* ticks also transmit *T. hirci* and *T. ovis*, causing relatively benign disease, and *Babesia canis*.

Rhipicephalus

Rhipicephalus spp. are medium-sized ticks with short mouthparts and, apart from the kennel tick *R. sanguineus sanguineus*, which has become widespread among domestic dogs, they are restricted to Africa. However, they are not as well adapted as *Hyalomma* spp. to extreme environments. Most species are three-host ticks, which infest a wide variety of hosts. The most important species, *R. appendiculatus* and *R. evertsi evertsi*, are capable of feeding at any stage of their life-cycle on a wide variety of domestic and wild ruminants. *R. evertsi* is a two-host tick, the nymphs of which infest the ears of cattle. In severe infestations, the adults of *R. appendiculatus*, preferring to feed on the ears, destroy the ear pinna of cattle and predispose them to infestation by myiasis flies. *R. appendiculatus* has been shown experimentally to cause a 4.0-g reduction in gain of liveweight in cattle for every engorging female tick that can be counted (i.e. standard females). These female counts also take into account the effect of the immature stages and the adult males. As with *Boophilus*, most of this loss is thought to be due to anorexia, the rest due to blood loss. In severe infestations, an indistinct toxic syndrome occurs, known as rhipicephaline toxicosis. Such toxaemias are more frequent with heavy infestations of *R. evertsi evertsi*. In some instances, a paralytic syndrome occurs in lambs infested with the same species.

R. *appendiculatus* is notorious as the vector of *Theileria parva*, the causative agent of East Coast fever. Although other species have been incriminated – *R. evertsi evertsi* can sometimes be important epidemiologically – *R. appendiculatus* is almost exclusively the vector throughout the range of the disease, i.e. East, Central and southern Africa. The pathogen has a very similar biology to *T. annulata*, but the mortality rate, particularly in calves, is much higher. East Coast fever is a major constraint on the use use of exotic livestock, typically highly susceptible to both the tick and the diseases. *R. appendiculatus* also transmits *T. lawrenci*, the causative organism of corridor or buffalo disease, and it has been associated with the transmission of *Babesia*, though this is not yet clear. However, it does transmit the Nairobi sheep disease virus to sheep in East Africa and the rickettsia of tick typhus, *R. conori*, to humans.

Argasidae

This is a small family, but it contains some ticks that are of great local importance. They are called soft ticks because they do not have a hard shiny scutum. However, they are extremely tough and the adult stages are adapted for survival in hot, dry conditions for long periods without food. Their life-cycle and feeding pattern are different from hard ticks. In general, there are repeated immature stages and repeated small meals of blood to support the transition from one stage to the next. Similarly, the females take repeated small blood meals to support the production of repeated small batches of eggs. Feeding can last from a few minutes to hours, though the ticks do not use cement to attach themselves to their host and they do not create large feeding lesions. There are, however, complex immune reactions in the skin of hosts to the feeding of these ticks, and the pruritus that results is a major cause of production losses. The ticks are typically adapted to having a complete life-cycle in the housing, nest or burrow of their host (i.e. nidicolous habit). However, the genus *Otobious* causes problems to cattle more typical of hard ticks.

Argas

These are the fowl ticks, important in poultry houses and around domestic housing where poultry are kept throughout the tropics. The ticks hide in crevices within the housing structure or in dry soil. *Argas persicus* is a vector of the spirocheate pathogen of poultry *Borellia anserina*, which is transmitted both trans-stadially and transovarially and occurs sporadically throughout the tropics. Massive infestations of *Argas* may build up in poultry houses and cause paralysis and death by stress and exsanguination.

Ornithodoros

Often spelt *Ornithodorus*, this genus is important locally in the tropics. *O. moubata* feeds on wild pig species and infests their burrows, but in association with domestic pigs it has become a peri-domestic species and will feed on man. *O. savignyi* lives in sandy soil at the shaded resting sites of livestock in semi-desert areas and feeds at night on the legs of cattle, sheep, goats and camels. Massive infestation of these ticks may build up and at night the ticks will seek out their hosts, which are often tethered or confined. Severe stress and blood loss can result. *O. moubata* is the vector of the virus of African swine fever and many *Ornithodoros* spp. transmit *Borellia recurrentis* varieties to humans, causing relapsing fever.

Otobius

Otobius megnini, the spinose ear tick, is widespread in the Americas and has spread to Africa and India. It feeds mainly on cattle and horses but also on sheep and goats. Infestations are associated with animal housing where the larvae can be found. The larvae attach within the ear canal of hosts, feeding like a hard tick and moulting on the host. Two nymphal stages are spent on the same host and ticks spend many weeks at the same site. The adults cannot feed and mating takes place off the host and the female lays a large batch of eggs. Heavy infestations in a host's ears lead to stress and damage and predisposition to myiasis fly attack.

Control of ticks

The conventional method for controlling hard ticks was developed at the turn of the century in the USA, South Africa and Australia for the control of babesiosis and theileriosis. The livestock are forced to jump into a long dipping bath and then swim to exit steps at the other end. The initial plunge into the bath soaks the head and the swim out soaks the coat, including the axillae and the peri-anal areas. On exiting, most of the dip wash drains off each animal back into the bath. The dip wash contains an acaricide as an emulsion or solution at a controlled concentration sufficient to kill any tick within hours. This method, using the very primitive and non-specific pesticide arsenic, and sometimes nicotine, was used to eradicate *Boophilus annulatus* from the USA and to control *Rhipicephalus appendiculatus* and East Coast fever successfully in the Republic of South Africa. With the discovery of the differential high toxicity of DDT to insects and acarines and low toxicity to humans, further research was undertaken to discover materials with good physical characters for use in dip baths. The use of lindane and toxaphene established the method of forming and maintaining a correct emulsion at the correct strength in the bath.

In many cattle ranching areas of the tropics, the dip bath (or spray race) is of central importance in ranch management. However, throughout the tropics there is a wide variety of tick types and management systems where conventional treatments are not appropriate or where they could be used more efficiently. Although the eradication of ticks has been achieved at the geographical limits of some species, in most tropical countries it is difficult to control ticks and tick-borne diseases to an acceptable level without spending more on the control than the problem costs. Intensive control is often only economic when exotic livestock are used in an attempt to improve productivity; these livestock tend to be more susceptible to ticks and disease but their higher productivity permits the cost of control.

Dip baths (plunge bath, dip-tank). A tank set in the ground, 1 m wide, 2 m deep and 4–6 m long, containing 12,000–15,000 litres of water plus acaricide (i.e. the dip-wash). The entrance has a vertical side and the exit has a ramp of steps. It is usually constructed of reinforced concrete, but glass-reinforced plastic (i.e. fibre glass) can be used. At the entrance, a splash wall up to 2 m high prevents the acaricide being wasted. It is essential that there is a system for catching the excess dip-wash from the livestock waiting after being dipped. Thus extensive and durable races and fences are required. A water storage tank or pump is essential for the regular topping up of the tank volume. The same dip-wash is usually used for 6 months or more, until the mud and faeces contaminating it reduces the efficiency of the acaricide. Then it is pumped out. A safe disposal site is essential, preferably a soak-away pit. Depending on the acaricide used, some system of monitoring its concentration is essential. A system of replenishment with acaricide and water based on the numbers of stock being treated can be used. Additionally, regular checks of the concentration of the acaricide in samples of the dip-wash are made by a laboratory. Some modern acaricides are soluble in water, which makes accurate replenishment much easier, because they are not removed from the dip-wash at a faster rate than the water is removed from the dip-wash (i.e. stripping).

Spray-races (mechanical sprays). These use the same acaricides, formulated in the same way, as dip-baths, and they are designed to give a high-volume acaricide wash at low pressure. A race of steel fencing directs the stock through hoops of steel pressure tubing with connecting tubes. About 40 spray nozzles are used to cover the whole animal. If a spray race is working well, it will soak all parts of each animal, but if the spray jets are blocked with mud or the pump engine is inefficient, then the ears and axillae may not be treated. Spray races are simpler to erect and easier to use with calves, pregnant cows or sensitive dairy cattle. Their biggest advantage is that only a small amount of fresh wash needs to be made up each time, and therefore it is much easier to use the correct concentration and avoid contamination. However, when large numbers of animals are being treated, the acaricide will only be used efficiently if there is provision for drainage of the excess wash from the animals back to the sump of the spray race pump and reservoir.

Hand-spraying. The effect of a spray race can be duplicated with small hand-operated or -powered spray nozzles on the end of a lance. This is suitable for farmers with a few cattle. However, it requires 10–15 litres of acaricide wash to soak a cow, and in a dip most of this is recovered and re-used; however, with hand-spraying, it is wasted. Often, only 1–2 litres of the older types of acaricides are used; this incomplete coverage gives incomplete control. If synthetic pyrethroids are used for hand-spraying, this may not be of such great importance because they spread well, last a long time on the coat and work at concentrations much lower than the normal working concentration. But the use of such acaricides may be limited by their cost and by regulations to control resistance to acaricides.

Hand-dressing (manual application). This varies from using a rag to apply conventional acaricide wash, painting a grease containing acaricide on to the ears and peri-anal region, or the pour-on and spot-on methods. Pour-on uses acaricides at a high concentration in oil, and a set volume per weight of the animal is poured along its back. A pyrethroid acaricide will spread superficially to give a fairly good coverage of the whole animal. Spot-on application uses a pump action applicator like a syringe to deliver a fixed small volume of oil, but this usually contains insecticide (see below).

Ear-tags and bands. Some pesticides can be incorporated into plastic, from which they slowly diffuse to have their effect. Synthetic pyrethroids are good for such an application on cattle because they spread well over the surface of the skin and are effective at very low concentrations, but organophosphorus compounds are also used. A conventional numbered ear-tag weighing 10 g can be formulated to contain 1 g of pesticide, and it will remain effective from several weeks to a few months. Obviously, they are very useful for the control of ear ticks; however, their effectiveness against ticks attached to the hind legs or tail is less clear. For this reason, bands around the neck or tail have been tested.

Environmental application. The experimental application of acaricides to pastures has shown that it is not economical and that it is more efficient to allow the livestock to collect the ticks and then kill them. However, such spraying is sometimes used for subsidized eradication schemes over limited areas. Soft ticks that infest animal housing and do not stay attached to their hosts may be controlled by spraying poultry houses and piggeries with acaricides that remain active in a residual deposit.

Injectables. The ivermectins can be injected to control a wide variety of parasites and they are sold as an aid to the control of one-host ticks. Currently, further research is required to make the injectable or rumenal bolus application of acaricides economical for tick control.

Vaccines. Currently, several laboratories have experimental vaccines against *Boophilus microplus* and *Rhipicephalus appendiculatus*. These are based on proteins from the gut of the tick. If they can be manufactured and then injected into cattle, the cattle will produce antibodies to these gut proteins. When the ticks feed, the large amount of blood they pass through will contain antibodies which react with gut proteins and damage the gut and the tick. Such vaccines may become commercially available, but only for ticks important over wide areas.

Timing. To control *Boophilus* ticks with a feeding period of about 21 days, treatment every 21 days is convenient and effective. The residual deposit of acaricide on the hair of the cattle will kill larvae attempting to attach for the next 2–5 days. Larvae attaching thereafter will feed through to nymphs and adults, but they will still be feeding by the next treatment and they will be killed before they can reproduce. This reduces the population that can infest the pastures, but permits some tick feeding. This is useful to maintain premunity against babesiosis and resistance against the ticks. To control all other types of two- or three-host ticks, the interval is usually once every 7 days. This may permit some larvae to feed for 2–3 days between the end of the residual period and the next treatment, but very few adults will feed and reproduce in this period. Treatment every 14 days is sometimes used in areas of low tick infestation, but adults will be able to maintain themselves. In the extreme case of the need to protect exotic cattle against severe threat of East Coast fever, it may be necessary to treat twice per week to prevent any nymphs or adults from even beginning to feed and thus transmitting *Theileria parva.*

Strategic treatment (strategic dipping). This is the planning in advance of the seasons in which it is most effective to make treatments. This contrasts with opportunistic or tactical treatments, which are carried out when a tick infestation is seen to be bad. The treatment intervals should remain the same as above, but the treatments should be carried out at the season when there is an increase in the numbers of reproducing adults. In the case of *Boophilus*, with several generations per year, it is necessary to know at what season the population of ticks starts to increase. Cattle are treated at 21-day intervals on 3–6 occasions during this period. Then the reduced population of ticks should not increase to problem levels for the remainder of the year. With three-host ticks, there may be a distinct seasonal rise of adults in relation to the end of a long dry season or the end of the cold season. Strategic dipping at weekly intervals is concentrated then so as to prevent each female laying thousand of eggs. However, the strategic treatment must be started before the ticks are an obvious problem, using accurate predictions of tick numbers according to climate. This requires good local experience or a lot of data for use in predictions or the computerized models (i.e. predictive equations) that are currently being developed. In wet tropical areas favourable to the ticks all year, strategic treatment may not be possible.

Threshold treatment. If it is known what is the loss of gain in liveweight due to the feeding of one tick, and what are the costs of treatment, it may be possible to calculate what number of ticks there need to be feeding on an animal at any one time for it to be economical to treat them. This occurs with any disease that can be controlled by drugs or vaccines. The number of ticks to be counted on the animal is the threshold number. It should be an aid to farmers in helping to decide whether or not it is cost-effective to treat the animals. However, it needs to be combined with consideration of strategic dipping and seasonal increases in numbers of feeding adult ticks. Information is only available on the loss of liveweight gain per tick for *B. microplus* (0.6 g), *R. appendiculatus* (4.0 g) and *A. varigatum* (approximately 50g).

Host resistance to ticks. This is the ability of individual cattle to acquire, during their development, the ability to reduce the numbers and weight of ticks feeding on them.

The mechanisms include behavioural avoidance, immediate hypersensitivity in the skin leading to grooming, delayed cutaneous hypersensitivity leading to interference with the feeding, and digestion of the ticks. Most individuals can acquire these responses to many species of ticks, but some individuals and some breeds are much better than others at doing so. In general, *Bos indicus* herds contain a much higher proportion of individuals with the ability to acquire resistance than *Bos taurus* herds. The practical application on a farm is to evaluate the economic advantages of using *Bos indicus* breeds for rotational cross-breeding so as to obtain a herd of 3:8–5:8 *Bos indicus*:*Bos taurus* for use in extensive ranching conditions for beef cattle. Two breeds of dairy cattle have been developed which incorporate the ability to acquire good resistance against *Boophilus microplus*, the Australian Milking Zebu and the Australian Friesian Sahiwal. In many tropical areas, the indigenous cattle will be of a type suitable for selection for resistance. Farmers can use host resistance in a simple form by noting which animals usually have heavy infestations of ticks and then to treat them with acaricide or to select them out for slaughter. It is a long-term task to select for resistance using bulls, but it may be useful in some areas. The best use of host resistance to ticks is in combination with strategic treatment and possible pasture management.

Pasture spelling (pasture rotation or management). For the control of *Boophilus microplus* in areas where it is the major tick problem, it is possible to kill many of the larvae while they are on the vegetation if the cattle are not allowed to graze such infested pastures. During hot, dry periods, a 6-week rotation of pastures, with acaricide treatment of cattle on transfer from one pasture to the next, will be enough to kill most larvae by starvation and desiccation. However, for this method to be successful, it must fit in with other management procedures and the pasture must not be allowed to deteriorate. This is difficult and the method is seldom used. Studies have been made on pasture plants that have a repellent or trapping effect on *Boophilus* larvae, such as the grass *Melinus minutiflora* and various species of the legume *Stylosanthes*. Usually, however, farmers prefer to use more productive or longlasting pasture plants and this method is rarely used. Pasture spelling will not work for three-host ticks where the nymphal and adult stages survive for months to years on the vegetation, and thus the potential application of these methods is only in Australia and South America.

Environmental control. The strict control of ticks with acaricides on cattle that are kept isolated in fenced pastures can result in the pastures having a very low infestation, and this may permit less intensive control. The rotation of crops, or the ploughing or re-seeding of such pastures, will also control most ticks. In open range-land, burning for the purpose of managing grass quality may kill some ticks, but not those at soil level. Zero grazing is commonly used in areas where *Hyalomma* ticks are a problem, but here the ticks that infest the cattle are found in the livestock housing. The construction of livestock housing so that it is easier to clean and has fewer cracks and crevices in which ticks can shelter, will reduce infestation by *Hyalomma*, *Argas* and *Otobious*.

INSECTS

Fleas

Order Siphonaptera

The fleas are notorious as vectors of bubonic plague to humans, but they are not usually a serious pest of livestock. However, severe infestations of fleas do accumulate in the housing of some domestic stock in the tropics under certain management systems. This causes anaemia and biting stress, resulting in loss of production and even death to young or poorly fed stock. Flea infestation leads to dermal hypersensitivity (types I and IV), increasing the effect of biting stress.

Fleas are advanced insects with a complete metamorphosis from larvae through pupa to the sexually mature adults. The female produces several eggs per day during a life-cycle of several months or more. The eggs hatch into legless larvae which feed on organic debris in the housing of their hosts. Pupation takes place in the same environment, and both the female and male fleas then repeatedly jump on and off their hosts to obtain blood meals through their fine piercing mouthparts. However, the sticktight flea of poultry, *Echidnophaga gallinacea*, remains attached at the feeding site, particularly on the head.

The most important species for domestic stock is *Ctenocephalides felis*, and to a lesser extent *C. canis*. While many fleas have a high host specificity, these cat and dog fleas have adapted to the domestic environment and accumulate in large numbers when livestock are confined in a peri-domestic environment. Transmission of disease is not important, but the dog tapeworm *Dipylidium caninum* is transmitted to dogs and cats when they ingest their own fleas.

Control of fleas

This can be carried out by improving the hygiene of animal housing, so as to destroy the larvae and pupae, but the construction of much animal housing in peri-domestic environments makes this uneconomic for smallholders. Many insecticides are effective against adult fleas, whether applied to the host as dusts, as pour-on or as collars of plastic impregnated with the insecticide. Because of the confined nature of the housing in which flea infestations are often found, it is sometimes feasible to spray or dust the animal bedding and flooring with insecticide.

Flies

Order Diptera

The Diptera are the true flies, with only one pair of wings and the back pair of wings modified into small balancing organs. They include typical flies, the mosquitoes and the specialized louse-flies or keds. A wide variety of problems are caused to livestock by flies and they are of major economic importance in many tropical areas. They are very advanced insects with a life-cycle of egg to larva to pupa to sexually mature adult, and they have an extremely wide range of physiological and ecological adaptations in relation to feeding on lifestock.

Blackflies

Family Simuliidae

These small bloodsucking flies are known as black flies because of their colour or buffalo flies because of their hump-shaped thorax. They are notorious as vectors of *Onchocerca volvulus*, which causes river blindness in humans. The eggs are laid in free-running clear water and the larvae are specialized for attaching to rocks or water plants and feeding by filtering organic debris. Pupation takes place at the water surface.

The male adults feed on plant sugars, but the females feed on blood. The skin of the host is pierced by coarse blade-like and saw-like mouthparts to form a blood pool in the skin from which whole blood is ingested (i.e. telmophagy). Such bites are painful, and because much saliva is required to maintain a flow of blood, hosts easily develop immediate hypersensitivity reactions to the flies.

The flies are often highly seasonal and localized and may occur in massive swarms. Exposed cattle suffer very severe biting stress, blood loss and immune shock, leading to death in extreme cases. Studies of such attacks have demonstrated that, on average, each cow is bitten 25,000 times a day. However, such massive swarms are more typical of temperate climates with a distinct summer season. In many tropical areas, there are insufficient breeding sites for these flies to be a major problem to livestock. The protozoan pathogen *Leucocytozoon* is transmitted to poultry by *Simulium* species, and non-pathogenic *Onchocerca linealis* and *O. gutturosa* are transmitted to cattle.

Control of Simuliidea

Insecticides are applied to rivers to try and control river blindness. This is also carried out in temperate regions where massive swarms of flies attack livestock, but extreme care has to be taken to prevent excessive contamination of the environment. This is rarely economically feasible or desirable for the control of biting attack on livestock in the tropics. Treatment of cattle with synthetic pyrethroids is effective if done sufficiently often, but it is expensive.

Keds or louse flies

Family Hippoboscidae

These are known as the louse flies or keds and may be mistaken for ticks when in a wingless form. In the genus *Hippobosca*, the adult flies are specialized for a semi-ectoparasitic life, remaining in very close contact with their hosts but able to fly rapidly from one host to another within a herd. Many host species have hippoboscids specific to them. The larval stage occurs within the female through to a pre-pupa which pupates immediately when extruded from its mother (i.e. larviparous). In the genus *Melophagus*, the pupae attach to the hairs of the host. Pupae of the genus *Hippobosca* develop off the host. Both sexes are blood feeders and feed several times each day. With such a life-cycle, the rate of survival is high, but reproduction is very slow and large populations do not accumulate. Biting stress presumably occurs, but it appears not to be severe. In cool climates, the sheep ked, *Melophagus ovinus*, is a wingless type which remains ectoparasitic on one host and transfers to new hosts by crawling. Severe infestations of this species lead to spoilt wool. The transmission of disease is not important and there are no control measures which are practised specifically for Hippoboscidae; however, control measures against ticks, scab mites or lice will also control keds.

Midges

Family Ceratopogonidae

These are known as biting midges in most areas. The genus *Culicoides* contains most of the species important to livestock. They are very small, but they have a feeding method similar to the Simuliidae and they are thus painful. Nocturnal swarms of *Culicoides* which cause biting stress are a problem to humans and livestock in temperate countries during the summer, but in the tropics the role of *Culicoides* in biting stress and blood loss has not been well documented, although thousands of bites per cow per night have been recorded. The larvae live in mud, damp soil or wet vegetation. In the tropics, breeding is continuous, dependent on the availability of wet habitats, but the adults are likely to be found in greatest numbers during and after rainy seasons.

Culicoides have been incriminated in the transmission of the viruses which cause African horse sickness, ephemeral fever and Rift Valley fever. They also transmit *Leucocytozoon* to poultry, *Dipetalonema* spp. of filarial nematode to man and some livestock, and *Onchocerca cervicalis* to horses. The bluetongue virus of sheep and cattle is transmitted by *Culicoides* spp. and is found throughout the tropics and the warm temperate regions of the world. Outbreaks are sporadic, depending on the varying susceptibility of livestock to the virus, wind-borne spread of the small adult flies, and the availability of suitable breeding sites. Biting midges cause a pruritic dermatitis in horses, called sweet itch, involving type I hypersensitivity.

Control of Ceratopogonidae

Owing to the diffuse nature of their larval habitats, it is difficult to control midges. The use of insecticides to prevent biting attack is rarely used, but the same principles as for other biting flies apply. At night, flocks of sheep susceptible to bluetongue may be provided with partial protection from *Culicoides* by either keeping them in exposed windy sites, in roofed housing or in close proximity to cattle on which the *Culicoides* prefer to feed.

Mosquitoes

Family Culicidae

The mosquitoes are biting pests of man and vectors of malaria and yellow fever and are common throughout the tropics wherever there is free-standing water, which provides a habitat for the larvae. Pupation takes place at the surface of the water. Both adult sexes seek meals of nectar or plant sap containing sugar, but it is only the females who seek blood meals from a very wide variety of hosts, although individual species are often fairly host-specific. The females feed by piercing the skin and then a capillary with a very fine fascicle and then they ingest a large meal of whole blood (i.e. solenophagy). After one large meal, the female rests and develops a batch of several hundred eggs. These are laid on or near water and the female seeks another blood meal to support further egg production. This is known as a gonotrophic cycle and in a favourable environment may be repeated at intervals of 4–5 days many times over. In favourable seasons and environments, populations of mosquitoes can accumulate to enormous nocturnal swarms. If livestock, particularly cattle, are available, then the problem of blood loss and biting stress can be severe, leading to death by exsanguination and shock in some cases. Such problems tend to be highly local and highly seasonal. Milk yields are reduced immediately and if the problem is prolonged there is loss of gain in liveweight. This has been demonstrated in many studies in the USA.

Mosquitoes are vectors of many pathogens to man and livestock. Although they have never gained the notoriety of tsetse flies as vectors of disease to livestock, the massive epizootics of Rift Valley fever indicate their importance. Rift Valley fever virus is transmitted by at least 10 species of mosquitoes throughout Africa. In most respects, it behaves like a true arbovirus (arthropod-borne virus), but it can be transmitted to humans dealing with infected animal carcases. The Venezuelan equine encephalitis virus has been found to be transmitted to horses by about 30 species of mosquitoes in Central and South America. The viruses of both Western and Eastern equine encephalomyelitis are similarly transmitted to horses in the USA and Canada by a variety of mosquitoes, but these are not economically important to livestock rearers in the tropics. About 70 mosquito species are known to transmit *Dirofilaria immitis*, the dog heartworm.

Control of mosquitoes

This is very highly developed in relation to the control of malaria, etc., but, as a live-stock pest, it is usually too expensive to control the larval habitats or prevent the feeding of mosquitoes by sheltering the livestock. The use of synthetic pyrethroids as sprays, pour-on or ear tag applications may assist, particularly if they protect against other types of fly attack. The pyrethroids are particularly suitable for this because they have a rapid knock-down effect at low concentrations and thus even in a brief contact between a mosquito and the treated hair coat of an animal, sufficient insecticide may transfer to the mosquito. The control of mosquitoes and all other types of biting fly can be carried out using several types of self-applicators, thus providing a constant supply of conventional insecticide in a dust or oil formulation. Repellents have been used experimentally, but they tend to be too expensive for maintaining control over a sufficiently long period.

Muscid flies

Family Muscidae

This diverse family contains flies important as biting pests, non-blood sucking flies of much nuisance, and tsetse which transmit trypanosomes.

HAEMATOBIA: HORN FLIES OR BUFFALO FLIES

This genus was formerly called *Lyperosia*. The subspecies *Haematobia irritans irritans*, the horn fly, is found in the Americas, North Africa and Europe. The subspecies *H. irritans exigua*, the buffalo fly, occurs throughout the Orient and in tropical Australia. In Africa south of the Sahara, *H. thirouxi potans* is found. Differences between the species are slight, and they are all highly adapted to life around and on cattle and buffaloes.

The eggs are laid on the fresh dung of their hosts, each batch containing up to 14 eggs but repeated batches are laid up to a total of 300–400 eggs. Pupation takes place in the dung pat and the emerging flies converge on their hosts for feeding and mating. The life-cycle can be less than 2 weeks. During warm wet seasons, which are favourable for adult activity and in which dung pats remain in a suitable condition, large populations may build up. The adults stay on the host, flying to take up different positions. Both sexes feed on blood and take repeated small meals every day. Infestations may see thousands of flies per animal, 10,000 having been recorded. Although the flies are small and they do not transmit serious pathogens, the loss of production due to biting stress and blood loss can be substantial, particularly in dairy herds.

Control of *Haematobia*

Most control measures are directed at applying insecticides to the cattle. Self-applicators containing dust or oil formulations and ear tags and tail bands impregnated with organophosphorus or synthetic pyrethroid insecticides are commonly used. Feed additives may be useful, containing systemic organophosphorus compounds to kill larvae in dung. Because the flies have such a rapid life cycle the development of resistance to insecticides (see below) has reduced the efficiency of ear tag type methods. Research is directed at the possible use of exotic dung beetles to destroy the dung or species of invertebrates that will parasitize the larvae, but there are no established methods for this yet.

MUSCA: HOUSE FLIES, BUSH FLIES, ETC

There are several species of *Musca* that are not blood feeders, but they are a severe nuisance to man and livestock. *Musca vetustissima*, the Australian bush fly, is a notorius nuisance pest of man and livestock. The face fly, *M. autumnalis*, is a nuisance to dairy cattle, and this species and *M. conducens* have been implicated as vectors of filarial nematodes of the genus *Stephanofilaria*, which causes hump sore in cattle. Horn flies and stables flies are also implicated in this disease. *Musca domestica* is extremely common throughout the world, and in the tropics it has an enormous potential for increasing its population rapidly and the ability to breed in a huge variety of materials. The economic loss is not due solely to loss of production due to irritation. The regulations concerning hygiene in egg production and in dairies tend to demand the stringent control of flies. The flies are not vectors of serious pathogens of livestock, but they are a potential means of transmission of numerous pathogens which contaminate human and livestock faeces. These are then transmitted back to humans and livestock and livestock products. Thus in dairies and poultry houses, fly control is of utmost importance. Though sometimes required by legislation, it is still cost-effective for livestock producers. Manure disposal and hygiene are fundamental for fly control. The various means of applying insecticides include aerosol misting, residual deposits, vapour dispensers, feed additives and the application of insecticide to larval habitats.

STOMOXYS: STABLE FLIES

The stable fly, *Stomoxys calcitrans*, is globally distributed, though it is more common in temperate zones than in the tropics. These flies are very similar in appearance to the non-biting houseflies, but they have a protruding proboscis. They attack cattle persistently and are a particular nuisance in dairies or other livestock housing. Milk yields may be reduced by 40–60% and the threshold for such a reduction has been estimated at only 25 flies per cow. Massive infestations have led to the death of both cattle and horses. Numerous other hosts, including poultry, are attacked. *S. nigra* has been recorded as forcing smallholders to keep dairy cows permanently under shelter and of inhibiting those undertaking artificial insemination of cattle. However, these flies are relatively unimportant in the transmission of diseases, although they may be involved in the transmission of *Anaplasma* and *Trypanosoma evansi* by mechanical means. The eggs are laid in a dung and vegetation mixture, typical of the surroundings of animal housing, or in many types of rotting vegetation. Pupation occurs at the surface of the larval habitat and the flies immediately start to feed and mate on their hosts. Both sexes feed on blood, taking 2–3 meals per day. The flies prefer to feed on the lower legs of cattle, causing constant irritation and restlessness. When they are not feeding, the flies are found resting in shade near their hosts.

Control of *Stomoxys*

The larval habitats of *Stomoxys* can be reduced by good hygiene and by using the dung and bedding for composting into manure. Good composting systems generate enough heat to kill the *Stomoxys* larvae. The application of insecticides to cattle is difficult because the lower legs, where the flies prefer to feed, are very inaccessible, and the flies spend little time on their hosts anyway. The spraying of residual insecticides to the resting sites of cattle housing can be used. Experimental methods include the use of visually attractive traps treated with synthetic pyrethroid and the addition of insecticides to cattle feed. Self-applicators may be useful, and repellents which may be cost-effective for dairy cattle have been tested.

Myiasis or flesh-feeding fly larvae

Myiasis is the infestation of animal tissues by the larvae of flies. It is an extremely varied type of parasitism that includes flies that sometimes exploit living flesh if accidentally laid in a wound or body cavity (*Calliphora* spp.: facultative myiasis) and the horse stomach bots which specifically infest the gastric mucosa of the stomach of horses (*Gasterophilus* spp.: obligate myiasis).

The myiasis flies are within the suborder of the Diptera known as the Cyclorrhapha which includes the family Muscidae, but nearly all the facultative and some of the obligate myiasis flies are within the family Calliphoridae, and the family Oestridae consists entirely of obligate myiasis flies. *Musca* spp. may sometimes become involved in accidental myiasis.

BLOW FLIES

Family Calliphoridae

The genera *Calliphora*, *Lucilia*, *Phaenicia* and *Phormia* are typical of the flies that cause distinct and regular problems to livestock owners. Only the larvae are problematic, as the adults do not feed on livestock. Wounds that are neglected and suppurating are attractive to the females for egg laying and the larvae will feed on necrotic tissue. In range-land livestock, the live flesh is likely to be invaded with much stress and damage to the host. Wool maggots belong to the same genera, and *Phaenicia* in particular is a major problem in Australia and other sheep-rearing areas. Breeds of sheep with folded skin and much wool around the back legs easily become soiled and the surface of the skin is very greasy due to excessive sebaceous and sweat secretions. This forms a food for the larvae and heavy infestations easily break through the skin to form large wounds.

Control of blow flies and wool maggots

Lipophilic insecticides tend to remain residual on sheep wool for a long period of time because of its greasy nature, and the typical organophosphorus compounds for application by spraying, showering or pour-on include trichlorfon, diazinon, chlorfenvinphos and fenthion. There are a variety of hygiene procedures used to overcome the susceptibility of sheep to these flies. Mule's operation consists of removing a strip of skin from the back legs and around the breech of lambs in order to produce a hairless scar, thereby reducing soiling.

OESTRIDAE: WARBLE FLIES AND BOTS

The warble flies, *Hypoderma* spp., are widely distributed throughout the tropics and temperate regions. They infest many species including man but, economically, cattle are the most important host. The eggs are laid on to the hair of the legs of cattle. When the larvae emerge, they burrow through the skin and slowly migrate through the musculature to below the skin suface on the back. Here they penetrate the skin to expose the spiracles, where they mature rapidly. When they have matured, they burrow through the skin, drop to the ground and pupate. The musculature is damaged by the tracks of the larvae, the hides are damaged and the cattle suffer stress leading to loss of production. However, the most dramatic loss associated with warble flies is the panic (i.e. gadding) experienced by cattle when they know the female flies are near. This is sometimes severe enough to lead to death by abortion, falling or drowning.

Control of warble flies

These have been eradicated in many temperate countries by the use of conventional insecticides such as coumaphos, applied by spraying or dipping. Recently, organophosphorus insecticides with a systemic action, such as fenthion or trichlorfon, have been used as pour-on applications. The ivermectins are also effective. An obvious difficulty with such treatments is the fate of the larvae within the host. Inflammatory reactions to the dead larvae can sometimes harm the host more than the live larvae. Therefore, timing is important so as to kill the larvae at their early developmental stages.

Dermatobia hominis

This fly is notorious throughout tropical South America as the torsalo or nuche. It is one of the most important ectoparasites of cattle in the region, and it infests a very wide variety of warm-blooded animals, including humans. The female lays its eggs on the legs of female mosquitoes. The eggs hatch immediately when the mosquito lands on a host to feed. (i.e. phoretic transfer) and the larvae burrow through the skin and establish individual infestation sites. The larvae do not burrow, but they tend to be clumped where many larvae have been deposited by a mosquito. The lesions are super-ficial, but the ruined hides and the stress caused by infestations reduce productivity.

Control of *Dermatobia*

The methods used are basically the same as for warble flies, but the problem is far more intractable than warble fly infestations in temperate countries, because in tropical South America *Dermatobia* is in the centre of its natural range and it does not occur in a distinct seasonal cycle. Methods of control are also directed at preventing mosquitoes from landing on cattle. Those control measures used for biting flies such as *Haematobia* are also relevant.

Nasal bot flies

There are numerous species of nasal bot flies, but *Oestrus ovis* is especially important throughout the world where sheep are raised. The female fly lays small batches of eggs in the nostrils of sheep. The larvae migrate into the nasal sinuses and attach to the mucous membranes. Mature larvae are sneezed out by the host and pupate in the ground. Infested animals have a purulent discharge from the nose, shake their heads a lot and suffer anorexia.

Control of nasal bots

Control is difficult because of the location of the larvae, but organophosphorus insecticide aerosols such as trichlorphon are effective. The spores of *Bacillus thuringiensis*, which is a natural pathogen of many insect larvae, are sold in various formulations (e.g. Thuringen) for pest control. There have been few veterinary applications, but aerosols of this agent can be effective against nasal bots.

Horse bots

The genus *Gasterophilus* is highly adapted for larval development in various regions of the gut of horses and other equines. The eggs are laid in a variety of sites, in some species actually on the vegetation which the horses feed on (*G. pecorum*). The larvae enter the mouth when the host feeds or grooms itself, and they migrate through the mucous membrane of the tongue and oesophagus to a specific maturation site such as the gastric mucosa. When they are mature, they pass out with the faeces and pupate in the soil. Infestations with small numbers appear to cause little harm, but large infestations can lead to intestinal blockage or rupture and to secondary infestations of the intestinal mucosa.

Control of horse bots

The application of carbon disulphide by stomach tube has been used effectively for a long time. Specific insecticides applied in the same way or as drenches include trichlorphon, dichlorvos and neguvon, which also has major anti-helminthic activity. Injectable ivermectins are also formulated for the combined control of *Gasterophilus* and helminths in horses.

SCREW-WORM FLIES

These flies have larvae which resemble a wood screw. They are found buried in the flesh of their hosts with their pointed head down, and with their air breathing spiracles exposed at the surface. The most notorious species are *Cochliomyia hominivorax*, the screw-worm of the New World (Americas), and *Chrysomyia bezziana*, the screw-worm of the Old World (Africa and Asia). One female lays a batch of 200–300 eggs on the edge of a wound. The hosts are typically cattle, but when there is a large population of flies, other stock and humans become infested. One batch of eggs forms a distinct lesion in the skin, and the larvae remain buried but exposed to the surface by their spiracles. When they are mature, the larvae crawl out and fall to the ground, bury themselves in the soil, pupate and then emerge as adults. The adults to not feed on or disturb livestock. Economic losses due to screw-worm in the Americas have been enormous.

Control of screw-worm

Screw-worm flies have been the subject of an eradication scheme which releases sterile males into the population. Though cost-effective, this technique has to be preceded by chemical control. One successful way of doing this is to use the bait Swormlure, which mimics the smell of necrosis. Attracted by the bait, the females die when they make contact with the dichlorvos or a similar insecticide contained in the bait (see below). Infestation lesions can be treated individually by dusting with coumaphos.

Tabanids

Family Tabanidae

The larvae of the horse flies or clegs live in diffuse habitats of moist soil and rotting vegetation. The larval stage may last for several years and pupation takes place at the surface of the soil. Adult males do not feed on blood. The females are large flies with strong flight and extremely good vision. They chase after their hosts during daylight hours. They rarely occur in large numbers but persistently follow livestock in search of a blood meal. Their mouthparts are exceptionally large and powerful, their cutting action forming a large lesion, and a lot of saliva is produced to promote blood flow. In addition, the mouthparts have a sponge-like labellum to assist in the ingestion of blood.

In many warm temperate regions, tabanid flies are important to livestock because their bites are painful. Both cattle and sheep form into protective groups as tightly packed as possible. Such formations may last for days without the animals grazing, drinking or sheltering properly. The resulting stress is known as fly syndrome and can occur with only small populations of tabanids. In addition, detailed studies of blood loss have shown that 500–1000 flies feeding on a cow in any one day results in a blood loss of 150–200 ml.

Because of their painful bites, interruptions in feeding are common, and there is a measurable quantity of blood that remains on the mouthparts after feeding. Thus mechanical transmission of pathogens occurs fairly readily. *Anaplasma marginale*, which causes anaplasmosis in cattle, may be transmitted by tabanids, but it is not clear how important these flies are as vectors compared with ticks. *Trypanosoma evansi*, the causative agent of surra in cattle, buffaloes and camels, is transmitted by numerous species of tabanid, but little is known of the epidemiology of transmission of this disease.

Control of tabanids

The very diffuse larval habits make control at this stage uneconomic. Self-application of insecticides to dairy cattle is probably the most cost-effective form of protection. For range-land animals, subject to fly syndrome, however, protection is more difficult. Thus the protection of animals to control anaplasmosis or surra is never likely to be practical because the fly attacks are too diffuse.

Tsetse

Genus Glossina

The tsetse flies are highly specialized and restricted to Africa south of the Sahara (i.e. the Afro-tropical or Ethiopian zoogeographic region). They are very important as vectors of human and livestock trypanosomes but, because of their low population density, they are rarely a serious biting pest. Though there are many species, those most important for the transmission of trypanosomes pathogenic to livestock are the savanna tsetse of the morsitans group. This is a taxonomic and ecological grouping which includes. *G. morsitans*, the most important vector, and *G. pallidipes*, the second most important vector on an Africa-wide basis. These tsetse inhabit savanna zones, characterized by open glassland with groups of trees to dry bushland. *G. austeni* is also in this group, but it is localized to the coastal forests in East Africa. Tsetse flies are highly dependent on suitable vegetation for their survival and feeding behaviour. Much effort has been spent on modifying habitats to render them unsuitable for tsetse flies.

Tsetse fly eggs are produced in very small numbers and retained within the female. The female mates only once and the sperm are stored within a spermatheca. The larvae are allowed to mature one at a time within the oviduct of the female. Repeated blood meals support the development of the larvae until each has a mass sufficient to support its further development into an adult without the need for further supplies of food (i.e. larviparous reproduction). A single fully grown larva is laid by the female on to loose sandy soil in a shady site. The larva burrows down and pupates. Pupal development takes 3–7 weeks in suitable temperatures. The adult which emerges from the pupa seeks a blood meal and mates within a few days. Both sexes are entirely dependent on blood. One female produces one larva every 10–11 days and in favourable environments will live 50–60 days. The rate of reproduction is very low, but the survival rate is very high and tsetse populations are persistent over repeated seasons. During the dry season, there is a contraction to more wooded areas to obtain the necessary shade.

Both sexes become infected with trypanosomes, which have an essential development phase in the tsetse fly. Thus even in *T. vivax*, which only occurs on the mouthparts of the tsetse fly, the transmission is truly biological. This is in contrast to the mechanical transmission of *T. evansi* by tabanid flies.

Control of tsetse flies

The main basis of the control of trypanosomosis is by chemotherapy of livestock at risk and, despite many efforts to develop vaccines against trypanosomes and the biological control of tsetse flies, drugs are likely to remain the most important defence against trypanosomosis. However, the control of tsetse flies by direct or indirect means has been shown to be feasible and cost-effective if run in conjunction with an effective land-use system. This is because the morsitans group tsetse flies usually do not re-invade areas that have been modified for domestic use by the cutting and burning of woodland and bushes.

A fully integrated scheme for tsetse control will cover a very large area and include some or most of the following methods. Barrier zones are created by the erection of fencing and the possible deforestation of strips of land at least 1 km wide. Within these barrier zones, game control is practised so as to preserve the fences and to reduce the number of hosts. However, the favourite hosts of *G. morsitans* are wild pigs and warthogs, which are difficult to hunt out. Within the barrier zone and possibly in conspicuous foci of infestation during the dry season, the vegetation is sprayed with residual insecticides. Dieldrin or DDT are used to give up to 3 months' residual action against adult flies seeking resting sites. Fixed-wing aircraft can be used to spray aerosol mists of short-acting insecticides (endosulphan or deltamethrin), which kill adult flies by direct contact. These treatments are repeated often enough to kill flies newly emerged from pupae in the ground. Recent experiments on the use of traps for the large-scale control of tsetse flies is entering commercial production (see below). Tsetse flies have been the subject of intensive research on the releasing of sterile males (see below).

Methods for the control of flies

The technical means for the control of flies affecting livestock are much more varied than for the conventional control of ticks. When dip baths or spray races are available, primarily for the control of ticks or mites, they will often be the most efficient means of applying insecticides to livestock. For example, although flumethrin pour-on is cheaper to apply and has a longer residual action on fly control than flumethrin dip wash, it may be more cost-effective for a farmer to use a dip bath or spray race for the combined control of *Boophilus* and *Dermatobia*, the most common combination of ectoparasites in South America. Methods specifically for the control of flies are listed below.

Showers. Sheep blowfly can be controlled by packing the sheep into a circular pen with an overhead shower boom for applying an insecticide wash.

Aerosol misters. A flow of hot gas or compressed air can be used to create an aerosol for fly control using the venturi effect to draw up insecticide from a reservoir. Spinning disc applicators can also be used, in which a fan creates an airflow and a spinning disc in the flow creates fine droplets of insecticide due to centrifugal spread from a central nozzle. This apparatus is hand-held and can be used in dairies and poultry houses. Synthetic pyrethroids are typical of the insecticides used.

Back-pack sprayers. There are two types of pressurized sprayers which have a reservoir of insecticide that can be carried on the operator's back. One is pressurized by manual pumping before use, whereas the other has a side-handle for operating the pump continuously while in use. These pumps have been used extensively in the control of tsetse flies. Residual deposits of insecticide are applied with very high specificity to the known resting sites of adult tsetse flies. Both types of pump can be used for applying insecticides to livestock and to breeding sites of flies, such as manure and waste piles.

Aerial spraying. This is a highly specialized operation carried out by a few commercial companies in Africa for the purpose of tsetse control. Small, twin-engined, fixed-wing aircraft are used, with the passenger space occupied by an insecticide reservoir. Insecticide at an ultra-low volume is supplied to two spraying booms bearing spinning cage applicators. The insecticide flows out over a metal mesh cylinder and is thrown from the spinning mesh to form an aerosol mist of droplets 30–50 μm in diameter. This drifts down between the vegetation to kill adult tsetse by direct contact. The mist only drifts into the vegetation when the air is still and the air near the ground is cool and the air above warm. Such conditions are found at night and around dawn. Because the spraying takes place at very low level, advanced navigation equipment is required. Ground teams mark out the flight paths, which are parallel to each other and several hundred metres apart. The spraying is repeated at intervals of several weeks to kill tsetse freshly emerged from pupae until local eradication is achieved.

Jetting. To apply insecticide to sheep, particularly woolled sheep, a pressurized jet of insecticide wash is applied manually to individual sheep via a tube with four or five nozzles like a large comb which is drawn through the wool.

Ear tags, pour-on and spot-on. These have been described under tick control for hand dressing cattle. These methods have great potential in the control of biting and nuisance flies and for repelling flies that produce myiasis larvae. Ear tags and pour-on incorporating synthetic pyrethroids are very effective against flies, and because they have a very rapid knock-down effect at low concentrations, they are sometimes mistaken for repellents. Spot-on applications are similar to pour-on, but a syringe-like applicator is used to deliver a set volume of oil-based insecticide along the back or between the horns. Pour-on formulations of organophosphorus compounds, available for the control of myiasis fly larvae, penetrate the skin and have a systemic action. Pour-on formulations of synthetic pyrethroids, available for tick and fly control, remain superficial, but they have a long-acting residual deposit. Users need to differentiate between these different modes of action for controlling myiasis larvae and for preventing adult flies from laying eggs.

Repellents. There are very few repellent chemicals of the type used by humans to repel mosquitoes and midges (diethyl toluamide) that can be applied to livestock. The problem is maintaining the repellent effect for long enough. They have been superseded by the synthetic pyrethroids, which have a long residual effect on the hair coat.

Self-applicators. These are often farm made, but some types are commercially available. They consist of a cloth sack which contains a dusting formulation of insecticide or that is soaked in an oil formulation of insecticide. They are hung near the water trough or salt lick areas of range cattle, where the livestock are able to gain relief from a biting fly attack by rubbing against the sack. Dairy cattle are able to apply the insecticide themselves by walking through a passage with a self-actuating switch to a pressurized aerosol sprayer with insecticide.

Traps and baits. Traps consist of an ultra-violet light which attracts flies past an electrocuting grid. Mosquitoes and midges are strongly attracted to these at night. However, despite their common use for controlling flies in commercial premises, they are not very attractive to day-flying muscid flies.

Muscid flies find baits more attractive. These granule formulations contain an aggregation pheromone (an externally released hormone), a feeding substrate and an insecticide. Similarly myiasis flies may be killed by baits formulated to smell like necrotic wounds, which are attractive to egg-laying females. The bait contains a contact insecticide. A type formulated for the control of *Cochliomyia hominivorax* is known as Swormlure. *Stomoxys* flies can be reduced in numbers by using traps which consist of translucent plastic panels coated with an adhesive or a residual deposit of insecticide such as a synthetic pyrethroid.

Traps for the control of tsetse flies have recently been developed for commercial production. They consist of a framed cloth screen about 2 metres square, set up close to ground level so that it can rotate and act as a visual attractant – black and blue have been found to be the most attractive colours. At the base of the screen bottles slowly release the attractants acetone and octenol (the latter is a synthetic food flavour). The screen is treated regularly with a residual deposit of a special formulation of the synthetic pyrethroid deltamethrin (Glossinex). These traps can be effective at densities as low as four per km² and they can be used together with aerial spraying, barrier zones, etc. Cattle can also be used as bait for the control of tsetse flies; a residual deposit of deltamethrin on the coat of the cattle will kill the flies on contact.

Pheromones. Pheromones, which are sexual attractants, have been developed successfully for the control of some crop pests. An aggregation pheromone attracts muscid flies to insecticide treated bait. Tsetse flies are attracted to a bait which is treated with a chemical sterilizing agent or insecticide; however, the cost and instability of the reagents limits application at present. Some species of ticks are attracted by dichlorophenol, which can be incorporated into an acaricidal bait. Finally, it appears that the most effective bait for controlling ticks on livestock is the hosts themselves.

Sterile male release. The idea of releasing sterile males into the population has been tried with tsetse flies, but it has been most successful in eradicating screw-worm flies (*Cochliomyia hominivorax*) from the USA and with eradication schemes in Latin America. The principle is to colonize large numbers of flies by feeding the larvae on proteinaceous material. The males are then treated with gamma radiation to sterilize them but which leaves them mobile and sexually active. (The same dose will also sterilize females in cases where the sexes cannot be separated on a large scale.) The natural population is reduced to a small percentage of its normal size by chemical control (baits, spraying stock, etc.), and then vast numbers of sterile flies are released over wide areas during the normal breeding season by aircraft. The flies are then dispersed further by their own flight. If the sterilized flies outnumber the unsterilized flies, then a sufficient number of the matings will take place with sterilized males to produce sterile eggs. It then follows that the population will not be able to be sustained naturally. Eradication is thus achieved, and it is sustained by maintaining barrier zones for the *ad hoc* release of sterile flies and chemical control to prevent re-invasion. Thus geographical barriers are most important.

To control tsetse flies in the same way is much more expensive. This is because (1) the flies must be fed on fresh blood from goats or through a membrane, (2) they have a very low reproductive capacity, and (3) there are less distinct geographical barrier zones in Africa than in Latin America. Studies have been carried out to control ticks in this way, but although they have an extremely high reproductive capacity, they are even more expensive to colonize and they are immobile in the environment.

Biological control. Studies have been carried out on the control of many ectoparasites of veterinary importance by using natural predators or pathogens, but there has been little success. Bacterial spores (see below) are commercially available but they have limited veterinary applications. The nuisance and biting flies in Australia, *Musca vetustissima* and *Haematobia irritans exigua*, have been subject to control by the introduction of dung beetles from Africa. These dung beetles have a better ability to remove cattle dung from pastures· than the indigenous beetles, which specialize in using the dung of marsupials and herbivores. However, the scheme has had only limited success. Biological control is a proven commercial success for some pests of greenhouse crops. To apply such principles to livestock in pastures is fundamentally difficult and extremely expensive.

Lice

Order Phthiraptera (Siphunculata)

These are the lice and are divided into two suborders, the Anoplura and the Mallophaga.

Anoplura

These are the sucking lice and have mouthparts adapted for piercing the skin of their host and sucking blood through a fine fascicle or bundle of components of the mouthparts. This penetrates a blood capillary and whole blood is ingested (i.e. solenophagy). The entire life-cycle is completed on the host. Lice cannot survive for long off a host and transfer to new hosts is by body contact, particularly under conditions of close confinement. Female lice feed and mate repeatedly, and the eggs (nits) are laid and glued on the hairs of the host. Eggs are laid over the life-span of the female, i.e. 20–50 days. The eggs hatch within 1–2 weeks to produce nymphs, which are like the adults and feed repeatedly and moult several times until they reach adult size and sexual maturity. A typical number of generations per year is 10.

Although blood loss due to an individual louse is not great, very heavy infestations can accumulate on cattle and pigs leading to anaemia, biting stress and anorexia. The loss of condition can be serious if the whole herd becomes infested. Sucking lice are notorious for the transmission of typhus and relapsing fever to humans, but they do not transmit serious pathogens to livestock.

The genus *Haematopinus* contains species which parasitize cattle, pigs and horses. *Linognathus* spp. typically parasitize cattle and sheep, and *Solenoptes* spp. are found on cattle.

Mallophaga

These are known as the biting or chewing lice because they do not have penetrating bloodsucking mouthparts; instead, they chew at the surface and at the base of feathers on poultry. If the skin is broken by the chewing, then leaking blood may be ingested. Because they are common on birds, and the Anoplura do not occur on birds, the

Mallophaga are often called bird lice. The life-cycle and ecology of Mallophaga are similar to Anoplura. The entire life-cycle is spent on the host. The life-cycle is short, there are many generations in a year and there is usually potential for massive accumulations of lice on individual hosts.

The chicken body louse, *Monopon gallinae*, is distributed worldwide, and *Goniodes gigas* is prevalent on poultry in the tropics. Heavy infestations cause irritation and loss of productivity in poultry. There are numerous species infesting sheep and cattle, typically of the genera *Damalinia*, *Bovicola* and *Trichodectes*, but the effects on health and productivity are usually less than with poultry. However, heavy louse infestations of wool sheep cause a reduction in the sale value of the wool.

The Mallophaga are not important in the transmission of diseases to livestock, but the filarial nematode *Dipetalonema reconditum* can be transmitted to dogs when they ingest the louse *Heterodoxus spiniger* which is infesting them.

Control of lice

This consists mainly of applying a wide variety of insecticides to the hosts which lice are susceptible to. Acaricides used for tick and mite control, such as lindane or dioxathion, will also control lice. Thus, if available, dip baths or sprays used for tick and mite control may be the best way of applying insecticides for the control of lice on cattle and sheep. This is particularly important considering the need to treat the whole herd, as a low infestation not noticed on a few individuals can spread by contact to the whole herd. Pour-on treatments are also suitable for cattle and sheep and self-applicators, as used for fly control, will assist in the control of lice. Hand sprays or pour-ons are most convenient for applications to pigs. Sucking lice are susceptible to the systematic avermectins, but chewing lice are less exposed to the toxic component.

The application of insecticides to poultry is difficult, and for economic reasons lice control may be combined with treatments to reduce attacks by mites. Dust formulations of carbaryl, coumaphos and malathion are typical for treating poultry against Mallophaga. Modern poultry houses and management methods are less conducive to heavy louse infestations, but breeder hens and roosters remain the most susceptible. Lousiness is usually worse in poorly nourished livestock and young animals are most susceptible.

PESTICIDES

Insecticides and acaricides used for the control of livestock ectoparasites are of numerous chemical varieties, most of which are formulated by different chemical companies under different brand names. The following list is an arbitrary selection of some commonly used pesticides, listed by their common (generic) chemical name, though some selected brand names are given. The term residual refers to the required length of time the pesticide is to be effective as a deposit placed where it is meant to work, e.g. on the hair coat of livestock or on branches where tsetse flies rest. Persistence refers to the chemical stability of the pesticide in the environment, either at the site of application or as an environmental contaminant. The term residue refers to the contaminating effect of any pesticide in or on livestock produce which may affect the consumers of that produce. The chemical principle of insecticides and acaricides is that they have extremely high toxicity for ectoparasites but low to negligible toxicity for humans and livestock. For example, DDT is less toxic than aspirin. However, the problems that have led to DDT being banned in many countries are that it is extremely persistent in the environment, it accumulates in the food chain and in the fatty tissue of predators, and there may be long-term harmful effects other than acute toxicity. On the other hand, the toxicity of some synthetic pyrethroids is so low it cannot be measured experimentally, and these chemicals are broken down rapidly in mammalian tissue and in the environment.

Organochlorine compounds

Lindane (also known as gamma benzene hexachloride, BHC or HCH) – "Gammatox". Often used in dips, sprays, hand dressings, etc., for the control of all types of ectoparasites. Moderate residual effect and fairly long persistence.

Toxaphene (also known as camphechlor) – "Coopertox", "Strobane". Very often used for tick and mite control in dips. Good residual effect, moderate persistence.

DDT – "Dicophane", "Neocid". The original synthetic pesticide, now restricted because of problems with extreme persistence, but still used for the selective residual spraying of the resting sites of tsetse flies.

Endosulphan – "Thiodan". Used often for aerial spraying against tsetse flies, it has a lower persistence than usual for organochlorine compounds.

Organophosphorus compounds

Coumaphos – "Asuntal", "Co-Ral". Often used against ticks with a good residual effect on wool to control myiasis fly attack. Also used in oil for back rubbers, etc.

Chlorfenvinphos – "Supona". Very commonly used for tick and fly control, but it has high mammalian toxicity and problems with residues.

Dioxathion – "Delnav", "Bercotox". Commonly used in dips and sprays for tick control, it has a moderate residual effect and moderate persistence.

Diazinon – "Neocidal". Widely used as a residual application to livestock and to buildings for fly control. Also used for mange control. No systemic action and moderate toxicity.

Phosmet – "Prolate". Used as a pour-on formulation for systemic action against myiasis larvae, mange mites and lice.

Malathion – "Cynthion". Commonly used for controlling mosquitoes and as dusting powders, etc., for flea and louse control because of very low toxicity.

Fenthion – "Tiguvon", "Baytex". Solution in oil as a pour-on for control of myiasis fly larvae by systemic effect.

Trichlorphon – "Dipterex", "Dylox". Commonly used as a pour-on for myiasis fly control or as "Neguvon" as an oral paste to control helminths and stomach bots.

Dichlorvos – "Vapona", "Equigard". Impregnated into plastic strips from where it evaporates to control flies, fleas, etc., and also as a stomach drench to control horse bots.

Famphur – "Warbex". Used as pour-on for systemic action through the skin to control myiasis fly larvae.

Tetrachlorvinphos (also known as stirofos) – "Rabon". Widely used as a spray for the control of muscid flies, or as a feed additive against poultry mites, and for incorporation into ear tags.

Carbamate compounds

Carbaryl – "Sevin", "Menaphtame". Very widely used against many insect and mite pests. Formulated as a dip wash, sprays and powders. Moderate toxicity and residual effect, low persistence.

Propoxur – "Baygon". Used for impregnation into collars, etc., for flea control.

Amidine compounds

Amitraz – "Tactic''", "Triatix". Formulated for tick control, it has a long residual effect and low persistence.'

Synthetic pyrethroids

The chemical structure of these is based on natural pyrethrum which is extracted from a plant and is used for domestic fly control.

Deltamethrin – "Butox", "Spoton", "Glossinex". Wide variety of applications from dipping to control ticks to aerial spraying against tsetse flies. Good residual effect, low toxicity, very low persistence.

Flumethrin – "Bayticol". Formulated as a dip wash concentrate or pour-on for tick and fly control (note that synthetic pyrethroids used as a pour-on only form a residual deposit on the epidermis, and do not penetrate the skin to have a systemic effect like the organophosphorus pour-ons). Very long residual effect, low persistence, negligible toxicity to mammals.

Permethrin – "Stomoxin", "Ectiban". Formulated in eartags and sprays for fly control and as a pour-on for the control of lice.

Fenvalerate – "Ectrin". Formulated in eartags and sprays for fly and tick control.

Miscellaneous compounds

Ivermectin – "Ivomec". The avermectins are produced from fungi (*Streptomyces avermitilis*) using similar methods to antibiotic production. Formulated as an injectable solution for the control of helminths, lice, mites and myiasis flies. However, "Ivomec" can only be used as an aid in the control of one-host ticks, and it is not efficient to use current formulations primarily for tick control.

Benzyl benzoate. Formulated as a soapy emulsion for the control of ear mites.

Bacillus thuringiensis – "Thuringen", "Bactimos". Spores of this natural pathogen of insect larvae are used for malaria control and may have veterinary applications such as nasal bot control.

Methoprene – "Viodat", "Altosid". An insect growth regulator administered as a feed additive to control biting and nuisance flies that breed in livestock dung.

Repellents

Diethyl toluamide – "Deet", "Off". Mainly used to protect humans, but dairy cattle can be protected from flies.
Dibutyl succinate – "Tabutrex". For the protection of dairy cattle against biting flies.

Resistance

Ticks and insects can develop the ability to survive normal doses of pesticides, which makes them inefficient or completely useless. Often, there is some degree of cross resistance within the same chemical class of pesticide, so that pests with resistance to one pesticide are resistant to a related pesticide even without prior exposure. Multiple resistance can occur within a population of pests, so that several chemical groups are ineffective. Control may become uneconomic or impossible.

This serious threat to pest control measures may be made worse by the loss of acquired resistance to vector-borne diseases that can occur in livestock previously well protected from ticks or insects. Resistance to pesticides is acquired over many generations by natural selection for metabolic mechanisms that detoxify or avoid the killing action of the pesticide. Once a resistant population is established, it will remain resistant for decades at least. The development of resistance appears inevitable. The faster the generation time of the pest the faster resistance develops, and thus *Musca* and *Haematobia* spp. develop resistance rapidly. However, resistance has not been recorded in tsetse flies to date.

The rate at which resistance develops in tick or insects populations in an area can be slowed down by reducing the numbers of times that the pesticide is used, together with making sure that the pesticide achieves the highest possible killing effect on the greatest number of pests. This is done by using a fresh, full-strength pesticide that is applied to give full coverage to all sites where the tick or insect will be found. When resistance does occur, it must be detected as soon as possible by the use of standardized testing systems (for ticks, by using larvae exposed to titrations of the suspect acaricide, followed by a count of the killed larvae). Often, the only way to resume effective control is to change to a new chemical grouping. e.g. from an organochlorine type to an organophosphorus type. Conservatism in the use of older (and cheaper) chemical groups can be economic if a system is applied nationally. Resistance already occurs to the new synthetic pyrethroids; it may be a mistaken policy to assume that chemical companies will be prepared to invest vast funds to develop new groups of pesticides for the control of livestock ticks, because the market for such compounds is small relative to that for crop pest control.

Further reading

Anonymous (1986). *The Merck veterinary manual*, 6th edn. Merck, Rahway.
Food and Agriculture Organization (1984). *Ticks and tick-borne disease control, a practical field manual*, Vols I and II. FAO, Rome.
Food and Agriculture Organization (undated). *Training manual for tsetse control personnel*, Vols 1, 2 and 3. FAO, Rome.
Harwood, R.F. and James, M.T. (1979). *Entomology in human and animal health*. Macmillan, New York.

Jordan A.M. (1986). *Trypanosomiasis control and African rural development*. Longman, London.
Kettle, D.S. (1984). *Medical and veterinary entomology*. Croom Helm, London.
Lancaster, J.L. and Meisch, M.V. (1986). *Arthropods in livestock and poultry production*. Ellis Horwood, Chichester.
Williams, R.E., Hall, R.D., Broce, A.B. and Scholl, P.J. (1985). *Livestock entomology*. John Wiley, Chichester.

Diseases caused by bacteria

R.M. Edelsten, R.N. Gourlay, G.H.K. Lawson, A.N. Morrow and
S. Ramachandran

ANTHRAX

Anthrax is a peracute, acute or subacute soil-borne infection of domestic and wild animals and man, characterized by bacteraemia and toxaemia.

Aetiology

Bacillus anthracis is – apart from its pathogenicity – a typical member of the genus *Bacillus*, resembling most closely *B. cereus* and *B. megaterium*. It forms large Gram-positive rods that are $0.75–1.0 \times 3.0–5.0$ μm in size. In animal tissues, it develops a prominent protective capsule of polyglutamic acid, which is not evident in culture unless suitable conditions are provided. The vegetative organism only sporulates in the presence of oxygen and when the ambient temperature is between 20 and 40°C, the humidity is above 60% and the pH is above 6.0. Under these conditions, spore formation starts within a few hours of excretion from the animal body.

Occurrence

Anthrax occurs all over the world and few countries are genuinely free of infection. In warm climates, the rapid production of resistant spores leads to contamination of soil and water. Spores may survive in certain soils and water holes for years, especially if the pH is slightly alkaline. In other situations, the organism appears to die out within a few weeks. Outbreaks of the disease occur when animals return to contaminated pastures or watering points; this often coincides with the local rainy season. Epidemics occur when an anthrax carcase is opened up by predators such as vultures or carnivores, and widespread contamination of an area takes place. Sporadic cases occur when spores are dispersed by the wind and predators, via contaminated feeds, fertilizers of animal origin and tannery effluent.

Species affected

All mammals, but most commonly herbivores, can be affected. Cattle, sheep and goats are most susceptible, followed by water buffalo, camels and equines. Pigs tend to be more resistant and carnivores even more so. Birds, especially scavengers, are usually refractory, but exceptions do occur, e.g. in zoos, where virtually any mammal or bird may be affected if fed by mistake on meat from an anthrax carcase. Outbreaks of disease are reported to occur sporadically in wild antelope. Man is susceptible to infection, but disease is less common than might be expected.

Transmission

The route of infection is usually by ingestion, and less commonly by aerosols or skin abrasions. In equines and camels, transmission by biting flies is often suspected and may be responsible for the oedematous lesions seen on the body and legs.

Anthrax is an occupational hazard for stockowners and people working with wool, hides and skins, infection occurring by skin abrasions or aerosols. In rural areas, it is often the custom to salvage carcases regardless of cause of death. Meat is usually cooked within a few hours and this rapidly destroys the vegetative form of *B. anthracis*, before the highly resistant spores have had a chance to develop.

Clinical features

In ruminants, especially sheep and goats, a peracute apoplectic type of anthrax is the most usual. Apparently healthy animals fall and death follows within a few minutes to several hours later. The disease may be less acute and animals, although febrile, linger for a week or more and occasionally recover. Such animals may show swellings in the throat or carbuncular lesions. Equines may show acute anthrax and die within 1–3 days. Others survive longer and show extensive oedema on the ventral aspects of the neck and body. In camels, the disease may take a subacute or chronic form, characterized by oedema. In pigs, the most common lesion is swelling of the throat, larynx and associated lymph nodes. In other outbreaks, the intestine is affected and animals show constipation or diarrhoea. Recovery is not infrequent. Severe inflammation of the throat, stomach and intestine is seen in carnivores, together with carbuncular lesions of the jowls.

Pathology

In peracute and acute cases, blood exudes from the natural openings and through the skin. Bloating and decomposition occur rapidly. The carcase, if accidentally opened, indicates septicaemia. The spleen often, but not always, is greatly enlarged, the pulp tarry. In equines and camels, subcutaneous oedema is seen along the ventral parts of the body and inguinal region. In pigs, inflammation of the throat, laryngeal and pharyngeal mucosa and lymph nodes is common. Haemorrhage and necrosis of the intestine and mesenteric lymph nodes may be seen.

Diagnosis

In tropical countries, the possibility of anthrax should be suspected in all cases of sudden death or where subcutaneous oedema and throat swellings are seen. Differential diagnosis should include blackleg, enterotoxaemia, pasteurellosis, lightning strike, snake bite and plant poisoning. Field officers should examine smears on the spot and, only if negative, proceed with a post-mortem examination. According to the distribution of lesions, smears should be made from blood, lymph node, abdominal fluid or subcutaenous oedema, in such a way that dissemination of infected material is minimal. The smears should be stained using a Romanowsky stain such as Giemsa. The polychrome methylene blue method is quicker but less efficient for putrefying cadavers. A search is made for large square-ended rods with a pink capsule. Organisms may be scanty in subacute or chronic cases. Capsules may appear unstained or partially disintegrate leaving "ghosts". This can occur in animals which have been treated or are partially immune.

Tissues or fluids should be submitted for culture or animal inoculation if smears are inconclusive. A piece of cartilaginous rib or skin may be useful if other tissues are not available. Tissues are best preserved by refrigeration, or immersion in 50% glycerol saline. The Ascoli precipitin test is not reliable and should not replace conventional methods of confirmation.

Treatment

B. anthracis is susceptible to penicillin, tetracyclines and some sulphonamides. These drugs are only effective when treatment is started early in the course of the disease. In the face of an outbreak in valuable animals, temperatures should be monitored for at least 2 weeks and antibiotics given to those showing fever. It must be remembered, however, that antibiotics will interfere with the action of the live spore vaccine, if used at this time. Animals must be revaccinated after the effects of the antibiotics have worn off.

Immunology

The anthrax bacillus produces a complex of antigens including a weak toxin, and filtrates of cultures grown on special media will immunize actively. The capsule, which is essential for the expression of virulence, plays no part in eliciting active immunity. Indeed, the most widely used vaccine, Sterne's spore vaccine, is prepared from a highly immunogenic strain which has lost its ability to form capsules.

Non-living vaccines are used to protect workers at special risk, but they are not sufficiently potent for use in animals.

Control

In endemic areas and on properties known to be infected, ruminants, equines and camels are protected by annual vaccination. Immunity wanes within 9–12 months and vaccination is therefore carried out a month before the peak risk period starts. Continued vaccination over a 4-to 5-year period eliminates some foci of infection but in other places infection persists for much longer. In some areas, one species of animal tends to be affected and not others; selective vaccination may be appropriate.

When anthrax is diagnosed, it is imperative that access to the carcase is prevented. Pending disposal, guards, thorn bushes or stones should be used to prevent predators from tearing the carcase open. Anthrax organisms die within a few days in an unopened carcase in the tropics. Burning of the carcase should only be carried out if it can be done effectively; otherwise, the carcase should be buried 1–2 m deep, and covered with lime.

The contaminated area around the carcase should be burnt; other surfaces should be treated with 10% caustic soda, 10% formalin solution or another approved disinfectant.

R.M.E.

BOVINE FARCY

A chronic disease of cattle previously known as bovine nocardiosis or tropical actinomycosis, bovine farcy affects the superficial lymphatic vessels and lymph nodes. The disease assumes importance because it resembles tuberculosis.

Aetiology

The current name of the organism most commonly isolated from lesions is *Nocardia farcinica*, a Gram-positive actinomycete, which is partially acid-fast and forms a delicate mycelium of branching filaments in tissues. *Mycobacterium farcinogenes* and *M. senegalense* have also been isolated from lesions of farcy. These organisms are closely related to *M. fortuitum*, a cause of skin tuberculosis. Their classification is the subject of continued taxonomic debate.

Occurrence

Farcy is reported sporadically from many countries, but it is most common in tropical areas. Its true prevalence is not known because it is often mistaken for tuberculosis. The prevalence of affected animals within herds is usually low. However, on occasions and for unknown reasons, the disease progressively spreads until almost a whole herd is affected.

Species affected

Only cattle are affected. A similar condition has been reported in Indonesian water buffalo; it is caused by an unclassified Mycobacterium and closely resembles leprosy in man.

Transmission

Transmission is by direct contact with affected animals or indirectly via contaminated bedding, harnesses and other fomites. *Amblyomma* ticks have been shown experimentally to be capable of transmitting infection transtadially, but it is not known if this occurs under natural conditions. In India, lice have been implicated in transmission.

Clinical features

The disease affects cattle of all ages. It appears initially as small subcutaneous nodules, most often on the medial aspect of the limbs and on the neck. The nodules develop slowly and some coalesce in the form of a large berry. They are firm and painless. Infection progresses towards the drainage lymph node over a period of weeks, the lymphatics appearing thickened or cord-like. Nodules show no tendency to rupture, even when the lesions are up to 10 cm across. Swellings may persist for years with no adverse effect upon the general health of the animal. Occasionally, metastasis to visceral organs occurs giving rise to cachexia and death of the animal.

A more acute, rapidly advancing disease is seen less often. Deeper tissues may be involved, accompanied by generalized swelling. In Asia, abscesses are reported to liquefy and ulcerate.

Pathology

Abscesses consist of caseous pus surrounded by a well-defined fibrous capsule. The lymphatic vessels are thickened and induration may extend to adjacent tissues. Lesions of varying sizes may be seen in internal organs, especially lung and associated lymph nodes. They resemble tuberculosis with white or yellowish pus which may calcify. The mammary gland may be affected. Ulcers in the trachea have also been reported.

Diagnosis

Bovine farcy closely resembles tuberculosis, especially when the internal organs are affected. Diagnosis should always be confirmed by laboratory examination. Smears of pus from unopened abscesses should be stained by Gram and Ziehl-Neelsen methods. *N. farcinica* is readily over-decolorized by acid-alcohol with the ZN method; 1–2% sulphuric acid is preferred. Nocardia grow well on routine media forming colonies within 3–5 days. Mycobacteria associated with farcy require specialized media and prolonged incubation for growth.

It should be noted that animals affected with farcy are sensitized to tuberculin. The response to avian tuberculin is usually greater than the response to mammalian tuberculin in a comparative interdermal test.

Treatment

The incision of abscesses and release of pus is only temporarily effective. Surgical removal of nodules may be successful if they are small and have not spread to the local lymph node. Antibiotics and other antibacterial substances have little effect on the course of the disease.

Control

Sporadic cases should be isolated where possible and severe cases should be slaughtered. Attention should be paid to yokes or harnesses which are abrading the skin. Tick and fly control may reduce the spread of infection.

R.M.E.

BOVINE GENITAL CAMPYLOBACTERIOSIS

Genital campylobacteriosis or vibriosis is a contagious disease. Infection is largely confined to the reproductive tract of the cow and the preputial sac of the bull and leads to irregular returns to service and occasional abortion.

Aetiology

The casual agent is *Campylobacter fetus*, a Gram-negative comma, S-shaped or spiral bacteria. Biochemical and serological variants named *C. fetus* subsp. *venerealis* and *C. fetus* subsp. *fetus* (*intestinalis*) are described, the first named agent being that most commonly associated with enzootic infertility and abortion. *C. fetus* subsp. *fetus*, at one time associated only with sporadic abortion in the bovine, is now on occasion recognized as a cause of infertility. Other non-pathogenic Campylobacters inhabit the genital tract of the cow and prepuce of the bull. *Campylobacter sputorum* subsp. *bubulus* and *Campylobacter faecalis* are closely similar and are important only in that they have to be differentiated from *C. fetus*.

Occurrence

The disease occurs worldwide.

Species affected

Traditional bovine enzootic infertility involving *C. fetus* subsp. *venerealis* is confined to cattle. *C. fetus* subsp. *fetus* strains are genitally transmitted between cattle but similar strains infect and cause abortion in sheep, and sporadic abortion in cattle. Interspecies transfer of subsp. *fetus* cannot therefore be totally excluded.

Transmission

The bull is generally responsible for the introduction of infection, both due to management practices and the total absence of clinical signs in the male animal. Infection may persist less readily in the prepuce of young rather than old animals. Infection is transferred to the female at coitus, or when infected semen is used for artificial insemination. Other routes of infection involving transfer by veterinarians or owners, flies or inanimate intermediaries may occur but are relatively less important.

Clinical features

Clinical signs, other than those of reproductive failure or abortion, are minimal or absent. The infection of females at conception results in establishment in the anterior vagina and subsequent spread to the endometrial surface and the fallopian tubes. The resultant endometritis persists for months and is unfavourable for the developing embryo, which dies. Infection is gradually eliminated from the uterus but persists for long periods in the anterior vagina and cervix. Embryonic death initiates cyclical activity in which the interval is irregular and prolonged, as endometritis resolves pregnancy may be maintained. The majority of infected animals are capable of maintaining pregnancy 4–5 months after infection, but some may still carry the infection. Abortions are an uncommon sequelae to infection and occur mainly after 2–6 months gestation; such animals conceive promptly if rebred.

Clinical signs in dairy herds which maintain adequate records of fertility are soon evident shortly after the introduction and use of an infected bull. In other cattle which are more extensively managed using natural service, infection may not be suspected until the calving pattern indicates a delay in conception and a reduced calf crop.

The presence of the disease is less remarkable where infection has been present for some time; in such a case, the signs will mainly be seen in heifers or calved heifers, with older animals that have experienced infection conceiving normally. Even here a few older animals may continue to show impaired fertility due to persisting salpingitis.

Vibriosis may be confused with *Trichomonas* infection and, moreover, the two diseases may co-exist. Where herd fertility is at all in question, particularly where natural service is used, it is important to confirm the absence of these two diseases before other factors are looked at in more detail. In severe outbreaks of these diseases, bulls serve females many more times than normal, with the result that they may be overworked and develop temporary infertility.

Pathology

C. fetus produces a diffuse mucopurulent endometritis. The placentitis associated with abortion is not specific and lesions are not present in infected males.

Diagnosis

Diagnosis can be based on mucus agglutination tests or culture. For the former, dioestral cervical mucus should be collected from 15 to 20 animals, concentrating on those females recently exposed to infection by service, open cows or those returning to their third or fourth service. The mucus should be collected by aspiration, by flushing out the anterior vagina with phosphate-buffered saline using a multiperforated tube and syringe or, in the case of beef herds, by tampons, and forwarded to the laboratory on ice. Because the antibodies persist for limited periods in animals following infection, the test is essentially a herd test, and occasional positive samples indicate the need for further examination including culture. The vaginal mucus agglutination response may be less marked in subsp. *fetus* infection.

Oestral mucus is best for culture and may be obtained by either of the first two methods already described. The viability of Campylobacters in mucus at ambient temperatures is poor, and washings in buffered saline should be chilled on ice or, alternatively, the samples should be diluted with specific transport media and maintained at ambient temperatures.

Preputial samples from bulls can be taken by a number of methods, all of which employ scraping or flushing the preputial cavity, the important feature being to ensure vigorous massage or contact with the preputial epithelium near the posterior fornix and rapid or appropriate transport to the laboratory.

Immunity

Infection in the female results in a local vaginal immune response which, initially, is incapable of eliminating the organism from that site. The elimination of organisms from the uterus occurs much earlier due to the presence both of immune IgA and IgG, whereas the vaginal secretion is limited to IgA. Conception, implantation and normal pregnancy can persist in the face of vaginal infection. Immunity can be stimulated in either male or female animals by inoculations of formalin-killed strains of *C. fetus* in oil adjuvant.

The vaccination of male animals is likely to be the method of choice in controlling established herd infection. Two subcutaneous inoculations of vaccine 1 month apart will eliminate infection from the preputial sac within 8 weeks of the commencement of immunization; although such animals might theoretically mechanically transfer infection from infected to clean animals, such occurrences are rare. Male vaccination may not eliminate infection from herds.

The vaccination of females is less convenient and probably only justified when multiple infections have recently taken place in a previously clean herd, and in such circumstances vaccination could be used to minimize the production loss.

Vaccinal immunity in male animals probably persists for up to 2 years, and thereafter should be reinforced as necessary.

Control

The method employed to control herd infections will depend on management practices and the availability of satisfactory vaccines. Intensively managed herds can be divided into infected and non-infected replacement animals; artificial insemination may be used with the former group, whereas natural service using bulls free of infection should be used with the latter. Such an approach depends a great deal on the quality of management, and one must be aware of the possibility of cross-infection taking place between infected and previously uninfected stock.

In addition to possible accidental transfer by infected bulls to females, it is thought that transfer occasionally takes place between bulls that are either in close contact or housed together. Artificial insemination aims to eliminate the infection from cows, and they can generally be considered clean when natural mating has not been used for two pregnancies. Bull vaccination is likely to be the method of choice in controlling infection in range cattle. Infection may persist in the female population, but the risk of transfer of infection from infected to uninfected females by vaccinated bulls is very limited. Effective vaccines are not always widely available.

In certain circumstances, it may be desirable to free bulls from infection by treating them with antibiotics, though such animals are of course susceptible to reinfection. Local treatment with penicillin and streptomycin or, preferably, clavulanate-potentiated amoxycillin, is the method of choice. Infected bulls produce infected semen for artificial insemination and the addition of antibiotics to the semen does not always eliminate the infection. Any such procedure used on semen from infected bulls must be carefully validated.

G.H.K.L.

BRUCELLOSIS

Brucellosis is the disease produced by infection with organisms of the genus *Brucella*, obligate, often intracellular parasites, which affect the reproductive organs of animals and which can also affect man.

Brucellosis in cattle (*Br. abortus*)

Brucellosis in cattle, previously called contagious abortion, has been recognized since ancient times. It is characterized by inflammatory changes in the foetal membranes, which lead to the premature expulsion of the foetus.

Aetiology

Br. abortus, of which nine biotypes are recognized, is the most frequent cause of bovine brucellosis. *Br. melitensis* infection may occur if cattle are grazed with infected sheep or goats. *Br. suis* infection is comparatively rare.

Occurrence

Brucellosis has been recognized in nearly all countries of the world where cattle are kept. It is most prevalent in areas of intensive cattle raising. As soon as cattle are housed or confined in any way – as often happens with dairy herds – the likelihood of transmission of the infection increases and the disease becomes more obvious. Under range conditions, the disease is often of low prevalence or absent. Brucellosis in cattle is primarily a disease of the sexually mature female, with bulls and immature animals often showing little or no clinical disease.

Species affected

Cattle are the main reservoir of *Br. abortus*. Water buffalo, yak and American bison are also highly susceptible to infection. Sheep, goats, pigs, equines, camels and dogs are occasionally infected but rarely act as a source of infection for cattle. Brucella organisms or antibodies have been detected in several species of wild herbivores, rodents and birds but they are also not regarded as true reservoirs of infection for cattle. Man is susceptible (see section on "Public health").

Transmission

The infected pregnant cow or heifer is the most important source of *Br. abortus*. The placenta, placental fluids and foetus from an aborting animal contain between 10^{12} and 10^{14} organisms, which contaminate the vulva, tail and legs of the animal and the surrounding environment. Excretion of organisms may occur for several days before abortion and a varying period of time after. This may be several weeks if a chronic endometritis develops. Infected animals which calve at full term may discharge large numbers of organisms; they are particularly dangerous because the infection is not apparent. Such animals may be cows which aborted in a previous gestation or heifers.

Brucella organisms can survive in contaminated material for days, even weeks if in the shade or protected within a foetus. Infection usually occurs from ingestion of contaminated pasture or water, or by licking a discharging animal, newborn calf or placenta. Predators can move a foetus or placenta for several kilometres and thus disseminate infection. Transmission can also occur via the conjunctiva or by inhalation.

Over 90% of cows and heifers excrete brucella in colostrum and milk during the first month of lactation. Intermittent excretion of organisms occurs in a decreasing proportion of animals thereafter. Calves are infected *in utero* or by sucking infected dams.

Venereal transmission rarely occurs in bovine brucellosis. However, artificial insemination with infected semen often results in transmission.

Clinical features

The course of brucellosis in cattle is governed primarily by the age of the animal when exposed to infection, and to a lesser extent by the severity of the challenge in terms of numbers of organisms and their virulence.

Pre-pubescent calves usually lose the infection once removed from the source of contamination. However, it is important in eradication campaigns to remember that occasionally heifer calves born to infected dams retain infection into maturity.

After puberty the chances of cattle becoming permanently infected increase greatly. Following entry to the body via a mucous membrane, organisms multiply in the local lymph node. A bacteraemia ensues and organisms colonize predilection sites such as mammary gland, testes, seminal vesicles and associated lymph nodes. Other sites are joints, bursae, liver and spleen. It is only where a placenta exists (i.e. second half of pregnancy) that the uterus is invaded and the classical signs of brucellosis are seen. The incubation period is about 6 weeks, and thus animals abort from the seventh month onwards. In less acute infection, cattle may give birth to a full-term but weak calf, or merely show a retained placenta. Infertility may occur, as a sequel to chronic metritis.

Mature non-pregnant animals, or animals in early pregnancy when exposed to infection, are more likely to develop immunity than show overt symptoms of disease.

Infected males show no clinical signs, though frequently there is testicular enlargement. There may be degenerative changes in semen with pus. Infection may or may not affect the fertility. Infected hygroma may occur in males, including steers, and also females, and in certain countries are regarded as highly indicative of infection.

Br. melitensis infection in cattle is a comparatively rare benign disease. Uterine invasion may be accompanied by abortion but more commonly infection is confined to the udder and supramammary lymph glands, and organisms are excreted in the milk. *Br. suis* infection in cattle is rare and self-limiting. The udder and associated lymph glands are the usual sites harbouring organisms.

Pathology

Lesions are seldom pathognomonic. A necrotic placentitis which may be acute or widespread is characteristic. The cells of the villi and the walls or the crypts become swollen and there is considerable leucocyte infiltration leading to necrosis. In bulls there may be seminal vesiculitis, epididymitis and orchitis, which may lead to abscess formation. In the udder, the lesions seldom progress as far as clinical mastitis but cellular counts are increased.

Diagnosis

Confirmation of brucellosis as the cause of abortion is made by demonstrating organisms in smears or by culture. Smears of placenta, foetal stomach or vaginal discharge are stained by the modified Ziehl-Neelsen or Koster methods; brucella may be confused with Q-fever organisms (*R. burnetti*). Tissues for culture include foetal stomach contents or lung, placenta, vaginal discharge, milk and semen. *Post mortem*, the best samples are mammary tissue and supramammary or iliac lymph nodes.

In eradication programmes, infected animals are detected by serological tests. The screening tests are the Rose Bengal and card tests carried out on drops of serum or whole blood, and the milk ring test made on milk from bulk tanks or individual cows. The ELISA test is also being used as a screening test in an increasing number of countries. These tests are very sensitive but not always specific, i.e. a definitive test must be carried out on animals which are positive to a screening test. Non-specific reactions are caused by vaccination and occasionally by infection with other Gram-negative bacteria such as *Yersinia* and *Salmonella*.

Of the definitive tests, the Complement Fixation Test (CFT) is by far the most sensitive and specific. It must be available if eradication of brucellosis is to be attempted on a large scale; however, it is difficult to carry out and requires skilled technical staff. The Serum Agglutination Test (SAT) is easier to carry out but is less sensitive and less specific than the CFT. It is difficult to interpret and cannot be recommended for use in herds where S19 vaccine has been used – in this situation, the CFT must be used to distinguish between reactions caused by vaccine and those due to infection.

As animals may be in the incubation stage of disease at the time of testing, a single negative result should not be taken as clear evidence of freedom from infection. A second test should be carried out 30–60 days later, or ideally about 14 days after calving when titres often rise rapidly.

Immunology

Pubescent and sexually mature but non-pregnant animals become immune to one degree or another following infection, in that they may never show clinical signs of disease. Animals which have aborted also become immune and do not usually abort again. However, many of the animals mentioned above are chronically infected and may excrete brucella at subsequent parturitions. The majority remain positive to the CFT, but a significant proportion become negative to SAT within a few months.

Good immunity is produced by vaccination with S19 *Br. abortus*, a live strain of low pathogenicity and high immunogenicity. A single inoculation of heifer calves between 3 and 8 months old confers life-long immunity against all but the heaviest challenge. Its disadvantage is that SAT antibodies persist in a few animals into adulthood. The full dose of vaccine is not recommended for use in older animals, as it causes persistent antibody titres (especially SAT) and will cause abortion in pregnant animals. Recently, however, it has been shown that vaccination with a greatly reduced dose of organisms is safe and effective in adults, and is recommended where calfhood vaccination has been missed. Administration of S19 by the intra-ocular route has also been shown to be safe and does not interfere with serological tests.

The inactivated 45–20 adjuvant vaccine is safe in all ages but annual revaccination is necessary. It interferes greatly with the interpretation of the CFT but little with the SAT. Its use has declined since it was shown to be safe to use reduced doses of S19 in adults.

Control

Control of brucellosis at farm level is based on a combination of good hygiene, management and vaccination. The most important husbandry procedure is the observation of pregnant animals, so that they can be isolated if an abortion appears imminent. Ideally, any animal about to calve should be isolated if suspicion of infection exists. Animals should remain isolated until uterine discharge has ceased.

Vaccination greatly reduces the risk of abortion and the excretion of organisms. It is the most appropriate control method where risk of infection is present. Vaccination will reduce the number of infected animals in a herd by over 90% if carried out for a period of about 5 years. Thus in countries with a high prevalence of brucellosis, large-scale vaccination is used as a first phase of control before test and slaughter procedures are adopted.

The detection and removal of infected animals should only be carried out if simultaneous efforts are made to prevent reinfection of tested herds. At least three clear tests of susceptible animals are needed before a herd is declared free of infection. On a national scale, the testing, certification and monitoring of a slaughter policy is a big undertaking, costly in compensation, field and laboratory operations, and should not be undertaken without careful planning.

Public health

Man becomes infected when in direct contact with cows at abortion, parturition or in the post-parturition period. Veterinarians and stockhandlers are particularly at risk from the splashing of infected droplets into the eye. Infection occurs in people who drink unpasteurized milk or milk products. Symptoms include recurrent bouts of pyrexia, headache, muscle and joint pains and general weakness. Brucellosis is easily confused with malaria and influenza.

The use of plastic arm sleeves and thorough disinfection of the vulva and tail of cattle helps greatly to reduce the risk of infection during obstetrical procedures. Pasteurization of milk and milk products renders them safe. Vaccines are considered unsafe to use in humans in many countries. Treatment using streptomycin and tetracycline combinations may effect a cure, but only if started early before chronic infection becomes established.

Brucellosis in sheep and goats (*Brucella melitensis* infection)

The disease is characteristically caused by *Br. melitensis*, an infection which is similar to *Br. abortus* infection of cattle. This section will be brief and only mention differences between the two infections.

    Br. ovis infection affects sheep only and is dealt with in a separate section. *Br. abortus* and *Br. suis* occasionally infect goats and sheep if kept in contact with cattle and pigs.

Aetiology

Br. melitensis share similar antigens to *Br. abortus* and *Br. suis*. Three biotypes exist.

Occurrence

The disease is endemic in many countries around the Mediterranean, the southern part of the USSR, the Middle and Far East, and it also occurs in the southern part of the USA and Latin America.

Species affected

Predominantly, goats and sheep. Cattle and other ruminants (domestic and wild) may become infected but pigs appear resistant. Man is highly susceptible and the organism causes Malta fever, the undulant fever first described by Bruce. Infection of European hares has been reported.

Transmission

As for *Br. abortus* in cattle. Poor hygiene in sheep and goat pens or houses is ideal for the survival of organisms and the transmission of infection.

Clinical features

Similar to cattle. In goats, the disease sometimes causes septicaemia and death. Sheep appear more resistant than goats. The incubation period ranges from 3 to 20 weeks, abortions usually occurring in the fourth or fifth month of gestation. Goats seldom abort more than once, but sheep may abort twice or produce stillborn lambs at the parturition following an abortion. In contrast to cattle, clinical mastitis is common and may represent the first sign of infection. Other symptoms include unthriftiness, bronchitis with a hacking cough, lameness and hygroma, and orchitis in males.

Pathology

As for cattle. Abscesses in the spleen and costochondral cartilage may occur and histologically granulomatous foci can be seen in parenchymatous organs.

Diagnosis

The same diagnostic methods as used in bovine brucellosis apply. However, the sensitivity and specificity of these tests are lower in sheep and goats than cattle. The milk ring test is unreliable because fat globules and the stained antigen tend to sink rather than rise in the test-tube. Several countries use "Brucellin" in an intradermal test for screening large numbers of animals. The test is best used to detect infected herds rather than individual animals. Its advantages are that identification of animals is not required and costly sampling and laboratory tests are avoided.

Control

As with bovine brucellosis, good husbandry is vital for the long-term control of the spread of infection. A live *Br. melitensis* vaccine, strain Rev. 1, is widely used and provides good immunity. The full dose is recommended for young animals, whereas adults should be vaccinated with a reduced dose.

Brucella ovis infection or ram epididymitis

Br. ovis gives rise to an atypical form of brucellosis which only affects sheep. It is primarily a disease of rams with ewes only occasionally showing clinical signs. *Br. ovis* is antigenically distinct from the other *Brucella* species, occurring only in the rough state.

The infection is most common in Australia and New Zealand, but is also reported from North and South America, East and Southern Africa, East and Central Europe. The reservoir of *Br. ovis* is the ram, which may or may not show obvious lesions. Infection is transmitted to ewes venereally, but the disease may be mild or inapparent in the female and infection does not usually persist. In affected flocks, however, lambing percentages and lamb viability may be lowered. Abortions occur only rarely.

Rams acquire infection by serving a ewe which was infected by another ram during the same oestrus. Infection occasionally occurs through homosexual activity or via contaminated shears. The incubation period is 6–8 weeks. The most consistent lesion is swelling of the epididymis which is often unilateral. Pyrexia, gross swelling of the scrotum and loss of libido may also occur. The disease tends to become chronic with abscessation of the spermatic cord and scrotum. Semen contains pus and fertility is decreased. Secondary infection with *Corynebacterium pseudo-tuberculosis* may occur.

The disease is confirmed by culture of the organism from lesions or semen, or by serological tests using *Br. ovis* antigens. Clinically, it can be confused with *Actinobacillus seminis* and *Chlamydia* infections.

The treatment of rams is not economically worthwhile. *Br. ovis* and *Br. melitensis* vaccines have had some effect in controlling the disease, otherwise, control rests upon the detection and removal of infected rams and segregation of young rams from those already used for breeding.

Brucellosis in pigs (*Br. suis* infection)

The disease in pigs is similar to that in cattle, but the male is more important in the epidemiology.

Aetiology

Three of the four biotypes of *Br. suis* are responsible for the disease. *Br. abortus* occasionally infects pigs but is seldom if ever transmitted to other animals.

Occurrence

The disease is important in the USA and is recognized in South America, Thailand, Hong Kong, several European countries and Australia.

Species affected

Br. suis biotypes 1 and 3 are primarily infections of pigs, although on occasions self-limiting infections of cattle, horses, dogs and poultry occur. The European hare has been incriminated as a natural host of biotype 2. Man is particularly susceptible to biotypes 1 and 3, but not 2.

Transmission

Boars are important carriers of infection, organisms can be transmitted venereally and are also excreted in urine and faeces. Sows and gilts liberate organisms in milk, foetuses, foetal membranes and vaginal discharges. Further spread occurs from ingestion of contaminated food and water; alimentary tract infection of young piglets is common.

Clinical features

When first introduced into a herd, the disease runs an acute course. It persists in chronic form in adult pigs but is evident as an acute condition in subsequent generations. The disease is characterized by abortions, stillborn or weak piglets, temporary or permanent infertility in both boar and sow, lameness and posterior paralysis.

Boars are usually infected at sexual maturity; there may be bilateral epididymo-orchitis, with great enlargement of the testes which contain purulent and calcifying foci. In sows, the gravid or non-gravid endometrium is frequently studded with pinpoint nodules containing caseous pus. The joints may be swollen and painful, contain increased fluid and may ankylose. Encapsulated abscesses 2–3 cm in diameter arise in the intervertebral discs or vertebrae of the lumbar and sacral area. Similar foci may be seen in internal organs or lymph nodes.

The disease, especially in small herds, may be clinically inapparent, abortions if they occur at all arising so early in pregnancy as to pass unnoticed. The disease is much more self-limiting than other *Brucella* infections and infections are occasionally eliminated.

Diagnosis

Tests similar to those used for bovine brucellosis are required to confirm the disease in pigs. Culture of blood is often productive, in addition to culture of reproductive organs or tissues containing abscesses. Serological tests have greater limitations in pigs than other animals, however, and interpretation is best made on herd tests and not on tests on individual animals. Animals known to be excreting brucella have on occasions been negative to both agglutination and complement fixation tests.

Control

Antibiotics and vaccines are of no practical use in preventing the spread of disease or curing infected animals. The most efficient method of eliminating infection from a farm is total slaughter of the pig herd and careful disinfection before restocking. Detection and slaughter of infected individuals is time-consuming and may be protracted. Retests should be carried out every 1–2 months and attempts should be made to rear a clean breeding herd separate from the infected group. Additions being brought into the herd should come from herds certified free of infection. The use of community boars is risky and should be avoided as much as possible.

Brucellosis in dogs (*Br. canis*)

Dogs cannot only act as mechanical vectors of brucellosis in other animals by transporting infected placentas and foetuses, but occasionally become infected with *Br. abortus, melitensis* and *suis*.

In recent years, a species named *Br. canis* has been reported from dogs. The infection appears to occur worldwide. Other animals are not susceptible. The disease has been reported most frequently in colonies of experimental animals and the beagle has been the breed primarily infected. The disease results in early or late abortions with prolonged vaginal discharge. The male may show epididymitis, testicular atrophy and dermatitis of the scrotum. A persistent bacteraemia is a constant feature of the disease. Infection may be detected with an agglutination test using a rough antigen; standard *Br. abortus* antigen is unsuitable. Successful vaccines have not been developed and chemotherapy has not been effective. Monthly bacteriological and serological tests are recommended for control in an infected colony of dogs.

Man is occasionally affected, usually by handling infected tissues in laboratories.

Further reading

Alton, G.G. (1973). Brucellosis in sheep and goats. *World Animal Review*, 5, 16–20.
Alton, G.G. (1981) The control of bovine brucellosis: Recent developments. *World Animal Review*, 39, 17–24.
Fensterbank, R. (1987). Brucellosis in cattle, sheep and goats. *O.I.E. Technical Series*, No. 6, pp. 9–35.
Kolar, J. (1984). Diagnosis and control of brucellosis in small ruminants. *Rev. Vet. Med.*, 2, 215–225.
Sutherland, S.S. (1980). Immunology of bovine brucellosis. *Vet. Bull.*, 50(5), 359–368.

R.M.E.

CLOSTRIDIAL INFECTIONS

Members of the genus *Clostridium* are widespread in the animal environment. The vegetative cells are large Gram-positive rods which multiply when the micro-environment is anaerobic. Resistant spores form under adverse conditions either in the soil or within animal tissues. They form part of the normal microflora of animal intestines and contaminate the body surface and natural orifices. Infections are usually soil-borne and the weight of infection increases with the level of faecal contamination; this occurs with more intensive husbandry on permanent pastures and in yards and houses. It is only under certain conditions that clostridia become invasive and produce powerful exotoxins. The factors which precipitate outbreaks of disease are not always clear, although tissue trauma and the sudden change to an improved diet are frequently implicated.

Cl. chauvoei, Cl. novyi and *Cl. perfringens* account for the majority of cases of gas gangrene and enterotoxaemias. Other clostridia acting as opportunists cause similar diseases sporadically. *Cl. tetani* and *Cl. botulinum* cause tetanus and botulism, respectively. However, the demonstration of any of these organisms in tissues has to be interpreted with caution, because they are ubiquitous and migrate rapidly from the gut *post mortem*. It is essential that fresh, well-preserved tissues are examined by competent laboratories for confirmatory diagnosis.

Excellent vaccines to combat clostridial diseases can be made by inactivating whole cultures or toxins. Oily adjuvants are now incorporated in many clostridial vaccines, thereby extending the duration of immunity to around 2 years. Mistakes in identifying the correct organism as the cause of disease are common, however, and the wrong antigens may be used in vaccines. Local strains should be used where possible, because cross-protection between strains may not be complete.

Gas gangrene

This term describes a fulminating invasion of living muscle resulting in myonecrosis, oedema and gas formation. It causes a profound toxaemia and death within 24–48 hours. The term includes blackquarter, malignant oedema and bighead of rams. The organisms responsible are *Cl. chauvoei, Cl. septicum, Cl. novyi* and occasionally other clostridia.

Blackquarter

Aetiology

The term blackquarter (blackleg) should be reserved for *Cl. chauvoei* infections. The organism produces haemolysins and several other toxins, some of which are anti-genically the same as *Cl. septicum* toxins.

Occurrence

Blackquarter occurs worldwide but its distribution is often restricted to certain areas, farms or even fields. In cattle, the disease is usually endogenous and restricted to animals between 2 months and 3 years old. Animals are often in good condition. In sheep, the disease affects all ages and is associated with obstetrical problems (post-parturient gas gangrene) and unhygienic surgical operations.

Species affected

Blackquarter is most common in cattle and sheep. It occasionally affects pigs and other animals.

Transmission

Cl. chauvoei survives best in soils rich in organic matter and water holes. Ingested spores pass in small numbers via the portal circulation into the liver and eventually into the muscles. They germinate when muscle is bruised or where necrosis occurs. Such infections are termed endogenous because there is no sign of an entry wound.

Alternatively, spores enter via broken skin. Serious outbreaks of blackquarter have resulted from contamination of vaccine containers or syringes and spread in mass inoculations, especially via the intramuscular route.

Clinical features

Typically, muscles of the hindquarter, less often forequarter, are affected. The swelling is hot, painful, oedematous and crepitant. Lameness and depression may be severe. The oedema spreads rapidly and death occurs within 18–48 hours. Often animals are found dead. The skin over the wounds is markedly darkened.

Pathology

In cattle, affected muscle shows a characteristic dark, almost black, dry, spongy-looking central area, containing small gas bubbles and surrounded by a yellow oedema of varying extent. There is always a pervading rancid odour which may be masked by the smell of putrefaction. Decomposition is rapid and greatly decreases any possibility of a confirmatory diagnosis.

In sheep, the skin is dark and may exude beads of bloody fluid. The lesion is swollen, oedematous and crepitant.

Diagnosis

It is difficult to distinguish clinically lesions caused by *Cl. chauvoei* and *Cl. septicum*. The latter is rare in cattle but more common in sheep and pigs. Blackquarter may also be confused with anthrax, bacillary haemoglobinuria and other clostridial infections. Smears of affected tissue should be submitted for fluorescent antibody staining which rapidly differentiates *Cl. chauvoei*, *Cl. septicum* and *Cl. novyi*. Where such staining is unavailable, or where other clostridia may be implicated, submit tissues for culture. They should be preserved by drying thin slices in air, or by packing in salt or glycerol saline.

Treatment

The early administration of large doses of penicillin has been recommended. In practice, it is rarely possible to start treatment soon enough to be effective. However, it is worth trying during the course of an outbreak where it may be possible to recognize and abort early cases.

Immunology

Under suitable conditions, a toxin can be produced with an LD_{50} for mice of 0.1 to 0.005 ml. When inoculated intramuscularly, it evokes a dark appearance of the muscle which simulates that seen in the natural disease. However, antitoxin raised against this toxin does not protect against infection; nor can an active immunity be induced by inactivated toxin. A high-grade immunity to natural infection can be induced by sterile culture filtrates or by formolized cultures.

Control

The annual vaccination of cattle and sheep with an effective vaccine will give adequate protection. It is not usually necessary to continue vaccinating cattle for more than 3 years. Avoid carrying out surgical or obstetrical procedures or inoculations on ground likely to be heavily contaminated unless the animals are known to have been well immunized.

Other gas gangrene infections

Anaerobic cellulitis

This condition occurs sporadically in different species of animal when skin or muscle wounds are heavily infected with *Cl. perfringens* type A. The organism is a common inhabitant of the intestine. Outbreaks of disease are associated with poor hygiene. Clinical signs and *post mortem* lesions are similar to those of blackquarter, but cases may linger for several days and occasionally recover. Penicillin and antitoxin may assist recovery. Commercial vaccines are not available. Control is based on improving hygiene.

Bighead

This is a condition in rams caused by *Cl. novyi* type A. It has been reported from Australia and South Africa where it occurs sporadically in young stud rams which have been butting one another. Oedematous swellings develop suddenly around the ears, eyelids, nose and lower jaw. Occlusion of the nasal passages may cause snoring, and fluid may exude through the skin. *Post mortem* there is massive oedema but little or no gas. There may be a slightly foul acrid odour. The fluorescent antibody test is used to identify the organism in tissue smears. Large doses of penicillin and antitoxin may be justified for treating valuable animals. Black disease vaccine is used to protect animals at risk; it is prepared from *Cl. novyi* type B, which shares a common α-toxin with type A.

Malignant oedema

The causal organism is *Cl. septicum*, which is antigenically related to *Cl. chauvoei*. Although the organism is ubiquitous, malignant oedema occurs only sporadically. The extent of its occurrence is exaggerated because *Cl. septicum* is one of the most common *post mortem* invaders and is mistakenly identified as the cause of gas gangrene. In temperate climates, the organism causes a rapidly fatal abomasitis in sheep, called braxy.

Infection in ruminants usually occurs via an obvious wound, and in pigs it is often endogenous. The disease resembles blackquarter but the oedema is more extensive and haemolysis more marked. The characteristic rancid odour may be overlaid by the putrid smell induced by other contaminating organisms. *Cl. septicum* should only be confirmed as the cause of disease if it can be demonstrated in tissues from a fresh cadaver. It can be quickly identified by fluorescence antibody staining.

Because disease caused by *Cl. septicum* is quite rare, it is usually uneconomic to vaccinate animals routinely. In practice, however, *Cl. septicum* anacultures are often included in polyvalent clostridial vaccines.

Cl. sordellii *infection*

Cl. sordellii is a very proteolytic member of the genus which occasionally causes gas gangrene when it contaminates wounds. The disease has been reported in sheep in the arid areas of North and South America and the Middle East. It has been associated with surgical procedures and sometimes liver fluke infections of cattle and sheep. The muscles appear redder than usual and the gelatinous oedema is tinged pink. The organism has to be cultured for identification. No vaccine is available for prevention of infection.

The enterotoxaemias

This term covers clostridial diseases which involve primarily part of the intestinal tract and often the liver. They are characterized by bacteraemia and toxaemia. The notes at the beginning of this chapter apply equally to the enterotoxaemias. *Cl. novyi* types B and D and *Cl. perfringens* types B, C and D are usually implicated.

Black disease (bradsot or infectious necrotic hepatitis)

Aetiology

Cl. novyi type B (*Cl. oedematiens* type B, *Bacillus gigas*) is an organism exacting in its requirements for anaerobiasis. It produces a powerful α-toxin, identical with the lethal toxin of *Cl. novyi* type A, and a β-lecithinase.

Occurrence

The disease has been reported in Europe, the USA, Australia and New Zealand. It is most prevalent in summer and autumn, particularly in badly drained low-lying areas, and associated with infestation by liver fluke.

Species affected

Cattle and adult sheep.

Transmission

In areas where the disease occurs, the organism can – with suitable techniques – be isolated from the livers of a considerable proportion of healthy sheep. The disease process is initiated by growth of the organism in the lesions produced by migrating liver fluke larvae. A similar mechanism may occur in cattle.

Clinical features

Sheep are very often found dead. Sick animals are dull and lethargic and die quietly within 1–2 hours of first showing symptoms. Cattle may survive 1–2 days before dying.

Pathology

There is usually an extensive clear subcutaneous oedema and a marked injection and darkening of the subcutaneous vessels, which is responsible for the name "black disease". The characteristic features are the extensive peritoneal, pleural and pericardial effusions which become blood stained as the cadaver putrefies. The liver invariably shows several pale necrotic foci 1–5 cm in diameter, usually on the diaphragmatic surface. In sheep, but not in cattle, tracks of fluke larvae are apparent.

Diagnosis

Based on the history, *post mortem* appearance and association with liver fluke infection. The demonstration of large Gram-positive rods in smears from necrotic liver foci in the fresh cadaver indicates a clostridial infection, which can be confirmed specifically by fluorescent antibody staining. The confirmation can be strengthened by demonstrating β-lecithinase in effusions or the lethal toxin in extracts from the foci in the liver.

Treatment

In the case of valuable sheep and cattle, it might be worth trying large doses of specific α-antitoxin with penicillin. The prognosis is poor.

Immunology

There is no evidence of naturally acquired immunity, but vaccines stimulate effective immunity.

Control

The incidence of black disease can be reduced by controlling the uptake of liver fluke but the most important means of control is by active immunization. The treatment of liver fluke infestation is valuable in itself, but will not, unaided, prevent the disease.

Bacillary haemoglobinuria

Aetiology

The causal organism *Cl. novyi* type D resembles *Cl. novyi* type B but is even less tolerant of free oxygen and more exacting in its growth requirements. Its clinical effects are mainly due to the very large amounts of β-lecithinase (haemolysin) it produces.

Occurrence

It is most common in summer in parts of North and South America, particularly in low-lying moist areas where infestation with liver fluke is heavy. At times, the mortality rates in cattle herds may be high. Sporadic cases of the disease have been recognized in Europe, the Middle East and New Zealand.

Species affected

Mainly cattle, less often sheep.

Transmission

The very resistant spores are found in contaminated water, urine, faeces and infected cadavers. Inapparent carriers of infection in kidneys and liver may shed organisms in faeces and urine. Ingested spores pass via the portal circulation to the liver.

Clinical features

The signs range from sudden death in peracute cases to virtually inapparent subclinical carrier cases. Typical features include high fever with abdominal pain, pale or icteric membranes, bile or haemoglobin-stained faeces, and haemoglobinuria. Death is the rule in such cases.

Pathology

The primary lesions are in the liver, usually at sites damaged by liver fluke larvae. *Post mortem*, pale necrotic areas 5–15 cm in diameter demarcated by a purplish zone of congestion are usual. The small intestine may be intensely reddened and large extravasations may occur into the large bowel. The endocardium and kidneys may show numerous petechiae and the bladder is often filled with red urine. The subcutaneous tissues may show haemorrhages and icteric staining and oedema. Pericardial and pleural effusions are common.

Diagnosis

The disease may be confused with other types of haemoglobinuria caused by babesiosis, anaplasmosis, post-parturient aphosphorosis, leptospirosis and, in some circumstances, by cystic haematuria and bracken poisoning. Smears from necrotic foci show large rods which stain specifically with fluorochrome-labelled antiserum; β-lecithinase can be demonstrated in peritoneal effusions or cultures of liver.

Treatment

Early administration of wide-spectrum antibiotics is often very helpful.

Immunology

The organism shows no α-toxin but produces a lethal necrotizing haemolytic lecithinase identical with the β-toxin of type B. Immunity can be produced by the use of inactivated culture vaccines.

Control

Vaccination plus control of liver fluke infestation. Burning or deep burial of carcases of affected animals. Because infection can be spread by symptomless carriers, caution should be exercised when moving animals from known infected areas to clean areas.

Pulpy kidney disease and "enterotoxaemia" (overeating disease)

Aetiology

Cl. perfringens type D which secretes α-and ϵ-toxins. The ϵ-toxin is produced as a prototoxin which is activated by trypsin. It is resistant to inactivation by other enzymes.

Occurrence

Found wherever sheep are kept. The disease is most common in 3 to 12-week-old lambs and in fattening lambs 6–12 months old. In endemic areas, the incidence in older sheep is negligible because animals acquire natural immunity. Adult animals are, however, fully susceptible to infection which is newly introduced into a region. In Nepal, it is known as 6-month disease because it coincides with moves between high-and low-altitude pastures.

Species affected

Mainly sheep, to a lesser extent goats and occasionally cattle.

Transmission

By ingestion from contaminated grazing. In endemic areas, the organism can be isolated from the intestinal contents of most sheep. If animals are suddenly changed from a poor to a rich diet – from grass to grain for instance – acidosis may occur and result in paresis of the forestomachs. The consequent passage of undigested starch grains into the small intestine provides excellent conditions for the multiplication of the organism and toxin production.

Clinical features

Onset is sudden, dullness and uneasiness being succeeded by convulsive movements in which the legs are stretched out and the head and neck thrown back. Death follows within an hour of the symptoms appearing. As a rule, the animals – usually those in good condition – are simply found dead.

The course is less acute in goats and cattle. Convulsions are not always prominent in goats.

Pathology

The ε-toxin increases capillary permeability, especially in intestinal mucosa and kidney, leading to renal damage, hyperglycaemia, hypertension and oedema of internal organs. Shortly after death, the carcase becomes bloated and the kidney cortex becomes friable ("pulpy"). The pericardium contains excess fluid and ecchymoses are seen in the endocardium.

Diagnosis

The convulsions seen before death may resemble hypomagnesaemia, but the *post mortem* picture is characteristic. Diagnosis is confirmed by demonstrating large numbers of stout Gram-positive rods in films of ileal mucosa and ε-toxin in gut contents.

Treatment

Treatment is ineffective, but further cases may be prevented by immediately restricting the food supply.

Immunology

In endemic areas, many sheep have *Cl. perfringens* type D in the gut actively producing toxin. These animals have a good acquired resistance. Toxoid vaccines provide good artificial immunity.

Control

Avoid sudden changes in diet which are likely to result in acidosis. A sudden outbreak in a susceptible flock can be controlled by passive immunization using antiserum. Lambs are protected in the first critical week of life by immunizing the ewes in pregnancy. Older animals need to be vaccinated.

Other *Cl. perfringens* infections

Cl. perfringens *type B*

The cause of lamb dysentery, which is restricted to lambs in the first 2 weeks of life. β- and ϵ-toxins are produced. The β-toxin is inactivated by enzymes, especially trypsin, in older animals. Affected lambs show acute abdominal pain and a yellow diarrhoea or dysentery. Death follows rapidly. The proximal small intestine is haemorrhagic with ulcers which may coalesce and perforate, resulting in adhesions between loops of intestine and peritonitis. Smears from lesions show large Gram-positive rods. The disease is confirmed by demonstrating β-and ϵ-toxins in intestinal contents or cultures. Lambs can be protected by vaccinating ewes in pregnancy, or by using antiserum.

   Cl. perfringens type B has also been isolated from cases of enterotoxaemia of adult sheep and goats in the Middle East and South Africa.

Cl. perfringens *type C*

This disease has been reported from many countries and several animal species and man. The most common syndrome, "struck", affects young ewes that are in a good condition. It resembles other enterotoxaemias and animals may also be lame. *Post mortem*, one sees an acute necrotic enteritis, sometimes with abomasitis, and effusions into the body cavities and pericardium. β-toxin, but not ϵ-toxin, can be demonstrated in exudates or culture. Type C antiserum and vaccines give excellent protection. Type B vaccine offers some cross-protection because it also contains β-toxin.

Cl. perfringens *type A*

This organism is present in the intestinal tract of most animals and man. It grows rapidly in culture, overgrowing other organisms. These features make it difficult to prove a causal relationship with any condition under investigation. It has been associated with the following:

1. In Peru, sudden deaths in extensively grazed cattle and sheep. Outbreaks occurred a month after the rains when protein content was high in grass. The best fed animals were usually affected. Almost no lesions were observed *post mortem*.
2. Also in Peru, intensively fed cattle on high protein or urea supplemented diets. Carcases appeared normal except for a deep red staining in the kidneys.
3. In west Java, enterotoxaemia in water buffaloes. Lungs were oedematous, excess fluid was seen in body cavities and haemorrhages in gastrointestinal tract.

In man, *Cl. perfringens* type A food poisoning is caused by the release of an enterotoxin from disintegrating cells. The condition has not been confirmed in animals.

Intoxication of the nervous system

Tetanus

Tetanus is an intoxication by the neurotoxin of *Cl. tetani*, characterized by muscular spasms.

Aetiology

Cl. tetani is a slender Gram-positive rod which quickly becomes Gram-negative as the culture ages. The spores are round and terminal.

Occurrence

Worldwide. More common on well-manured land and usually associated with surgical procedures. Cases are usually sporadic, but occasionally outbreaks occur which involve many animals.

Species affected

A variety of animals and man are susceptible. Horses, sheep and goats are very susceptible; dogs and cats less so; cattle and pigs are fairly resistant; birds are relatively insusceptible.

Transmission

Cl. tetani is common in faeces and in heavily manured soil. It can grow in the depth of quite insignificant wounds or on surface injuries in the presence of aerobic organisms producing a low oxidation-reduction potential. It enters through wounds, during surgical procedures with improperly sterilized instruments, sutures or dressings, and during crude farm surgery such as docking, castration, dehorning, shearing, etc.

Clinical features

Early or slight cases show little more than a little stiffness, anxiety and an exaggerated response to external stimuli. Later, the characteristic rigidity, spasms, opisthotonous and protrusions of the nictitating membrane develop. Finally, continuous convulsions end in respiratory arrest and death.

Pathology

No specific changes are observable.

Diagnosis

The diagnosis is mainly clinical. The detection of organisms resembling *Cl. tetani* in wounds is suggestive evidence only, even if a precise recognition can be made by using specific fluorochrome-coupled antiserum. The symptoms resemble those of strychnine poisoning.

Treatment

Affected wounds should be cleaned and well drained. Antitoxin given subcutaneously and intravenously will neutralize toxin not yet fixed, but will have little effect on any already bound. Acetyl promazine or other sedatives can be used to treat symptomatically.

Immunology

Animals can be immunized passively with antitoxin or via the colostrum. The latter procedure is used in practice to protect very young lambs. Active immunization with formol toxoid is widely used to protect horses.

Control

Avoid surgery in a heavily contaminated environment, and avoid the use of unsterilized instruments and dressings. Where there exists a constant risk inherent in farm procedures, immunize actively, particularly in the case of valuable animals.

Botulism

Botulism is an often deadly food poisoning, characterized by a flaccid paralysis of the voluntary muscles.

Aetiology

Cl. botulinum species is divided into seven types on the basis of seven serologically distinct toxins, all of which produce similar pharmacological effects. Botulism is almost invariably caused by the ingestion of food in which the organism has grown and produced toxin.

Lethal doses of the different toxins vary for different animal species. For example, types C and D toxins are highly lethal for equidae and ruminants, but far less so for primates. Type A, on the other hand, is highly lethal for primates.

While types A, B and E are easily grown in artificial media, surface cultures of types C and D require far more exacting conditions.

Occurrence

Worldwide. Usually sporadic, but outbreaks can reach epidemic proportions in arid areas where nutritional deficiencies (especially of phosphorus) occur. This provokes a craving in animals for cadaver material, which may be highly toxic consequent on the growth in it of *Cl. botulinum*. Sporadic cases follow ingestion of fodder in which rodents have died and become toxic. Occasionally, serious local outbreaks have followed the feeding of improperly sterilized swill. Large-scale intoxications of wild fowl have occurred when local conditions favour the development of *Cl. botulinum* in algae and weed.

Species affected

A variety of animals and birds are susceptible. Species vary widely in susceptibility to the various types of *Cl. botulinum*. Carnivores and pigs tend to be less susceptible.

Clinical features

Typically, botulism presents as a slowly developing flaccid paralysis. The animal finally collapses and rests on its sternum or lies on its side, unable to lift its head. The posture in bovines resembles that in milk fever. Salivation is often present because of paralysis of the muscles of deglutition. Large doses of toxin considerably shorten the time to death, which may be as short as a few hours and be accompanied by spasms and an appearance of rigidity.

Pathology

Insignificant.

Diagnosis

Depends on clinical observation and history. Care should be taken to consider rabies in differential diagnosis. The demonstration of toxin in food known to have been eaten is helpful. Occasionally, when a relatively resistant species has ingested a large amount of toxin, this may be detectable in the blood. The finding of *Cl. botulinum* in food, intestinal contents and cadavers in regions where botulism is endemic, is not by itself conclusive evidence that the case being investigated suffered from botulism.

Treatment

Symptomatic and supportive, if the value of the animal justifies this. Complete recovery takes a long time.

Immunology

The toxins are distinguished by neutralization tests, usually in mice, against specific antitoxin. Some types of *Cl. botulinum* produce small amounts of heterologous toxin. This has to be taken into consideration when typing.

Control

In regions where the organism is known to occur, the feeding of preparations (swills, etc.) which favour the growth of *Cl. botulinum* should be avoided. Where toxic cadaver material is eaten, any underlying nutritional deficiency should be remedied, e.g. correct phosphorus deficiency by bone meal supplementation. The most certain method of protection is by active immunization against the prevalent types.

Further reading

Niilo, L. (1980). *Clostridia perfringens* in animal disease: A review of current knowledge. *Canadian Veterinary Journal*, **21**, 141–148.

Smith, L.D. and Holdeman, L.V. (1968). *The pathogenic anaerobic bacteria*. Charles C. Thomas, Springfield, Ill.

Sterne, M. and Batty I. (1975). *Pathogenic Clostridia*. Butterworths, London.

R.M.E.

CONTAGIOUS BOVINE PLEUROPNEUMONIA

Contagious bovine pleuropneumonia (CBPP) is an acute, subacute or chronic disease of cattle characterized by pneumonia, serofibrinous pleurisy and oedema of the interlobular septae of the lungs.

Aetiology

The disease is caused by *Mycoplasma mycoides* subsp. *mycoides* (small colony biotype), the type species of the genus *Mycoplasma*. This organism is a pleomorphic prokaryote that lacks a cell wall and is bounded by a plasma membrane only. Its shape varies from small coccal bodies (0.3–0.8 μm in diameter) to long slender branched filaments. A well-defined capsular layer, apparently consisting of polysaccharide galactan, can be demonstrated by electron microscopy. The organism may be stained in a number of ways, for example by Giemsa, but are best observed by microscopy with darkground illumination when they appear non-motile. They can be isolated from the blood and most organs, but particularly from lung and thoracic exudates ("lymph"), nasal and bronchial secretions, and from thoracic lymph nodes, and can be cultivated in various types of serum broth. There is, however, no evidence for the existence of more than one antigenic type.

Occurrence

The disease is widespread in Africa, mainly in the semi-arid countries lying south of the Sahara from Somalia to West Africa. The disease is also said to occur in India (Assam), China (Tibet, Inner-Mongolia, Sinkiang and Szechuan), Mongolia, Burma and Bhutan. Sporadic outbreaks have occurred in Egypt (1969), Jordan (1971), Zambia (1970), France and Spain (1967, 1980, 1982), Portugal (1983), and also in Kuwait and Bahrain.

Species affected

Natural infection is confined to cattle and water buffaloes. Experimental infections have been achieved in cattle, sheep, goats, rabbits, mice and embryonated eggs.

Transmission

Under natural conditions, infection is contracted by inhalation of the organisms expelled by an infected animal, and there is no evidence of intermediate hosts. A most serious aspect of the disease is the carrier animal or "lunger", which appears clinically healthy but has a localized focus of infection in its lungs. The focus is surrounded by fibrous tissue in the form of a sequestrum which may vary in size from a pea to a large orange. So long as the fibrous capsule persists, the carrier animal does not disseminate infection, but in time, perhaps after many months, the capsule may break down, allowing the still viable organisms to escape through the bronchi and so infect susceptible in-contact animals. The apparently healthy carrier animal, therefore, is mainly responsible for the perpetuation of the disease.

Spread of infection through a herd is relatively slow and mortality may vary between 10 and 50%. The incubation period is usually between 3 and 6 weeks.

Experimental transmission is difficult, for the parenteral inoculation of infective material does not usually cause classical pleuropneumonia but a flat, plaque-like, painful swelling (Willems reaction), which may spread considerably and cause death from a generalized toxaemia in 2–4 weeks. In order to obtain true lung involvement, the use of infective material in aerosols or administered by endobronchial intubation is necessary. Cattle infected experimentally by these methods may be used as donors to infect susceptible animals when closely confined together.

Clinical features

The acute form of bovine pleuropneumonia is characterized by a rise in temperature, accelerated respiration, anorexia, a rough coat, and a generally dejected appearance. Subsequently, a cough develops, which is at first dry and then becomes moist, the breathing becomes laboured and expiration may be accompanied by grunting. A characteristic stance is assumed in which the animal faces the wind with its head extended and its elbows turned out. Auscultation and percussion should reveal the affected areas of lung. In fatal cases, death occurs 2–3 weeks after the onset of symptoms, and may be preceded by a muco-purulent nasal discharge and an oedematous infiltration of the lower part of the chest.

In subacute and chronic cases, signs are much less marked and may even escape detection, although usually a cough can be induced by making the animal run after a period of rest.

A considerable number of animals recover but some retain infected sequestra in their lungs and remain potentially dangerous carriers. Infection in young calves may be complicated by severe specific arthritis and synovitis, but this is not usual in Africa.

Pathology

Lesions are commonly confined to one lung, with adhesion of the affected parts to the chest wall by a yellow spongy mass of tissue. In addition to fibrinous pleurisy, there is oedema of the mediastinum, with variable amounts of straw-coloured or turbid exudate in the pleural cavity. This exudate, in which may be found yellowish flecks of fibrin, clots on exposure.

The lesions in the lung take the form of pneumonic areas, which may be small or extensive, in various stages of hepatization and consolidation. A typically marbled appearance in various colours is thus presented. At the time, the interlobular septae become grossly thickened and their lymph spaces distended with fluid, causing a beaded appearance. The cut surface exudes a clear yellow fluid. The interlobular septae are eventually converted to firm connective tissue and the lobules lying within become grey or brown or, if necrosis has taken place, yellow.

In animals that recover, sequestra may develop, consisting of an affected portion of lung surrounded by a thick fibrous capsule. This may eventually be absorbed, or calcified, or it may become liquefied, having the appearance of an abscess. In old cases, the only evidence of past infection may be a thickening of the pleura with adhesions between the lung and chest wall together with thickening of the adjacent fibrous septae.

An occult form of the disease with no obvious lesion sometimes occurs and can only be confirmed by the isolation of the organisms from one or other of the thoracic lymph nodes, or from tonsils.

Diagnosis

Clinical diagnosis can present many difficulties, owing to the number of atypical cases, subclinical infections and apparently recovered animals which occur. However, a provisional diagnosis can usually be made from a post-mortem examination of either a dead or a slaughtered animal. The mosaic or marbled appearance of affected lobules, divided from each other by grossly distended septae containing beads of lymph, pleurisy with adhesions and the presence of quantities of straw-coloured fluid in the thorax, are the characteristic lesions of contagious bovine pleuropneumonia.

For laboratory examination, portions of affected lung preserved in 50% glycerine, together with "lymph" collected from the chest cavity, should be forwarded so that attempts to isolate the causal organism in culture may be made. Specimens of lung preserved in formalin should also be forwarded for histological examination. In East Coast fever areas, the lung of an animal which died of this disease may simulate contagious bovine pleuropneumonia and in cases of doubt an examination for the presence of *Theileria parva* should be made. Subacute pasteurellosis may also occasionally cause confusion, but this may be differentiated by demonstration of the causal pasteurella.

A number of serological tests may be used to aid diagnosis, although none is absolutely satisfactory on grounds either of sensitivity for all stages of the disease or of specificity.

The complement-fixation test is regarded generally as the most reliable for the examination of sera from individual animals and techniques for the screening of large numbers of samples have been developed.

Agglutination tests, performed either in tubes or as a rapid slide technique, in which a stained culture antigen suspension is mixed with either whole blood or serum, have been developed. Reports have indicated that false reactions may occur, particularly with the slide technique, which, although convenient for use in the field, is now used only as a screening procedure to select animals for further investigation. The indirect haemagglutination test has been used experimentally.

Tests for precipitating antibodies have not proved of much value, but precipitation tests, in particular the agar gel diffusion precipitation technique in which samples of lung tissue, lymph node or pleural exudate are examined for specific *M. mycoides* antigens against hyperimmune sera, have proved a useful aid. Positive reactions may be obtained with tissues too putrid for cultural examination, and also with tissues preserved in formalin or glycerine. Circulating antigens may also be demonstrated in sera at some stages of acute infection when tests for antibodies may give negative reactions.

The greatest proportion of positive reactions is, therefore, likely to be detected by applying a number of serological tests, including a precipitation reaction to detect antigen.

Treatment

Treatment is rarely justified because of the risks of converting active infection into the apparent carrier state. Treatment can also mask the clinical signs, serological responses and autopsy findings, all of which are important in diagnosis.

Immunology

The duration of immunity following recovery from the natural disease is not well understood, but must last for a considerable period, as there is good evidence that some vaccines provide a serviceable protection for up to 2 years. In addition to induced immunity, some animals display a marked natural resistance.

Broth vaccines have been produced by attenuation of a mild strain of the organism by serial passage in culture media. The problem is to produce a vaccine which is safe to use but immunizes effectively. The safest but least immunogenic vaccine in KH3/J, which has been widely used in parts of West Africa and also the Sudan since 1930, but even this vaccine will sometimes cause adverse reactions when given subcutaneously.

The T1 broth vaccine developed in Kenya is rather less attenuated and should be given in the tail-tip where adverse reactions are less important. A third vaccine made from a naturally mild strain of the organism (V_5) was widely used in Australia. It was given in the tip of the tail but is considered to be too virulent for use in Africa.

The T1 vaccine has how been lyophilized and can be stored. This is of considerable importance as broth vaccines in Africa have a shelf-life of not more than 30 days.

Little success has followed the use of killed vaccines owing to the poor quality of immunity engendered. These products may be of some value for immunizing highly susceptible animals as a preliminary to giving a booster dose of living organisms.

Control

In countries where bovine pleuropneumonia does not normally exist, the prompt slaughter of affected and in-contact animals is imperative. In endemic areas, the immediate imposition of a slaughter policy is usually impractical because of the resistance of nomadic cattle owners. Reliance must be placed on the control of cattle movement, the imposition of quarantines, the recognition and elimination of carriers and subclinical cases by serological tests, and the creation of an overall high level of immunity by intensive vaccination campaigns. The present policy in most African countries is to vaccinate all cattle twice in the first year of the campaign and once a year thereafter.

Such measures will generally lead to substantial reductions in incidence until, provided attention is paid to the sociological problems and education of cattle owners, the gradual introduction of a slaughter programme with adequate compensation to owners may become practicable, economically justified, and acceptable as is already the case in some African countries.

Because animals in the incubative stages of the disease may prove negative to the complement-fixation test, it is unwise to pronounce animals free from infection until at least two successive negative results at monthly intervals have been obtained. Cattle previously infected but recovering may also be positive to the test, but subsequent tests will show a gradual decline in the antibody level. The same applies to recently vaccinated animals in which complement-fixing and agglutination antibodies usually disappear within 1–2 months.

Where examination of large numbers of animals for the presence of pleuropneumonia is required, e.g. prior to some large-scale movement, and particularly when the animals are situated in remote areas, the rapid slide agglutination test should prove of particular value as a method of preliminary screening, the positive or doubtful sera being sent on to the laboratory for confirmation by the complement-fixation test.

Further reading

Reports of Joint FAO/OIE/CCTA Expert Panel on contagious bovine pleuropneumonia (1960, 1964,1967, 1971). F.A.O., Rome.

Hall, S.A. (1983). The diagnosis of contagious bovine pleuropneumonia and other infections with *Mycoplasma mycoides* subspecies *mycoides*. Document No. EUR 8654 of the Commission of the European Communities.

Hudson, J.R. (1971). Contagious bovine pleuropneumonia. *F.A.O. Agricultural Studies*, No. 86.

R.N.G.

CONTAGIOUS CAPRINE PLEUROPNEUMONIA

Contagious caprine pleuropneumonia (CCPP) is a peracute, acute or chronic contagious disease of goats characterized by a fibrinous pneumonia, pleurisy and profuse pleural exudate.

Aetiology

Mycoplasma mycoides subsp. *capri* has long been regarded as the aetiological agent of CCPP.This mycoplasma can indeed induce experimental pleuropneumonia in goats. However, there is now convincing evidence that "classical" CCPP, first described by Hutcheon over a century ago, is really caused by an as yet unclassified and unnamed mycoplasma, represented by the F38 strain which has so far only been isolated in Kenya, Sudan, Libya, Tunisia and Yemen. It appears that *M. mycoides* subsp. *capri* is probably the cause of only sporadic cases of caprine pleuropneumonia. Another mycoplasma, *M. mycoides* subsp. *mycoides* (large-colony biotype), serologically similar but biologically different from the causal agent of contagious bovine pleuropneumonia, has in recent years been isolated from goats in many countries of Africa, the Middle East and Europe, and also the USA and Australia: many of these countries do not have "classical" CCPP. This mycoplasma can also cause caprine pleuropneumonia, but is more commonly associated with other disease manifestations including polyarthritis, mastitits, keratoconjunctivitis and septicaemia, particularly in young kids. Thus, the situation is complex and made more difficult by the fact that mycoplasmas that cause "classical" CCPP, represented by the F38 strain, are more fastidious in their growth requirements and are therefore more difficult to isolate than the *M. mycoides* subspecies.

Species affected

Natural disease induced by the F38-type mycoplasmas is confined to goats and is readily contagious to susceptible goats. However, local oedematous reactions are not induced in goats following subcutaneous inoculation. *M. mycoides* subspp. *capri* and *mycoides* (large-colony biotype) can induce disease in goats and less commonly in sheep. In contrast to the F38-type mycoplasmas, inoculation of these subspecies subcutaneously into goats results in massive cellulitis at the inoculation site, pyrexia and even death. Pleuropneumonia due to these two mycoplasmas is not readily contagious to in-contact susceptible goats.

Transmission

Natural infection occurs by direct contact, probably via the respiratory tract. Several workers have transmitted the disease by the intratracheal inoculation of infective material or by in-contact exposure.

Clinical features

In the peracute and acute forms of CCPP, characteristic signs of pneumonia are easily recognized. In peracute cases, there is a rapid course (3–5 days) and death may occur even within 24 hours of the onset of clinical signs. In fact, sudden death with little or nothing in the way of premonitory signs is by no means unusual. Mortality rates of 60–100% are common.

In the chronic form, the characteristic signs are nasal cattarh and chronic cough, enteritis, general debility and emaciation. Because the chronic stage of the disease is non-infective to susceptible goats, it represents more accurately a phase of slow convalescence following recovery from a previous acute infection. This is borne out by the observation that some chronic cases may suddenly relapse and develop acute signs, indicating that little or no immunity was acquired from the first attack.

The incubation period in natural infection is generally considered to be 3–5 weeks; rather less if transmission is effected by artificial means.

Pathology

Lesions in acute cases consist of unilateral or bilateral pneumonia with varying degrees of consolidation and pleurisy; sections of lung present a variegated mosaic appearance. Affected areas of lung are commonly covered with a lemon-yellow deposit containing much pleural exudate in the lacunae. A clear, straw-coloured exudate, which may measure as much as 500 ml, is almost invariably present. In less acute cases, soft gelatinous adhesions between the parietal and visceral pleurae may be found. The bronchial lymph nodes are swollen and moist.

In chronic cases, the lungs are found to be in various stages of resolution with encapsulation of acute lesions. In contrast to contagious bovine pleuropneumonia, fully developed sequestra are not recognized in uncomplicated infection. Firm fibrinous adhesions attaching the lung to the chest wall are commonly seen.

Diagnosis

In typical outbreaks, it is not difficult to arrive at a tentative diagnosis of CCPP. The characteristic signs of severe nasal catarrh, respiratory distress, coughing and general weakness, especially if there is a history of spread through the herd, are more than indicative in endemic countries. Significant corroboration can be obtained from post-mortem examinations. Laboratory tests may be necessary, however, to confirm the diagnosis and eliminate the possibility of pneumonia due to other causes. These consist of the recognition of mycoplasmas in pleural exudate by darkground microscopy and isolation by appropriate cultural methods. Species and strains vary in their adaptability to growth in culture, which can prove exceedingly difficult at times, even when microscopy has given evidence of the existence of pleuropneumonia-like organisms.

For laboratory examination, fresh material such as pleural exudate, mediastinal lymph nodes and diseased lung tissue should be submitted, preserved in 50% glycerine if necessary. A technique for the aspiration of exudate from the pleural cavity of living goats has been reported. Lung tissue preserved in formalin should also be induced for histological examination.

The complement-fixation test is said to be satisfactory.

Treatment

Treatment with tylosin tartrate is said to be effective and other broad-spectrum antibiotics have also been used with some success. Treatment should not be attempted if eradication of the disease is envisaged.

Immunology

In the past, vaccines against CCPP were reported to give varying success. These included formalin-inactivated vaccines, attenuated live vaccines and fully virulent organisms in the form of fresh pleural fluid ("lymph"). These vaccines were prepared against *M. mycoides* subsp. *capri* and perhaps *M. mycoides* subsp. *mycoides* (large-colony biotype), but not against the F38-type mycoplasmas. However, some of the pleural fluids may have, unknowingly, contained the F38-type mycoplasmas.

Little information is yet available on immunity to the F38 strain of mycoplasma. The exposure of goats to an attenuated strain of this organism is reported to have induced immunity to experimental contact challenge. Recent work has also shown that vaccines made from sonicated organisms in incomplete Freund's adjuvant or lyophilized organisms, together with saponin as adjuvant, can confer immunity to experimental challenge.

Control

In countries where CCPP does not normally exist, the prompt slaughter of affected and in-contact goats may prove to be the most economic policy provided action can be taken before the disease becomes widespread. Where the disease is endemic, however, control can usually be attempted only on a herd basis. Restriction of movements by the imposition of quarantines should help to prevent dissemination and, because infection spreads by direct contact, the prompt removal and isolation or preferably destruction of all affected animals should be carried out. So far as possible, the herding together of goats at night in cramped, confined quarters should be avoided. Wet, cold conditions are predisposing factors. Chemotherapeutic treatment may be attempted, and dead vaccines, if used on a sufficiently widespread and frequent basis, may help materially in reducing the incidence of the disease.

R.N.G.

DERMATOPHILUS INFECTION

Dermatophilosis (cutaneous streptothricosis) is an acute or chronic, and sometimes fatal, exudative dermatitis characterized by thick scab formation.

Aetiology

Dermatophilus congolensis, a branching filamentous organism belonging to the genus Dermatophilaceae of the order Actinomycetales, is present in skin lesions. It is a Gram-positive, non-acid-fast aerobic or microaerophilic bacterium. The filaments are composed of parallel rows of cocci which under moist conditions are released as motile zoospores.

Occurrence

The infection occurs worldwide but is particularly severe in parts of the humid tropics, especially West and Central Africa, Madagascar and a number of the Caribbean islands where the disease in cattle is of major economic importance. Its occurrence as lumpy wool disease of sheep is also of considerable importance, especially in Australia.

The disease is seasonal in incidence, most cases occurring during the rainy season.

Species affected

The disease occurs in a wide range of domesticated and wild animals and man. Of the domesticated species, it is of greatest importance in cattle, sheep, goats and horses. Certain breeds of cattle are more susceptible, especially exotic European breeds, while N'Dama, Mutura, Dinka and West African shorthorns are much less affected.

Transmission

Infected animals, including symptomless carriers, are the major source of infection. The organism can survive for years in dried scab material from which motile zoospores are released following wetting. However, the disease is probably not contagious in the ordinary sense, because it is not possible to produce the progressive form of the disease by simply infecting skin with the organism.

It appears necessary for the skin to be damaged before infection can take place. There are three natural barriers to infection: the hair or wool, the film of sebaceous wax on the skin, and the *stratum corneum*. Damage may be caused in many different ways, but the two major ones are prolonged wetting, which emulsifies the sebaceous wax and macerates the *stratum corneum*, and mechanical damage by ticks, biting flies, thorns or other wounds. The susceptibility of the host is also increased by intercurrent diseases, which depress cellular immunity, and pregnancy. The occurrence of a severe form of the disease in the tropics is often associated with infestation with *Amblyomma variegatum* ticks.

Transmission of the organism between animals may occur by direct or indirect contact, and both biting and surface-feeding flies have also been implicated. In some animals, the infection persists and the scabs remaining attached to the hairs provide a reservoir of infection which is reactivated during the next wet season.

Clinical features

The predominant clinical feature is an exudative dermatitis which varies with regard to the site affected and the extent of skin involvement. In many cases in cattle, the dorsal surface would appear to be the predilection site for early lesions, but in other cases it appears to start on the hairless parts of the body. Oral lesions affecting the hard palate, upper and lower gums and both sides of the tongue have been reported in cattle. The most common sites of infection in goats appear to be the face, ears and legs. Lesions on horses may be extensive or restricted to the face or lower limbs, especially behind the pastern.

The lesions commence as papules and pustules which coalesce into extensive scab formations. Where haired skin is involved, the serous exudate coagulates causing the hairs to stick together and stand erect giving the so-called "paint brush" effect. Subsequently, the lesions increase in size and thick irregular scabs are formed. Often adjacent lesions become confluent, and in severe infections of cattle more than 50% of the body surface may become covered with scabs. In acute cases, such generalized infection can occur in as little as 2 weeks, whereas in others it may take several months to develop. The scabs are usually firmly attached to the skin, especially at the edges, and undersurfaces are covered with a yellow-grey or cream-coloured exudate. The underlying skin is reddened and has a coarsely granular appearance and is often haemorrhagic. The scabs separate from the skin surface in healing lesions but remain attached to the hairs.

The disease may often become static and limited to certain areas and it invariably regresses during the dry season.

Pathology

D. congolensis filaments penetrating the epidermis induce an acute inflammatory response which is characterized by congestion, oedema and infiltration of the site with neutrophils. Alternate layers of inflammatory cells, epidermal keratinocytes and exudate gives the scab a distinct lamellar structure. There is proliferation of the prickle cells, resulting in the stratum malpighi becoming thickened with enlargement of the interpapillary pegs. The more superficial cells may show evidence of hydrophic change, while on the surface there is a loose hyperkeratosis with a variable degree of parakeratosis. Infiltration of the epidermis with mononuclear cells may also occur. The causal organisms may be observed in association with inflammatory cells either within hair follicles or in the epidermis, and in large numbers in the scab material.

A few internal lesions may be associated with the condition, such as hyperplasia of lymph nodes, a toxic hepatitis and nephritis.

Diagnosis

The macroscopic appearance of the skin lesions together with the seasonal occurrence of the disease in an endemic area are characteristic. Confirmation of the diagnosis is obtained by making smears either directly from the underside of the scab or from a piece of scab which has been emulsified in water. The smear is stained by Gram's method, Giemsa or methylene blue, and examined for the presence of branching filaments composed of multiple parallel rows of coccoid cells. For a specific diagnosis, filaments having rows of four or more cocci should be present.

Where filaments have been completely converted to zoospores, identification of the organism requires the use of fluorescent antibody techniques or its culture and subsequent identification on smear preparations.

The organism is usually successfully isolated from scab material by inoculating blood agar plates containing aerosporin (100,000 i.u./ml), which inhibits most contaminants, both pathogens and commensals. Similar results may be obtained using Colombia Agar CNA with 7% sheep blood added. The organism is slow growing and produces β-haemolysis. Some colonies are leathery in texture with a ridged appearance, whereas others are mucoid.

Experimental lesions may be established in laboratory animals at scarified skin sites using a suspension of the organism obtained from scab material or cultures.

Treatment

External treatment necessitates the removal of the scabs to be effective. The organism is susceptible to many antibacterial substances. Parenterally administered antibacterials must be given in very high doses to obtain effective concentrations in the epidermis. Injection with long-acting oxytetracycline or penicillin and streptomycin, on three consecutive days, is usually effective. However, some animals, especially those that relapse following earlier treatment, fail to respond to antibiotic therapy.

Immunology

Recovery from the natural infection does not confer immunity. Reports in the literature indicate the presence of antibodies to *D. congolensis* in serum and skin washings following infection, but these do not appear to be protective. A delayed hypersensitivity reaction has been demonstrated in sheep and rabbits following vaccination and experimental infection. This is seen as an accelerated cellular infiltration around secondary experimental lesions, limiting the penetration of filaments and promoting earlier healing. It is probable, therefore, that resistance to *Dermatophilus* infection is dependent on cellular rather than humoral immunity.

Attempts to produce immunity by vaccination have been unsuccessful.

Control

It is important to identify and eliminate those factors which predispose to the disease. Animals should be treated regularly with acaricide to keep them free from ticks, especially *A. variegatum*; measures to reduce the number of flies or to protect animals from them may be beneficial; thorny plants should be removed from grazing areas; sheep should not be sheared in wet weather when transmission of the infection is facilitated; and the provision of shelter from rain for animals at night, especially for horses, is also helpful.

Care should be taken to prevent excessive build-up of the organism in contaminated sheep dipping tanks. Aluminium sulphate has been used as a method of control in sheep, either in a dip or as dusting powder during the wet season.

In preventing the disease in cattle, the greatest benefit results from the control of *A. variegatum* ticks. It is also possible to increase herd resistance by selective breeding from resistant individuals.

Intercurrent disease, such as demodectic mange, lumpy skin disease, globidiosis and trypanosomosis should also be treated and controlled.

Further reading

Hyslop, N.St.G.(1980). Dermatophilosis (streptothricosis) in animals and man. *Comparative Immunology, Microbiology and Infectious Diseases*, **2**, 389–404.

Lloyd, D.H. and Sellers, K.C. (eds) (1975). *Dermatophilus infection in animals and man*. London, Academic Press.

Stewart, G.H. (1972). Dermatophilosis: A skin disease of animals and man. Parts I and II. *The Veterinary Record*, **91**, 537–544, 555–561.

A.N.M.

GLANDERS

Glanders is a contagious disease of solipeds that can also affect man and other animals. It is characterized by the formation of fibrocaseous nodules in the upper respiratory tract, lungs and skin.

Aetiology

The disease is caused by *Pseudomonas mallei*, a non-sporing Gram-negative bacillus which is only slightly resistant to adverse influences and is unlikely to survive for more than 2–3 months outside the body.

Occurrence

Glanders is now found only in the Middle East, India, Pakistan and the Far East where its incidence is described as low and sporadic, and in Mongolia where it is widespread.

Species affected

The horse is the most commonly affected animal and the disease in this species is frequently chronic, whereas in the donkey and mule it is often acute. In man and carnivores, infection is rare. Cattle and pigs are not susceptible. Of the laboratory animals, the guinea-pig in particular and also the mouse are highly susceptible.

Transmission

Transmission follows ingestion of contaminated food or water, although it is considered by some that inhalation may play a part. Indirect transmission by fomites such as harnesses or stable utensils can occur. In man, infection is thought to be by contamination of cuts and abrasions. Carnivores may contract the disease by eating infected carcases.

Clinical features

The incubation period is very variable. It may be as short as 2 weeks but is often several months, and in many cases infection remains subclinical. It is probable that complete recovery can occur.

Clinical forms of glanders are described as pulmonary, nasal and cutaneous (farcy), but all may co-exist. In the acute disease there is fever, coughing, and a nasal discharge which may periodically be "snorted" from the nostrils. The submaxillary gland is enlarged and painful. There are signs of respiratory distress, and death may occur within 2 weeks. The acute form is commonly seen in donkeys and mules but is rare in horses, and when it does occur is usually secondary to the chronic form, being activated by stress conditions.

In the chronic form the onset is insidious, with general malaise, coughing, unthriftiness and intermittent fever, followed in some cases by nasal and farcy lesions and enlargement of the submaxillary glands. Sometimes with rest and good feeding a temporary improvement occurs.

The earliest sign of nasal lesions is a thin glairy discharge from one or both nostrils which later becomes purulent and often bloodstained. Nodules on the nasal mucosa rupture to produce ulcers which may coalesce to form eroded areas. These in the process of healing leave star-shaped scars on the nasal septum, which in extreme cases may be perforated.

In farcy, one or both hind legs are usually affected but lesions may occur elsewhere. Farcy buds are found along the course of the lymphatics under the skin. The nodules, which are pea-sized, soon rupture, discharging a yellowish grey oily pus and leaving ulcers. Nodules, ulcers and neighbouring lymph nodes are connected by thickened lymphatics which can be felt under the skin, and the affected limb becomes markedly swollen and painful.

Pathology

Lung lesions are found in almost all cases. In the uncut lung, nodules that are pea-size or smaller can be felt or seen. On section, these nodules in the early stage are red in colour, but later develop a yellowish centre which increases in size until a pearly-yellow lesion is formed. Old nodules may have a definite capsule. Similar lesions may be found in the liver and spleen.

In the larynx and trachea and on the nasal mucosa the characteristic lesions are ulcers. Of the lymph nodes, the most commonly affected are the submaxillary, but the bronchial and thoracic may also be involved. They are enlarged and oedematous and may show nodules on sectioning but rarely burst.

Diagnosis

Various methods of diagnosis are available, including serological and biological tests (Strauss reaction). The method used in the field, however, to confirm a clinical diagnosis and to screen in-contact animals, is the extremely efficient intradermo-palpebral mallein test in which 0.1 ml of concentrated mallein is injected into the skin 5 mm below the lower eye-lid; a positive reaction results in local swelling and a muco-purulent discharge which reaches its height within 24 hours and lasts for 2–3 days. Subcutaneous, cutaneous and ophthalmic tests are also available.

Clinically cutaneous glanders can be confused with epizootic lymphangitis and ulcerative lymphangitis and acute glanders can be confused with strangles. The use of the mallein test or demonstration of the causal organisms will differentiate them.

Treatment

If an attempt is to be made to eradicate the disease, treatment should not be permitted. In countries where the disease is endemic, some success has been claimed for sulphadimidine, nitrofurans and polymyxin, but there is the danger that treated animals may become subclinical carriers.

Immunity

No immunity appears to be produced.

Control

The destruction of clinical cases alone will not eradicate glanders, because subclinical cases continue to disseminate infection. If an outbreak occurs, all in-contact equines must be quarantined and mallein tested at 28-day intervals and the reactors slaughtered. As the disease is transmitted by fomites, care must be paid to stable management and communal water troughs must be avoided. The buildings and all grooming kit, equipment and nosebags, water troughs and mangers should be disinfected and bedding and debris destroyed.

The rational use of the mallein test with effective quarantine will result in the eradication of the disease from any country where the necessary cooperation of horse owners can be assured and where suitable replacement animals are available.

R.M.E.

HAEMORRHAGIC SEPTICAEMIA

Haemorrhagic septicaemia (HS) is a form of acute pasteurellosis of water buffalo and cattle.

Aetiology

By definition, haemorrhagic septicaemia is caused by *Pasteurella multocida* serotypes 6B and 6E (Namioka and Murata's classification). Type B, known as type I in Carter's classification, is more commonly isolated in Asia, whereas type E is the usual isolate in Africa. Outbreaks of acute pasteurellosis caused by other serotypes of *P. multocida* or by *P. haemolytica* should not be called haemorrhagic septicaemia, even though septicaemia may be a feature.

Occurrence

Haemorrhagic septicaemia is endemic in south and east Asia. Sporadic outbreaks occur in Africa, southern Europe and the Near East.

In Asia, the disease appears annually with the monsoon rains and is considered to be the most important infection of water buffalo and cattle. It is prevalent in the river valleys and deltas where animals are used for rice cultivation. The factors which influence the onset and spread of disease are not always obvious. Just before the monsoon, animals are in poor condition, and are working hard preparing the land for the planting of crops. These stress factors, coupled perhaps with viral or other infections, weaken host defences and predispose animals to pasteurella. In endemic areas, animals over 1 year old have often acquired immunity from previous outbreaks and disease is more common in the young stock. Outside endemic areas, clinical cases are seen in all age groups. Morbidity rates vary from low to high therefore, but in general case mortality rates are over 50% and may approach 100%.

In Africa, the predisposing factors in outbreaks of HS are even less obvious. The disease may suddenly appear in a location and may not reappear for many years. Most of the reports of disease are not confirmed by laboratory tests and the true prevalence of HS is therefore not known. Outbreaks which have been investigated in detail suggest that the transport and herding of animals together, e.g. in vaccination campaigns, may trigger the first cases of disease. Spread within a group occurs at night when animals are enclosed and between groups via communal watering points.

Species affected

Water buffalo are the most susceptible species, followed by cattle. It is only these species which are regularly affected by the disease. Sporadic, often unconfirmed, cases of pasteurellosis resembling HS have been reported from many other domestic and wild ruminants, pigs, horses and camels.

Transmission

In endemic areas, small numbers of healthy water buffalo or cattle carry organisms, in the nasopharynx or tonsils. These animals act as the reservoir of infection between outbreaks of disease. Organisms are spread via the aerosol route. During an outbreak, sick animals excrete large numbers of bacteria in nasal discharges, saliva and faeces. The bacteria can survive for several hours in moist conditions but die rapidly if exposed to sunlight or dessication. Indirect transmission of infection is possible and undoubtedly occurs. For several weeks after an outbreak, between 20 and 50% of animals carry the organism and are capable of infecting susceptible in-contact animals.

The same epidemiological pattern appears to exist in areas where the disease occurs sporadically.

Clinical features

The majority of cases in both water buffalo and cattle are acute or peracute with death occurring within 24 hours of the onset of illness. The first symptoms are dullness, reluctance to move and fever. Excess salivation and a clear nasal discharge appear. A common feature is oedema of the laryngeal region, which spreads down to the brisket and up to the parotid region, sometimes right around the head. The tongue may swell and protrude and mucous membranes are congested. Respiratory distress is apparent to varying degrees. Some animals remain sick for several days, but recovery from true HS is rare, especially in buffaloes. Death is caused by the release of endotoxins and toxaemia or suffocation.

Pathology

The first lesion to be observed is usually oedema of the head, throat and brisket. The fluid is straw-coloured and infiltration may extend from subcutaneous tissue into muscle. There are scattered petechiae. Pharyngeal cervical lymph nodes are swollen and may be haemorrhagic. Excess blood-tinged fluid is present in the thoracic, abdominal and pericardial cavities. Pneumonia with oedema and thickening of interlobular septae may be seen in animals where the disease has lasted several days. Well-established bronchopneumonia is more likely to be caused by other serotypes of *P. multocida* or *P. haemolytica*. Petechiae are seen under serous membranes throughout the body. Some animals, particularly calves, may show haemorrhagic gastroenteritis, ranging from small lesions to widespread frank haemorrhage. Apart from a few petechiae the spleen is unchanged. Atypical cases occur which show little or no throat swelling.

Diagnosis

Outbreaks of HS in endemic areas are easily recognized, but individual cases or outbreaks in non-endemic areas will require culture of organisms and serotyping to confirm that the disease is HS. The rapid course of illness and the presence of throat swellings are suggestive of HS. Anthrax, gas gangrene caused by clostridial species and certain snake bites occasionally give rise to similar lesions. Other *Pasteurella* infections may be characterized by haemorrhages, but lesions are often more pronounced in the lungs. Contagious bovine pleuropneumonia lesions are confined to the lungs but can closely resemble HS.

The best tissues for smears and culture are blood, lung, liver and spleen. A long bone should be submitted if the animal has been dead for more than 8 hours. The organism is a small coccobacillus which shows bipolar staining with Giemsa, methylene blue or equivalent stains. *P. multocida* grows well on routine laboratory media and can be identified to species level by simple biochemical tests. Serotyping, however, is the work of a reference laboratory. Haemagglutination tests detecting somatic antigens or mouse protection tests which detect capsular antigens are the most reliable.

Treatment

As with other rapidly progressing bacterial diseases, treatment is only successful if started in the very early stages of illness. It has little value once animals appear shocked and may in fact precipitate a terminal crisis, by causing death of organisms and release of endotoxin. Antiserum in theory should be therapeutic but is rarely available. Sulphadimidine or tetracyclines are the drugs of choice.

Immunity

Naturally acquired immunity exists in endemically infected herds, in which morbidity and mortality rates are substantially lower than herds not previously affected. Immune animals, however, can carry and presumably transmit infection. Immunity is thought to be humoral rather than cell-mediated.

Artificial immunity is provided by use of formalin-killed vaccines. Plain bacterin protects for about 6 weeks, alum-precipitated vaccine for up to 5 months and oil-adjuvant vaccine for 8–12 months. The duration of immunity can be increased by larger doses than normal, but the risk of toxicity goes up correspondingly. Cross-protection between serotypes is poor and it is important that vaccines are manufactured from appropriate isolates.

Control

In endemic areas, the only realistic method of control is annual prophylaxis using the oil-adjuvant vaccine. Immunity takes 2 weeks to develop and vaccinations should therefore be made about 1 month before the onset of the monsoon.

In non-endemic areas, it is difficult to justify the use of regular vaccination on economic grounds. Vaccination in the face of an outbreak can be worthwhile and funds would be better spent on logistical support for emergency programmes rather than routine campaigns of doubtful value. In this situation, it is recommended that plain bacterin is used, because onset of effective immunity is quicker. It can be used simultaneously with oil-adjuvant vaccine if available.

Herd quarantine, the segregation of sick animals from healthy ones and routine disinfection all help to slow the spread of the disease between and within herds.

Further reading

Bain, R.V.S, de Alwis, M.C.L., Carter, G.R. and Gupta, B.K. (1982). Haemorrhage septicaemia *F.A.O. Animal Production and Health Paper*, No. 33. F.A.O., Rome.
de Alwis, M.C.L. (1981). Mortality among cattle and buffaloes in Sri Lanka due to haemorrhagic septicaemia. *Tropical Animal Health and Production,* **13**, 195–202.

R.M.E.

JOHNE'S DISEASE

Johne's disease (paratuberculosis) is an infectious, contagious and almost invariably fatal enteritis caused by *Mycobacterium paratuberculosis*. The disease is characterized by a chronic course with wasting and diarrhoea, and at autopsy thickening of the intestinal mucosa.

Aetiology

The disease is caused by *M. paratuberculosis (M. johnei)*, a small acid-fast bacillus which is relatively slow growing in the laboratory and which requires mycobactin, a growth factor obtained from other mycobacteria. The organism is relatively resistant to adverse environmental influences and can survive for many months in faeces, water and soil, but only about 7 days in urine.

Occurrence

The disease has a worldwide distribution and may occur either sporadically or as a minor epidemic within a herd. It usually occurs in areas of high cattle density and appears to be more prevalent in more temperate and wetter zones than in hotter and drier climates.

Species affected

Cattle, sheep and goats are the species most commonly affected, but in the Middle East and Asia the disease has been reported in camels, yaks and buffaloes. Cases have been reported in llamas and in a variety of species of antelope and deer. A closely related mycobactin-dependent mycobacterium has been isolated from human patients with Crohn's disease.

Transmission

Infection is normally acquired by ingestion of milk, water or food contaminated by infected faeces. Some clinically infected animals excrete *M. paratuberculosis* in the milk and the organism has also been isolated from the semen of infected bulls. However, venereal transmission is thought not to be important. The organism may be isolated from the foetuses of infected dams, especially those in an advanced stage of the disease, but intra-uterine transmission of paratuberculosis does not appear to be a significant cause of natural infection.

Animals less than 30 days old are most susceptible to infection. Infection acquired when young is more likely to develop into clinical disease, while older animals may become carriers without developing the disease overtly.

Clinical features

Many animals harbour and excrete the causal organism without showing signs of the disease. The annual rate of clinical cases in an infected herd varies between 1 and 5%, but the infection rate can be greater than 50%. Clinical disease is the terminal stage of a slow chronic subclinical infection and may be precipitated by stress factors. The disease in cattle rarely manifests itself before the age of 2 years, but may occur at any age thereafter. Subclinically infected animals show decreased productivity and increased infertility and susceptibility to other infections including mastitis. In the early stages, affected cattle lose condition and even prior to that may not attain expected milk yields. Diarrhoea is intermittent at first but terminally is constantly present. In the later stages, emaciation becomes progressive despite an unimpaired appetite leading eventually to prostration and death. The clinical course may last from 3 to 6 months.

In sheep, diarrhoea is not a feature, although the faeces may be softer than normal. Otherwise, the disease is one of chronic wasting and clinically indistinguishable from the other sheep diseases which have similar presenting features.

Pathology

If the disease is sufficiently advanced, specific macroscopic lesions may be seen in the intestinal walls of the lower part of the small intestine and extending into the large intestine. The mucosa is thickened and corrugated and has a "Morocco-leather"-like appearance. Confirmation can be made by examination for the characteristic small acid-fast bacilli in mucosal scrapings, but bacilli may be absent or few in number even in the presence of extensive lesions in some cases. Confirmation can best be made by histological examination of the mucous membrane and the draining mesenteric lymph nodes. The lesions are characterized by diffuse granulomatous changes with infiltration of the *lamina propria* and submucosa of the intestine and cortices of the nodes with endothelioid and, less commonly, giant cells. Macrophages and giant cells are usually filled with acid-fast bacilli. Lesions found elsewhere include focal granulomas in the liver and vascular changes. There is no tendency to necrosis, encapsulation or calcification in cattle, although these changes may be found in sheep and goats.

In sheep, thickening of the intestinal mucosa is not a feature and mesenteric lymph node enlargement is not always present. Lesions found on histological examination may be very extensive, even in the absence of gross changes.

Diagnosis

The disease can be confused with other chronic wasting diseases, but the history and clinical signs are usually suggestive as is a positive complement fixation test in advanced cases. The finding of clumps of acid-fast bacilli in the faeces provides confirmation of the disease, but not all cases can be confirmed by this means. At autopsy an examination for the presence of microscopic lesions in the intestinal wall and mesenteric lymph nodes from which *M. paratuberculosis* can be isolated, is the best method of establishing a definitive diagnosis. Diagnosis in the preclinical stages of the disease is more difficult. The use of immunologic methods for diagnostic testing of individual animals is of limited value, but on a herd basis they have some diagnostic merit. Allergic and single serological tests (either complement fixation or immunofluorescence) are largely unreliable. An enzyme-linked immunosorbent assay (ELISA) using *M. phlei* absorbed serum gives improved results with earlier detection of infected animals and fewer false positives.

Faecal culture is probably the best available method but it takes at least 2 months for a result to be obtained. Again, not all infected animals are detected at a single test. An examination of mesenteric lymph node biopsies from the region of the terminal ileum is reported to give very accurate results but is less practical.

Treatment

The disease is incurable even by drugs which have a high *in vitro* activity against *M. paratuberculosis*. Animals exhibiting clinical signs of the disease should be isolated and slaughtered as soon as possible, because their presence is a danger to the rest of the herd or flock.

Immunology

M. paratuberculosis has shared antigens with most organisms in the order Actinomycetales, especially *M. avium* with which it is antigenically very closely related. Anergy develops usually during the terminal stages of the disease and humoral responses may eventually disappear also.

Vaccination with attenuated strains or heat-killed *M. paratuberculosis* in an oil adjuvant markedly reduces the number of clinical cases and also the number of animals excreting the organism, but does not confer absolute immunity or prevent a carrier state. Unfortunately, vaccination causes some interference with tuberculin testing and precludes future allergic or serological tests for Johne's disease itself.

Control

Control is difficult because of the insidious nature of the disease, the presence of clinically normal carriers of infection and the lack of a satisfactory test for early diagnosis. Elimination of infection from an infected herd involves identification and culling of infected animals, improved hygiene and vaccination of replacements. Adult animals should be tested by faecal culture every 6 months and all positive animals sent to slaughter. The introduction of infection into a herd or into a country is almost invariably by means of latently infected animals, and therefore the limitations of diagnostic tests and even of lengthy quarantine should be borne in mind.

Strict attention should be paid to hygiene in an infected herd and aimed at preventing transmission to the more susceptible young animals. Calves should be separated from their mothers at birth and reared separately using pasteurized milk. Steps should be taken to prevent contamination of food or water supplies with faeces and infected pastures should be kept free of ruminants for at least a year. *M. paratuberculosis* is resistant to many disinfectants, but those that are effective include 5% formalin, phenol (1:40 dilution), cresylic disinfectants (1:32) and calcium hypochlorite (1:50).

Vaccination, if practised, should take place in the first month of life. Revaccination is not recommended as a decrease in resistance is likely to result.

Further reading

Chiodini, R.J., van Kruiningen, H.J. and Merkal, R.S. (1984). Ruminant paratuberculosis (Johne's disease): The current status and future prospects. *The Cornell Veterinarian*, **74**, 218–262.
Julian, R.J. (1975). A short review and some observations on Johne's disease with recommendations for control. *Canadian Veterinary Journal*, **16**, 33–43.
Merkal, R.S. (1973). Laboratory diagnosis of bovine paratuberculosis. *Journal of the American Veterinary Medical Association*, **163**, 1100–1102.

A.N.M.

LEPTOSPIROSIS

Leptospirosis is the disease produced by infection with pathogenic serovars of the genus *Leptospira*. Most infections appear to be subclinical, but severe disease characterized by haemolytic anaemia leading to jaundice, haemoglobinuria, and occasionally death, or milder forms with fever, agalactia, often described as atypical mastitis, and abortion, may occur. The available evidence suggests that it is the cause of enormous economic loss in tropical and subtropical countries.

Aetiology

Leptospires belong to a single species, *Leptospira interrogans*, containing two major groups, the saprophytic complex containing the free-living leptospires and the pathogenic complex containing leptospires that may be strict parasites. There are now 26 recognized serogroups and approximately 200 serovars have been identified. In theory, any parasitic leptospire may infect any animal species, but in practice only a small number of serovars will be endemic in any particular region, while each serovar tends to be maintained in specific maintenance hosts. Therefore, in any animal species, infection may arise from (a) strains adapted to and maintained in that species, or (b) strains maintained by other species of domestic and wild animals.

Occurrence

Leptospires have been widely reported in livestock especially in Europe, North America, South East Asia and Australia, and there is also widespread serological evidence of infection of cattle throughout the tropical and subtropical regions of Africa and South and Central America.

The optimum environment for leptospires is warm, wet conditions with a pH value close to neutral. These conditions occur all the year round in parts of the tropics and in the later summer and autumn in more temperate zones. Incidental infections are therefore relatively more important in the tropics. Where rainfall is seasonal, transmission of incidental infections may also be seasonal. Leptospires cannot tolerate desiccation, excessive sunlight, pH values other than near neutral, salinity and many kinds of chemical pollution.

Species affected

Leptospirosis is a common zoonotic disease which can affect most mammals. All domestic animals are susceptible. In cattle, infections by strains belonging to the Sejroe serogroup almost always predominate. These are mostly of the cattle-adapted strain serovar *hardjo*. *L. pomona* appears to be the most prevalent serotype associated with the acute form of the infection in cattle. Other serotypes occur less commonly but may cause clinical disease and even death, e.g. *L. australis* and *L. icterohaemorrhagiae*.

In sheep and goats, haemolytic anaemia caused by *L. pomona* is seen in lambs and death may occur from *L. grippotyphosa*.

In pigs, *L. pomona* may cause infertility and abortion. Similar problems may occur with *L. tarassovi*, *L. canicola* and *L. lora*, and piglets may die from infection with *L. icterohaemorrhagiae*.

Horses appear to be susceptible to a wide range of serotypes. Infection may lead to abortion, death of young animals and possibly moon blindness (periodic opthalmia; uveitis).

Dogs may act as a reservoir of *L. canicola* infection and they are also susceptible to infection with other serotypes, *L. icterohaemorrhagiae* being most frequently recorded. Cats appear to be relatively resistant to leptospirosis.

Man is susceptible to a wide range of leptospiral infections and usually becomes infected from domestic or wild animals. Although severe cases occur with *L. icterohaemorrhagiae*, most cases are milder. The disease should be suspected in any case of pyrexia of unknown origin if there are suspicious circumstances.

The largest reservoir of leptospires is in wild animals. Rodentia including rats, voles, mice and gerbils appear most important, but other orders that have been found to be infected are Insectivora, Carnivora (foxes, jackals, mongoose, civets, skunks and racoons) and Marsupiolia (bandicoots and opossums). Chiroptera (bats), Artiodactyla (deer) and Lagomorpha (hares and rabbits) appear less important.

Transmission

Leptospires are excreted in urine for a variable period, depending on the infecting serovar and the age of the animal. In incidental infections urinary excretion usually only lasts for several weeks, but with the cattle-maintained strains (serovar *hardjo*) excretion can last for at least 18 months and possibly for the animal's lifetime. The organism is also found in post-calving uterine discharge for up to 8 days. Rats have been shown to excrete *L. icterohaemorrhagiae* for at least 220 days.

Direct infection may occur when animals are herded together. However, infection usually arises from contact with a contaminated environment, infected water playing an important role in the transmission cycle. The organism may survive for months in water-saturated soil.

Leptospires may enter a new host through the skin, especially if this is damaged, or through the mucosa of the muzzle, mouth or conjunctiva.

Other routes of infection are bites from rodents, venereal spread (leptospires have been isolated from bulls' semen), predation, where animals hunt and kill infected prey, and transplacental infection of the foetus.

Clinical signs

The clinical signs of leptospirosis vary considerably in severity, with infection being inapparent in the majority of cases. Clinical bovine leptospirosis can be divided into two distinct phases: first, an acute phase whose onset coincides with the bacteraemic phase of infection and, secondly, a chronic phase which occurs much later and whose affects are mostly noticeable on the reproductive tract. The most severe form is usually observed in young animals, although outbreaks do occur when mortality is high even among adults, particularly when *L. pomona*, *L. grippotyphosa*, *L. icterohaemorrhagiae* and *L. automnalis* are involved.

The incubation period is usually 5–7 days. The clinical signs are those of severe septicaemia with pyrexia, anorexia, an acute haemolytic anaemia, haemoglobinuria and jaundice. When animals recover there is a prolonged convalescence period. A necrotic dermatitis may occur in some animals infected with *L. grippotyphosa* strains and occasional cases may be characterized by signs of meningitis. A synovitis has also been recorded in some affected animals. The degree of jaundice varies considerably and may be difficult to detect.

The most noticeable sign is often discolouration of the urine, which varies in colour from bright red to almost black in cases of *L. pomona* and *L. grippotyphosa* infection.

In the mildest form of acute infection which is seen in adult dairy cattle there is pyrexia, which is often undetected, and a marked drop in milk production. The milk is thickened in consistency similar to colostrum and may be tinged with red or yellow. It contains clots and has a high white cell count. All four quarters of the udder are affected. The changes are usually transient and the secretion returns to normal after several days. There is no inflammation of the udder which usually appears flaccid.

The incidence of leptospirosis in a population will vary. In susceptible herds 50% or more may become infected within a 2-month period, whereas only sporadic cases will occur in endemically infected herds.

The most important chronic sequelae of leptospirosis are seen in pregnant animals where foetal infection with resultant abortion, stillbirths and premature live births of weak calves may occur up to 3 months, and occasionally longer, after the acute phase of infection.

Pathology

At post-mortem examination, severe jaundice, when present, is striking as the entire carcase may appear very yellow. In some species, particularly dogs, a haemorrhagic gastroenteritis is prominent with haemorrhages throughout the organs but particularly the lungs and heart. There may be ulcers and haemorrhages in the abomasal mucosa in cattle. In all species, the liver may be swollen, and the pattern of lobulation may be abnormally distinct, the kidneys may be enlarged and the cortex a reddish brown mottled colour. Urine in the bladder may be coloured red or black. Histologically, there is focal or diffuse interstitial nephritis and centrilobular hepatic necrosis.

In chronic cases in all species, the kidneys may contain innumerable white foci level with the surface or larger lesions with the appearance of infarcts. Histologically, this appears as a periarteriolar lymphocytic infiltration of the intestinal tissue leading to compression of the nephron: syncytia and giant cells may be seen. Tubules in the medulla may be dilated and contain hyaline casts.

Diagnosis

Leptospires may be detected in plasma, urine or organs including foetal tissue by dark field microscopy, fluorescent antibody techniques or by a number of silver staining methods. A variety of artefacts in fresh preparations examined by dark field and silver stained preparations can make diagnosis difficult. The identity of the infecting leptospires cannot be determined by microscopic methods alone. The isolation of the infecting strain either by direct culture or the inoculation of laboratory animals is to be preferred. Leptospires are very fragile and do not survive long in a decomposing carcase. Cultures are most readily obtained from the liver and kidneys of an animal recently dead or slaughtered for examination. Fluorescent antibody techniques may be applied to cultures or infected urine to differentiate the serotypes involved.

A selective medium (EMJH) containing flurouracil is beneficial in isolation of the organism from urine. Leptospiral infection in aborted foetuses may be demonstrated by a combination of foetal serology, isolation of leptospires and immunofluorescence. The kidneys, lungs and pleural fluid of the aborted foetus should be examined for the presence of the organism.

The demonstration of antibodies remains the usual method of confirming a diagnosis. A variety of tests are available, but the microscopic agglutination test using either live or formolized antigens is most commonly undertaken. A presumptive diagnosis may be made on the basis of a rising titre of antibodies in paired serum samples taken 7–10 days apart.

Serological tests are not specific for the whole genus and will generally only detect infection by closely related strains within a serogroup. Advice on the selection of suitable antigen strains should be obtained from a reference laboratory.

Differential diagnosis in cattle consists of distinguishing the acute form of the disease from other causes of jaundice and haemoglobinuria including anaplasmosis and babesiosis which may be intercurrent or secondary; *Clostridium haemolyticum* infection may also present a similar picture. The kidney lesions in cattle resemble those of some cases of East Coast fever. Similar conditions in other species such as azoturia and infectious equine anaemia in horses, babesiosis and anaplasmosis in sheep, and poisoning by a variety of toxic plants in all species should be considered.

The main sign in less acute cases in cattle, pigs and occasionally horses is abortion, and a laboratory examination is necessary to distinguish leptospirosis from the many other possible causes.

Treatment

Treatment of leptospirosis should be started early to prevent irreparable damage to the liver and kidneys and to prevent the development of the carrier state.

Streptomycin is the drug of choice in the control of infection, but one of the tetracyclines may also be effective. In acute infections, streptomycin is given for three consecutive days at the rate of 25 mg/kg daily. A single injection of 25 mg/kg dihydrostreptomycin is effective in eliminating urinary tract infections. Oxytetracycline added to the feed (800 g/tonne) for 10 days is also claimed to eliminate a carrier state in pig herds. No form of treatment is successful once a haemolytic crisis has developed, but whole blood transfusion can be attempted in valuable animals.

Treatment of periodic ophthalmia in horses with streptomycin and cortisone has been recommended but has little effect on the course of the disease.

Immunology

Leptospiral infection induces a rapid production of antibody which assists in the removal of leptospires from all organs except the kidney tubules where the leptospires may persist for weeks or even years. As in most infections, the early production of IgM is replaced by IgG, the level of which may remain high for a prolonged period, possibly due to periodic antigenic stimulation by reinvasion from the kidney tubules.

The microscopic and macroscopic agglutination tests principally measure the relatively short-lived IgM antibodies. This is useful in tracing the development of natural infection in a population of animals. Antibodies may also be detected in milk and urine. The detection of IgG antibodies which are protective, requires additional tests such as the hamster protection test, the passive haemagglutination test or the growth inhibition test.

Successful immunization requires the specific identification of the resident serotypes, because vaccination against one serotype may not give protection against others, even where they exhibit antigenic relationships *in vitro*.

The pathogenesis of periodic opthalmia appears to involve partial antigenic identity between equine cornea and leptospiral organisms.

Control

Vaccination with and without supplementary antibiotic therapy (dihydrostreptomycin at 25 mg/kg) offers the only effective method of controlling and preventing clinical leptospirosis in cattle herds. In closed herds, vaccination of all members of the herd should be carried out annually whereas in open herds all members should be revaccinated every 6 months. The vaccine used should be a multivalent bacterin containing the serovars endemic in the region. In a few animals, vaccination may fail to prevent colonization of the renal tubules and the development of a carrier state. Live avirulent vaccines, where available, appear to be more effective.

Further reading

Amaaredjo, A. and Campbell, R.S.F. (1975). Bovine leptospirosis. *Veterinary Bulletin*, **43**, 875–891.
Ellis, W.A. (1984). Bovine leptospirosis in the tropics: Prevalence, pathogenesis and control. *Preventive Veterinary Medicine*, **2**, 411–421.
Turner, L.H. (1967). Leptospirosis I. *Transactions of the Royal Society of Tropical Medicine and Hygiene*, **61**, 842–855.
Turner, L.H. (1968). Leptospirosis II: Serology. *Transactions of the Royal Society of Tropical Medicine and Hygiene*, **62**, 880–899.
Turner, L.H. (1970). Leptospirosis III: Maintenance, isolation and demonstration of leptospires. *Transactions of the Royal Society of Tropical Medicine and Hygiene*, **64**, 623–646.

A.N.M.

MELIOIDOSIS

Melioidosis is a glanders-like disease of animals and man.

Aetiology

The causal organism is *Pseudomonas pseudomallei*, a highly virulent pathogenic organism which can survive for considerable periods in soil and water.

Occurrence

Until 1949, melioidosis was recognized as a sporadic disease in South East Asia only, but it is now reported from Australia, Malaysia, Papua New Guinea, Niger and France.

It is reported as endemic in some piggeries in Australia. It is possible that single cases in Africa and Europe are contracted from men who have developed the disease in South East Asia.

Species affected

The disease is regarded as a natural infection of rodents and other wild animals with sporadic accidental infection of man and domestic animals. Sheep, goats, horses and pigs are most commonly affected, cases in cattle being extremely rare. Dogs are also susceptible.

Transmission

Infection is said to be due mainly to ingestion of water or food contaminated with the organism passed in the faeces of infected rodents, but it can also occur through skin abrasions and the respiratory tract. There is, however, considerable confusion as to the reservoir and mode of infection. Some are of the opinion that the disease is often absent from rodents in areas where the disease is endemic in man and consider that infection by ingestion is not usual. However, it is agreed that the organism can live in water for several weeks and that contaminated water is the chief source of infection. It has been suggested that bloodsucking arthropods may also transmit the disease.

Clinical features

These include intermittent fever, cough, nasal and ocular discharges. The course of the acute form of the disease in domestic animals can vary from 2 to 8 weeks. Chronic and symptomless infection is common and apparent recoveries occur.

Pathology

Multiple abscesses varying in size from small miliary lesions to ones over 1 inch in diameter are found in the lungs, liver and spleen, and in associated lymph nodes. In pigs, the submandibular lymph node is the most common infection site.

Diagnosis

The disease in horses can be confused with glanders and in sheep with caseous lymphadenitis, but cultural and serological diagnostic methods for differentiation are available. The causal agent should be demonstrated in pathological material such as pus, nasal-pharyngeal discharges or infected blood. Melioidin (analogous to mallein) is used in sheep and goats for diagnosis, but in horses does not differentiate from glanders. Its usefulness has not yet been fully evaluated.

Treatment

It is difficult to cure chronic cases of melioidosis. Chloramphenicol is said to be effective in subacute cases in horses and man.

Control

If the disease has been recently introduced, all infected animals should be slaughtered and disposed of by burning or deep burial and, depending on the circumstances, in-contact animals should also be slaughtered. In countries where the disease is endemic and symptomless cases are common, no control policy has been evolved.

R.M.E.

MINOR MYCOPLASMA INFECTIONS

Apart from the causal agents of the classical syndromes of contagious bovine and caprine pleuropneumonia, about 20 species of the genus *Mycoplasma* of moderate to high virulence have been isolated from a variety of clinical conditions in small and large ruminants. The more widespread and adequately characterized of these are contagious mastitis or agalactia, polyarthritis and kerato conjunctivitis. Also, other mollicutes such as acholeplasmas and ureaplasmas of mild or no pathogenic potential have been demonstrated in a wide range of urogenital and respiratory disorders in these species.

Contagious agalactia

Aetiology

The classical syndrome consisting of mastitis, arthritis and keratitis is attributed to *M. agalactiae*, the first mollicute to be isolated and characterized. An almost identical syndrome of an acute nature and shorter course and dominated by pulmonary lesions is widespread in France, southern Germany, Spain, Portugal and Israel, and is caused by *M. mycoides* spp. *mycoides* of the large-colony caprine biotype and less frequently by *M. capricolum* or *M. putrefaciens*. "Sparta disease" of goats in Greece, previously regarded as an atypical, fulminant form of agalactia, is now known to be caused by an, as yet, unclassified serovar of mycoplasma having a marked serologic cross-reactivity with *M. mycoides* spp. *mycoides* (L.C) *caprine biotype* and *M. mycoides* spp. *capri* (PG-3).

Occurrence

Mycoplasma mastitis of bovine, sheep and goat dairy herds is an important disease entity in many countries. The classical disease "Contagious agalactia", first recognized in Italy more than 170 years ago, is now endemic in at least 23 countries and no continent seems free from it.

Species affected

The disease affects only sheep and goats under natural conditions.

Epidemiology

The term agalactia is unfortunate because the lesions are not strictly limited to the udder, but also occur in the joints and/or eyes in lactating ewes and does and in the external genitalia of males. Young animals are more severely affected and case fatality rates are high. Goats seem more prone than sheep under identical natural conditions. Pregnant ewes in the third semester of gestation are especially vulnerable. In both species, the disease is seasonal, prevalence rates being significantly high in the spring and summer months.

Agalactia is manifested at the time of parturition and spreads through the herd quickly. Following clinical recovery, the agent persists in the udder tissue and other anatomical sites for long periods. Periodical recrudescences of infection are therefore common in newly introduced populations. Mycoplasmas also persist in the external ear of goats. Ectoparasites such as ticks and mites are suspected of having a potential role in the maintenance and transfer of infection.

Transmission

It occurs directly by contact with infective exudates and milk and is effective by inhalation and ingestion. Neonates are infected by sucking colostrum or milk and adults through milkers' hands or contaminated fomites. Mycoplasmas survive for nearly 3 years in the soil under low temperatures and anaerobic conditions.

Clinicopathological features

Both acute and chronic forms of the disease occur, but the latter is more common. In the acute phase, there is mycoplasmemia, which synchronizes with general malaise and is followed by fever, anorexia and prostration. Pregnant animals may abort full-term. Mastitis is often bilateral and of an acute, catarrhal or parenchymatous type causing greatly reduced lactation or total agalactia. Infected milk is thick, alkaline, yellowish-green and contains clots which may obstruct the teat canal. Cell counts are high, and dominated by neutrophils and acinar cells.

Mycoplasmemia results in ocular, articular and pulmonary localizations. The most commonly affected joints are the tarsus, carpus and hock which are hot and oedematous. Lesions may progress from uncomplicated synovitis to fibrinous or suppurative arthritis, erosion of the synovial membrane, periarthritis and ankylosis.

Ocular lesions are characterized by conjunctivitis, copious lacrymation and photophobia followed by corneal opacity, and vascularization. In severe cases, the changes mature into parenchymatous keratitis, hypopyon, iridocyclitis and extrusion of aqueous humour and iris. In young animals, pneumonia and pleurisy are the dominant signs and cause high mortalities. Other recorded lesions are enteritis, fibrinous pericarditis, metritis, vulvovaginitis and balanoposthitis.

Diagnosis

Clinical diagnosis is unreliable. Pulmonary forms of *M. agalactiae* infection are difficult to differentiate from pneumopathies due to *M. ovipneumoniae* and *M. arginini*. Infections caused by *M. capricolum* and *M. mycoides* spp. *mycoides* (L.C) are usually acute or hyperacute with a shorter course and severe lung pathology. In *M. putrefaciens* mastitis, the milk has a strong putrid odour.

Laboratory diagnosis ensures the identity of the causal mycoplasma and is based on cultural, biochemical and serologic procedures. Lesions may be colonized by more than one type of mycoplasma, thus causing diagnostic confusion. The complement fixation test is widely applied in the diagnosis of herd infections and is reliable.

Treatment

The consensus is that it is not likely to be effective unless applied at the onset of the first clinical signs. Symptoms may be ameliorated by correct doses of tylosine, tiamulin or tetracyclines, but organisms are not eliminated and the carrier state is therefore not prevented.

Prophylaxis

Recovered animals resist reinfection. Two types of vaccines are in use, the chick-embryo passaged, live, attenuated vaccine and the formalin-inactivated adjuvanted culture suspensions of *M. agalactiae*. Two doses are necessary. Trials in Iran, Turkey, Israel and Italy have given satisfactory results.

Control

Standard sanitary procedures such as isolation, quarantine, restriction of animal movement and disinfection of infected premises are effective. Heat-treated colostrums fed to neonates in the first 1–3 days provide passive protection without the risk of alimentary infection. Bought-in stock may be serologically tested to identify and eliminate carriers. Periodic vaccination and culling of infected animals are other appropriate measures.

Bovine mycoplasmal mastitis

Several species of mycoplasmas and a few acholeplasmas and ureaplasmas are implicated. Of the proven pathogens, *M. bovis* is widespread. Large-scale outbreaks have been described in Europe, the USA, Canada, South America, Japan and recently in China. *M. bovis* mastitis is also recognized in buffaloes in India. Other pathogenic species are *M. californicum, M. canadense, M. capricolum* and unnamed strains of Leach's serogroup 7 (bovine). In addition, *M. bovigenitalium, M. alkalescens, M. arginini, Acholeplasma laidlawii* and ureaplasmas, which occur as normal resident flora may, on occasions, induce or exacerbate mastitis in concert with bacterial pathogens.

The main source of infection is the carrier cow. The transfer of infection occurs during milking. Semen, respiratory and urogenital discharges are the other major sources.

There is considerable variation in the severity and duration of bovine mycoplasma mastitis. *M. bovis* and *M. californicum* infections are severe and characterized by marked swelling and firmness of the udder. In infections due to other mycoplasmas, the mastitis is painless and asymptomatic, although infective titres may be high.

Diagnosis is readily established by standard laboratory procedures. Treatment is notoriously ineffective. Control relies on routine sanitary measures, the detection of carrier-cows by serologic tests and slaughter of the infected.

Infectious kerato conjunctivitis of sheep and goats

Also known as "pink-eye", it has been reported in 43 countries.

Aetiology

The causal agents are bacteria belonging to the genera *Moraxella, Listeria* and *Branhamella, Chlamydia psittaci* and mycoplasma species. The principal mycoplasmal cause is *M. conjunctivae*. Others less frequently recovered from the lesions in goats are *M. agalactiae* in Italy and the USA and *M. capricolum* in France. *M. mycoides* spp. *mycoides* (small-colony, PG-1 caprine type) has been sporadically isolated from sheep in different countries. In both species, opportunist mycoplasma such as *M. arginini, M. ovipneumoniae, Acholeplasma oculi* and ureaplasms have been frequently demonstrated in the lesions.

Epidemiology

Outbreaks can be traced to carriers. The disease spreads rapidly through the herd, is self-limiting and generally runs a short course.

Clinicopathological features

Ocular lesions begin as intense hyperaemia and swelling of the palpebral conjunctiva, and are accompanied by profuse lacrymal discharge, blepharospasm and epiphora. In due course, there is corneal vascularization and pannus. Severe cases manifest corneal ulceration, and panophthalmitis. There is frequent pulmonary and arthritic involvement. The organisms persist for several weeks in the eyes of recovered animals.

In chamois, which are raised with sheep in some alpine regions of Europe, *M. conjunctivae* causes a devastating form of disease characterized by parenchymatous keratitis, corneal ulceration and complete blindness.

Diagnosis

The causal mycoplasms can be detected in conjunctival smears by indirect immunofluorescent testing using specific antisera. Confirmatory diagnosis relies on cultural isolation and serologic identification. Mycoplasmal keratitis is non-follicular and can be differentiated histologically from the *Chlamydia*-induced follicular type.

Treatment

It is of little avail, but topical application of ointments incorporating tetracyclines, polymyxin-B and ethidium bromide may help reduce the severity of the lesions.

Bovine keratitis

Its aetiology is complex. Several species of bacteria, some helminths and viruses are involved. The most common cause is _Moraxella bovis_, but mycoplasmal association markedly enhances concomitant bacterial infections. The potentiating effect seems restricted to _Mycoplasma bovoculi_ and not shared by other ocular mollicutes such as _Mycoplasma bovis_, _M. bovirhinis_, _M. verecundum_, _Acholeplasma oculi_ and _Urea-plasma diversum_, which frequently colonize the lesions. Infections due to _M. bovoculi_ are far more prevalent than with any other species and colonization levels are also high.

Calves are severely affected and _M. bovoculi_ establishes a persistent infection. Adult cattle show trivial clinical signs and relapses are uncommon.

Polyarthritis

Mycoplasmal arthritis is often recognized as a distinct clinical entity resulting from neonatal mycoplasmemia or as a part of the pathology of systemic mycoplasmosis, conjunctivitis and pneumonia. The condition is widely prevalent in USA and Australia and to a lesser extent in several other countries. The causal agents in most instances are _M. mycoides_ spp. _mycoides_ (L.C. biotype) and _M. capricolum_. In sporadic cases, _M. agalactiae_, _M. mycoides_ spp. _mycoides_ (S.C. PG-1, caprine biotype) and an unclassified strain, designated as 2D caprine biotype, have been recovered.

The clinical disease is a septicaemia with moderate to severe hyperthemia, polyarthritis and polyserositis. Mortalities are excessive in lambs and kids. Adults have marked pulmonary lesions, pleurisy and peritonitis.

A severe form of primary mycoplasmal arthritis due to _M. bovis_ has been reported in calves in Bulgaria.

Genital mycoplasmosis

The association of different classes of mollicutes with a wide range of genital disorders in both sexes, and also with abortions and stillbirths in cattle, buffaloes, sheep and goats is well documented. Mycoplasmal contamination of bovine semen seems ubiquitous. Several species have been identified and those with reported high isolation rates are _M. bovigenitalium_, _M. bovis_ and _M. canadense_. Infected semen may be a principal means of domestic and international dissemination of these organisms.

Mycoplasmal attachment to bull spermatozoa and to the _zona pellucida_ of bovine morulae has been reported. Though structural damage was not detected in the electron microscope, there was evidence of impaired motility of frozen-thawed sperms. Use of infected semen has been shown to cause a reduction in conception rates, uterine inflammatory changes, prolonged diestrous and increased calving intervals.

Vulvo-vaginitis in sheep and goats is frequently associated with *M. agalactiae*, *M. capricolum* and *M. mycoides* spp. *mycoides* (L.C). In India, *M. agalactiae* has been isolated from stillbirths and premature kids. The frequent recovery of ureaplasmas in the genital lesions of cows and aborted bovine foetuses should be considered significant. Of the different species identified, *Ureaplasma diversum* had high isolation rates from preputial and vaginal swabs and urine samples in Australia and Japan. The addition of lincomycin, spectinomycin and tylosine to bovine semen was effective in the elimination of mycoplasma and saw a marked reduction in titres of acholeplasmas and ureoplasmas.

S.R.

SALMONELLOSIS

Salmonellosis is an infectious disease of man and animals caused by organisms of the genus Salmonella. These bacteria are primarily intestinal organisms. Sometimes, therefore, either as a consequence of clinical disease or subclinical infection, they may be found in farm effluents, human sewage or in any material subject to faecal contamination.

Aetiology

Approximately 1800 different salmonella serotypes have been described. All members of the genus are considered to be potentially pathogenic. They do, however, vary in their host specificity, virulence and the pathological syndromes they produce. Some serotypes are relatively host-specific, thus *Salmonella typhi* infects only man who is also the principal host of *S. paratyphi*. *S. pullorum* and *S. gallinarum* are confined to poultry, *S. cholerae-suis* and *S. dublin* are mainly restricted to pigs and cattle, respectively. *S. abortus-ovis* and *S. abortus-equi* are mainly restricted to sheep and horses, respectively. In contrast, *S. typhimurium* is frequently encountered in all species of animals, birds and man, although certain phage types appear somewhat restricted in their range.

Occurrence

Salmonellosis has been recognized in all countries of the world. It is most prevalent in areas of intensive animal husbandry, especially of poultry and pigs. Under conditions of extensive range husbandry, the disease is most likely to manifest itself when the animals are gathered or at parturition. A seasonal incidence associated with the hot rainy season has been described in some countries.

Species affected

Salmonellosis can affect all species of domestic animals. Young, debilitated and parturiant animals are most susceptible to clinical disease. Man is highly susceptible to infection, either by direct contact with infected animals or through their products.

Transmission and epidemiology

Salmonellosis is primarily an enteric disease and is transmitted principally by the faecal – oral route. Salmonellae are excreted in large numbers in the faeces of infected animals with consequent contamination of the environment. In any outbreak, the majority of animals will acquire infection by direct contact with faeces, or food, bedding or water contaminated by faeces.

The introduction of infection into uninfected premises may be by a variety of means, but principally by asymptomatic carrier animals, contaminated feedstuffs or polluted water supplies. Such introduced infection may either remain silent or develop into clinical disease, the outcome being influenced by both the species and the numbers of contaminating bacteria.

Physiological stress factors, nutrition, management and intercurrent disease are liable to render animals more susceptible to infection or to activate the latent carrier state. Conditions such as piroplasmosis, foot and mouth disease, fasciolosis and swine fever may demonstrate concurrent salmonellosis. In almost all infections, only a minority of animals will demonstrate clinical disease.

Although the factors influencing infection in poultry are fundamentally the same as those affecting other domestic animals, a point of difference is that the two host-adapted species (*S. pullorum* and *gallinarum*) may cause infection of the ovary and in some cases the contents of eggs become infected directly and not by passage of the organism through the shell.

Clinical features

Cattle. Clinical infection occurs most commonly in calves and post-parturient adults and often involves *S. dublin* or *S. typhimurium*. Signs in calves vary from acute septicaemia in neonates to acute enteritis, often with dysentery, along with fever and inappetance in animals 1 week of age or more. Affected calves quickly lose condition, become dehydrated and emaciated. Pneumonic signs may also be seen and chronic cases may show polyarthritis. Adult cows show fever, anorexia and enteritis, manifested by abdominal pain and dysentery in which the faecal matter may contain large amounts of clotted blood. While many adult infections are sporadic and related to calving, occasionally multiple case outbreaks occur in which the precipitating factor is a degree of starvation. Clinically affected animals may abort in the absence of other clinical signs. Recovery from clinical signs is often prolonged and some animals, particularly calves, show a dry gangrene of the extremities – ears, limbs and tail. Many infections, especially in adults, are totally asymptomatic.

Sheep and goats. The pattern of infection is similar to that seen in cattle with an emphasis on abortion, deaths in adults due to septicaemia and enteritis either before or after partuition, along with septicaemia but more commonly enteritis in young lambs or kids. Infections with *S. abortus-ovis* are generally asymptomatic, other than abortion in the last 6 weeks of gestation.

Pigs. Only young pigs, less than 4 months of age, are clinically affected. The acute form of the disease is manifested by anorexia, fever and a purple discolouration of the extremities, with a high mortality in untreated animals. Milder forms of the disease do not show discolouration, but penumonia or enteritis with fluctuating fever. The faeces are often bile stained and contain necrotic mucosal debris, rarely blood. Serotypes commonly associated with clinical disease are *S. cholerae-suis* and *S. typhimurium*, the former being involved in septicaemia, the latter more often in enteric-type disease.

Poultry. *Salmonella* infections in domestic hens result in three types of disease that differ clinically and epidemiologically. *S. pullorum* causes pullorum disease, mainly in young chicks and is a true egg infection. Paratyphoid also mainly infects young birds, but infection reaches young chicks mainly by faecal – egg shell contamination. Fowl typhoid is a disease of adult birds caused by *S. gallinarum*, but on occasion infection may mimic pullorum disease.

Chick infections may be manifest soon after hatching, reaching a peak mortality after 2–3 week of life, with lassitude, inappetance and the passage of white excreta; surviving birds grow poorly and some may show joint or synovial lesions. Fowl typhoid in adults presents as a sudden onset anorexia and fever with death taking place within 10 days.

Horses. The disease is only common in adults where infection coincides with stress, transport or overcrowding. The clinical signs in foals do not necessarily require these initiating factors. The predominant signs are those of diarrhoea, acute abdominal pain, fever and neutropenia. One should draw attention to the particular dangers associated with anaesthesia of subclinically affected animals and the risk of infection in veterinary hospitals. Abortions associated with *S. abortus-equi* show few other signs and are possibly primarily initiated by rhinopneumonitis.

Pathology

Cattle, sheep and goats. Lesions in calves or adults are essentially similar with the predominant changes affecting the gastrointestinal tract as a cattarhal to fibrinohaemorrhagic gastroenteritis with acute inflammation of the drainage lymph nodes. Changes are often present in liver and spleen, the former showing on occasion the typhoid nodule, pin-head foci of cells or necrosis in the substance; splenic changes vary from enlargement and congestion to those similar to the liver lesion. Antero-ventral pneumonic lesions of calves may yield *Salmonella* or culture along with other bacterial pathogens. Sheep and goats show lesions similar to those seen in cattle.

Pigs. A purple discolouration of the extremities is characteristic but not pathognomonic of septicaemic salmonellosis. Other changes include heavy, wet congested lungs, enlarged spleen and focal paratyphoid lesions in the liver. Petechial haemorrhages may be present but are often not a prominent feature of the uncomplicated disease. Gross intestinal changes typical of more chronic disease are generally confined to the large bowel and comprise a fibrino necrotic enteritis of the colon or caecum.

Horses. Characteristic lesions in acute cases are confined to the alimentary canal. The large intestine is most severely affected with a haemorrhagic inflammation of the mucosa and lymph nodes that leads to superficial necrosis of the epithelium. Chronic cases show less clear-cut changes, which may be restricted to a local ulceration or areas of fibrinous surface exudate.

Poultry. Acute disease in young chicks can only be diagnosed microbiologically. Chicks dying after some days of symptoms may show nodular necrosis or cellular foci in heart, liver, lungs, lower bowel or gizzard. Fowl typhoid in adults may show a similar lack of specific changes in acute deaths. More frequently, there is enlargement and congestion of liver, spleen and kidneys. After more prolonged symptoms, bronze to greenish brown discolouration of the enlarged liver with miliary cellular foci in both the myocardium or liver is characteristic. Chronic infection of adult hens by *S. pullorum* is demonstrated by misshapen and discoloured ova, sometimes associated with oviduct impaction and peritonitis.

Diagnosis

Clinical diagnosis can be substantiated by the cultural examination of faeces, which should be reliable for most serotypes. Serological diagnosis can only realistically be employed where the offending serotype has been identified and may be useful in evaluating the epidemiology and extent of previous infection on an infected premises.

The identification of carrier animals is more difficult. Because excretion by such animals may be irregular and at low levels, it is recommended that 3–5 separate faecal samples, examined by enrichment techniques, are obtained before considering an animal to have ceased excreting. Serological tests have not proved reliable in the detection of carrier animals.

Necropsy and culture of visceral and intestinal tract of cadavers or aborted foetuses provides conclusive evidence of infection. It should be remembered that many conventional enrichment techniques are unsuitable for the recovery of *S. abortus-ovis* and *S. cholerae-suis*. In clinical conditions in adult horses, recovery of the offending *Salmonella* is said sometimes to be difficult from either faeces or large bowel and recovery should be sought from the drainage lymph nodes of these sites.

Diagnosis of avian salmonellosis following chick mortality should not prove difficult using culture and selective media from intestinal tract and visceral tissues. The carrier state is much more difficult to detect in either pullorum disease/typhoid or paratyphoid. For the latter, the tissue of choice is the caecal contents or caecal tonsil. Where infection with the former is suspected, the culture of any lesions, visceral tissues using gram amounts and enrichment techniques are required to demonstrate infection. Serological tests are used extensively to control pullorum and fowl typhoid infections, mainly using stained antigen in tests with whole blood.

Treatment

Many antibiotics have been used with varying degrees of success, but in general ampicillin, chloramphenicol, nitrofurazones and trimethoprim-sulphonamide mixtures have proved most useful. Treatment rarely eliminates faecal excretion and antimicrobial therapy may extend the period of excretion. Fluid replacement is probably the most important and useful supportive therapy, and this may involve either intravenous or oral administration.

Immunity

Animals that have recovered from infections are generally immune to reinfection by the serotype. Most indications for vaccination require protection for young animals in the immediate post-natal period. Satisfactory immunity for these young animals often requires live vaccines to stimulate adequate protection, and such vaccines are available for *S. dublin* and *S. cholerae-suis*. Protection against *S. typhimurium* may be achieved using a killed vaccine, but the quality of the immunogen is of paramount importance. Effective vaccines against fowl typhoid involve live vaccine and the 9R strain.

Control

The prevention of salmonella infections in clean herds depends on the exclusion of these bacteria from both food and water, and that introduced animals are obtained from non-infected sources. Certain livestock producers will always find these criteria difficult to apply and must constantly face the risk of infection. Such risks may, however, be minimized by limiting the exposure of very young animals to infection, i.e. young calves or ruminants should be retained on the farm of birth until they are less susceptible to the clinical effects of infection. While many feral animals and birds have possibly been incriminated as sources of infection, the initial introduction more probably involves other sources; such wild animals pose a distinct threat by the local transfer of infection from an established outbreak.

   The appearance of clinical salmonellosis in intensive livestock units requires proper control, including the following:

1. Identify groups of animals that are infected and if possible the source.
2. Isolate all infected animals.
3. Minimize all movement or traffic, animal or human.
4. Careful disposal of infected bedding and carcases.
5. Thorough disinfection of infected areas before the introduction of susceptible animals.

Public health

Salmonellosis is one of the most common, widespread and important zoonoses of the temperate zones. Human infection with Salmonellae can derive from infected animals (whether or not they exhibit clinical disease) by either direct contact or indirectly from the consumption of animal products such as meat, offal or milk. Consequently, the prevention of human infection will depend on the reduced prevalence of infection in livestock, satisfactory abattoir facilities, the pasteurization of milk, sanitation and the provision of uncontaminated water supplies.

G.H.K.L.

TUBERCULOSIS

Aetiology

Mycobacterium bovis is the usual cause of tuberculosis in cattle and is equally pathogenic to other ruminants, pigs and man. _M. avium_ is a member of the heterogeneous _M. avium-intracellulare_ group and gives rise to disease in poultry. It is frequently isolated from pigs and is not uncommon in cattle. _M. tuberculosis_ is responsible for the majority of cases in man and is only occasionally isolated from farm animals.

Of the many other less pathogenic mycobacteria, _M. fortuitum_ is worthy of mention because it causes lymphadenitis or skin tuberculosis in cattle. _M. marinum_ causes tuberculosis in fish and "swimmers granuloma" in man.

The causative organisms appear as small slender rods, straight or slightly curved, without capsules and spores. They are acid-fast, a characteristic related to the presence of mycolic acid in the cell wall. The organism is resistant to desiccation, putrefaction and the action of certain disinfectants such as alkalis and phenols.

Occurrence

Tuberculosis is distributed worldwide, but its prevalence varies according to the type of husbandry and the efficacy of control measures. Bovine tuberculosis is of low prevalence in cattle kept extensively on pasture and not enclosed at night. Enclosing and in particular housing animals aids aerosol transmission and leads to high infection rates. The stress of repeated pregnancies and lactations weakens host defences, allowing the disease to develop progressively, until it becomes clinically significant. Hence tuberculosis is seen most often in housed dairy cattle, especially older animals, and where hygiene is poor. The disease has been almost eradicated from countries with well-organized meat inspection and quarantine services.

In contrast to bovine tuberculosis, avian tuberculosis occurs most frequently in extensively kept poultry and is rare in intensive units, where hygiene is usually excellent and the average life of birds is short.

Species affected

Cattle are affected most frequently by _M. bovis_. However, water buffalo are probably as susceptible as cattle kept under similar conditions. The disease is sporadic in other ruminants, camels and equines. Tuberculosis of one or more lymph nodes of the head is quite common in pigs and is caused by _M. avium_; however, progressive disease is rare. A wide range of wild mammals can become infected by _M. bovis_, but these infections assume importance only during the final stages of tuberculosis eradication programmes.

In addition to poultry and pigs, _M. avium_ sporadically affects a wide range of other domestic and wild birds.

Transmission

The entry of tubercle bacilli can occur by various routes. Cattle are much more susceptible to infection by inhalation of contaminated dust particles and droplets than by ingestion. However, milk is a common source of infection for calves. Depending on the site of lesions, organisms are excreted intermittently and in small numbers from the respiratory and alimentary tracts, milk, urine or uterine discharge. Tubercle bacilli survive for weeks or months on shaded pasture and yards or in houses, and indirect transmission is readily achieved. The organisms are rapidly killed by direct sunlight.

Poultry and pigs are usually infected by ingestion when feeding in a contaminated environment.

Clinical features

There are no clinical signs in the early stages of infection. Cattle with pulmonary lesions develop a persistent cough, anorexia and loss of body condition. There may be slight fever. The mammary gland, if infected, becomes enlarged, firm and nodular. Infected lymph nodes of the head, neck and forequarters become enlarged. Lesions in the intestine or other internal organs lead to gradual loss in condition.

Pathology

In animals, as in man, infection starts with the formation of a small cellular lesion in an organ, usually the lung in cattle, which then spreads to the drainage lymph node. This is known as the primary complex. Subsequently, the original lesions may disappear leaving an incomplete primary complex in the lymph node. If the mycobacteria overcome the host defences, lesions in the organs or lymph nodes will progressively enlarge. The abscesses so formed contain caseous pus which may calcify. The capsule varies from a thin incomplete shell to a thick fibrous mass permeating the lesion. In the former instance, mycobacteria escape periodically and infect adjacent tissue or organs, or pass via lymph and blood to other organs. In the pulmonary form, the infection progresses along the bronchi causing a bronchopneumonia.

Pathological changes found *post mortem* can vary from a single small well-calcified lesion, to a huge abscess containing semi-liquid pus, or widespread smaller lesions, the so-called miliary tuberculosis affecting peritoneum, pleura and many organs. Histopathological examination reveals a variety of structures depending on whether necrosis, exudation or proliferation predominates. Plasma cells, epithelial cells, giant cells, macrophages, fibroblasts and lymphocytes can all be seen. Giant cells often contain a variable number of organisms.

Diagnosis

In live animals, tuberculosis is diagnosed by demonstrating hypersensitivity to tuberculo-protein in the tuberculin test. Modern tuberculin is a purified protein derivative (PPD) produced by growing mycobacteria in a protein-free medium and precipitating a cell-free filtrate. The test is usually carried out by intradermal inoculation of tuberculin on one occasion, i.e. the single intradermal test. In cattle, the site of inoculation is the skin on the side of the back or the caudal fold; in pigs, the base of the ear is used and in poultry the wattle.

In cattle, bovine PPD (from *M. bovis*) is now preferred to human PPD (from *M. tuberculosis*). The reaction is read after 72 hours and the presence of any oedema is regarded as positive. A small firm circumscribed swelling of 2–3 mm without oedema is negative. For administrative purposes, the increase in skin thickness can be measured and recorded. The test in infected cattle is highly sensitive. Sensitivity usually develops within 4 weeks of infection; recently infected animals may therefore pass the test. Animals in advanced stages of tuberculosis may become anergic and also pass the test; such cases are usually emaciated and should be detected by clinical examination. Cows in the first month of lactation may be temporarily anergic.

False positive reactions occur relatively frequently in cattle and can be caused by one of the following: infections with *M. avium*, *M. johnei* or other mycobacteria; *Nocardia* species or other actinomycetes; and Johne's disease vaccination. The single intradermal *comparative* test is used in this situation to distinguish *M. bovis* infections from non-specific infections. Avian tuberculin is inoculated at one site and bovine tuberculin at a second site. A bovine reaction larger than the avian indicates *M. bovis* infection.

Post mortem, tuberculosis can resemble nocardiosis, actinomycosis and old parasite lesions. Ziehl-Neelsen staining may reveal acid-fasts but is not a sensitive technique. Otherwise, tissues should be submitted for culture or animal inoculation; mycobacteria grow only slowly and results will not be available for 4–8 weeks.

Treatment

Treatment of livestock has been tried experimentally and on a small scale in the field. For example, isoniazid fed to cattle over a period of several weeks reduced the number of animals with tuberculosis lesions at slaughter. However, the cost was high, not all of the animals were cured and reinfection was common. Because of these disadvantages and the danger of the disease to humans, treatment is not recommended.

Immunology

Spontaneous recovery once tuberculosis lesions have developed appears to be rare. Cell-mediated immunity may develop and the growth of lesions is arrested. More often, mycobacteria persist and multiply in the phagocytes which ingest them.

The attenuated strain of *M. bovis*, known as the Bacille Calmette Guerin or BCG vaccine, has been used experimentally in cattle. Even with huge doses of vaccine and revaccination every 6–12 months, immunity was never complete in a group of animals. At present, therefore, vaccination has no place in the control of animal tuberculosis.

Control

The control of bovine tuberculosis requires in the first place the prevention of spread of infection from animal to animal. In view of its public health significance, the elimination of the disease from individual herds, and ultimately the national herd, should be the aim. Tuberculosis eradication schemes are usually based on the method initiated by Bang, which aimed at the detection and elimination not only of animals with open forms of tuberculosis but of all infected animals, combined with cleaning and disinfection of premises. Remaining animals are retested after approximately 2 months and the process repeated until 2–3 clear tests are obtained.

When prevalence rates are low, traceback of cases detected at meat inspection is economic and worthwhile, but requires proper identification of all animals moving to slaughter.

The control of tuberculosis in pigs and poultry seldom presents major problems where intensive husbandry is practised, and is uneconomic in extensive production systems.

Public health

Man is equally susceptible to infection with *M. tuberculosis* and *M. bovis*. Unfortunately, identification to species level of isolates from human infection is not always carried out and medical authorities are often unaware of the possibility of animal sources of infection. Man usually becomes infected with *M. bovis* by the aerosol route or by drinking tuberculous milk. Pasteurization effectively kills mycobacteria. Meat inspection and condemnation of affected organs or parts of a carcase are important weapons for public health. The whole carcase should be condemned if miliary tuberculosis is seen.

Further reading

Collins, C.H. and Grange, J.M. (1983). A review – the bovine tubercle bacillus. *Journal of Applied Bacteriology*, **55**, (1), 13–29.
Francis, J. (1958). *Tuberculosis in animals and man*. Cassell, London.

R.M.E.

ULCERATIVE LYMPHANGITIS AND CASEOUS LYMPHADENITIS

Ulcerative lymphangitis and caseous lymphadenitis are infectious diseases of equids and small ruminants, respectively. The disease in equids is characterized by inflammation of the subcutaneous lymphatic vessels. In sheep and goats, it occurs as a chronic disease characterized by suppurating, necrotizing inflammation of one or more lymph nodes.

Aetiology

The causal organism is *Corynebacterium pseudotuberculosis* (sometimes referred to as *C. ovis*). Different strains of the organism are involved in the disease in equids and small ruminants.

Occurrence

Ulcerative lymphangitis occurs sporadically in many African countries, the Americas, the Middle East and the Indian subcontinent. Caseous lymphadenitis is prevalent in areas of the Americas, Australia, Asia and Africa and is reported occasionally in Europe.

Species affected

Horses and to a lesser extent mules and donkeys are susceptible to ulcerative lymphangitis. Caseous lymphadenitis affects sheep and goats, causing considerable economic loss in some areas. *C. pseudotuberculosis* has been isolated sporadically from suppurative processes in a variety of other species including cattle, deer, camels, swine, cheetah and a hedgehog. Several cases of human infection have also been recorded, usually involving individuals in contact with sheep.

Transmission

Spread of infection results from environmental contamination and the presence of skin abrasions, providing an entry point for the organism. The organism survives for long periods in soil contaminated with pus. In horses, the disease is more common when they have been standing in muddy conditions. Insects have been implicated, in some cases, in the transmission of infection among horses, but contaminated bedding and grooming utensils may also be involved with kicks, treads, shackle chafes and other injuries becoming infected. The infection in sheep is believed to result largely from contamination of shearing wounds, though contaminated sheep dips have also been implicated in its spread and the organism is claimed to be capable of penetrating intact skin. Skin abrasions, fighting wounds and rubbing against contaminated fencing posts are thought to be important in the transmission of infection in goats.

Cross-infection by the specific strains between horses and sheep and goats is thought not to be important.

Clinical features

In horses, the hind legs from the hock downwards is the most common site, the affected limb being swollen, hot and painful. Nodules form which rupture, discharging a creamy pus which may be bloodstained. These leave granulating ulcers which heal in 2–3 weeks, but other nodules form and adjacent lymphatics become corded. In some areas, the disease is characterized by the occurrence of deep abscesses in the pectoral and ventral abdominal regions. Very rarely the infection spreads to internal organs such as the kidneys. *C. pseudotuberculosis* may cause abortion in mares and the organism has been isolated from equine mastitis.

In sheep and goats, there is abscessation of lymph nodes, predominantly involving superficial nodes, but internal nodes and organs, especially the lungs, may also be involved causing a more severe form of the disease. Acute bronchopneumonia due to *C. pseudotuberculosis* has also been described. In goats, it is usually confined to the head and neck area with the parotid lymph node most commonly affected. In sheep, it is the precrural node that is most often involved. Abscessation of visceral lymph nodes is a major cause of ill-thrift among sheep in some parts of the world. The prevalence of lesions increases with age in both sheep and goats.

Pathology

On incision, affected nodes in sheep have a laminated appearance with layers of caseous materials separated by fibrous bands which are usually absent from lesions in goats. Lesions in the lungs of sheep and goats are characterized by areas of consolidation with raised subpleural or deep-rooted greenish-yellow encapsulated nodules. There is typical caseous necrosis with neutrophils, macrophages, lymphocytes and giant cells present. In acute cases, there is a fibrinous pleuritis with accumulation of exudate in the air passages. Abscesses were present in the lungs, liver and spleen of an aborted foal.

Diagnosis

Pus smears prepared from untreated lesions reveal the presence of short Gram-positive diphtheroid organisms in the characteristic "Chinese letter" configuration. The organism grows relatively slowly on blood agar producing yellow-white flat colonies surrounded by a narrow zone of haemolysis. Strains isolated from small ruminants tend not to reduce nitrate to nitrite, whereas isolates obtained from horses almost invariably do. Various serological tests have been used to aid diagnosis including the anti-haemolysin inhibition test, the synergistic haemolysis inhibition (SHI) test, an indirect haemagglutination test and an ELISA with the SHI test proving useful in the detection of infected carriers. Skin testing has also been used. Ulcerative lymphangitis is differentiated from epizootic lymphangitis by the demonstration of *Histoplasma farci minosum* in the latter and from cutaneous glanders by the Mallein test.

Treatment

C. pseudotuberculosis is sensitive to a wide range of antibacterials including ampicillin, erythromycin, chloramphenicol, gentamycin, tetracycline, penicillin and sulpha-methoxazole-trimethoprin. Treatment of ulcerative lymphangitis is by incision of the affected nodes, slight caretting of ulcers and irrigation with an iodine-based antiseptic fluid followed by the application of oxytetracycline dressings. Satisfactory results have also been obtained by treating daily with oxytetracycline for 5 days.

Immunology

Experimental vaccination of goats and lambs with killed whole organisms and especially with toxoid resulted in a decreased number of abscesses following experimental challenge. An attenuated live vaccine has also shown promising results. Sheep vaccinated with BCG showed a decreased incidence of the disease.

Control

All cases of ulcerative lymphangitis should be isolated and special care taken in the disposal of wound dressing. General hygienic measures and good stable management including manure disposal, fly control and wound prevention and protection must be enforced. Whenever possible standings should be used which can be disinfected and kept dry. Care should be taken to prevent contamination of sheep dipping fluid and it is important not to introduce infected animals into clean flocks.

Further reading

Brown, C.C. and Olander, H.J. (1987). Caseous lymphadenitis of goats and sheep: A review. *Veterinary Bulletin*, **57**, 1–11.

A.N.M.

Diseases caused by helminths

J.A. Hammond and M.M.H. Sewell

ANCYLOSTOMATIDOSIS

Infection with nematodes of the family Ancylostomatidae, including both ancylostomes and necators. Often termed hookworm disease. These are all bursate nematodes; those in carnivores and *Agriostomum* being up to 16 mm long, while *Bunostomum* and *Gaigeria* are up to 30 mm in length.

Ancylostoma have a clear notch on the posterior margin of the buccal cavity. *A. caninum* and *A. tubaeforme* have three pairs of teeth on the anterior margin of the buccal cavity, whereas *A. braziliense and A. ceylanicum* have only two and *Agriostomum vryburgi* has four. The necators, *Uncinaria, Bunostomum* and *Gaigeria*, have chitinous semilunar plates instead of these teeth and a dorsal cone instead of the notch. *G. pachyscelis* has long spicules and a bursa with a large, thick dorsal ray and small lateral lobes, while *B. trigonocephalum* has short spicules, an asymmetrical dorsal lobe and large lateral lobes. *B. phlebotomum* has long spicules but in *Agriostomum* they are short.

Aetiology

The adult hookworms are found in the small intestine, where they damage the mucosa. *A. caninum* and the ruminant hookworms suck blood. Disease commonly occurs in animals which are crowded together in a warm, moist environment.

Occurrence

With the exception of uncinarosis, all forms of hookworm disease are particularly prevalent in warm, humid climates or seasons.

Species affected

As well as the hosts shown in Table 1, these hookworms may also occur in wild carnivores. *A. braziliense* and *U. stenocephala* can also cause skin lesions (cutaneous *larva migrans*) in man.

Table 1　Hosts and distribution of hookworms of domestic animals

Species	Main hosts	Distribution
Ancylostoma caninum	Dogs ⎫	Tropics, subtropics
A. tubaeforme	Cats ⎬	and warm temperate
A. braziliense	Dogs, cats ⎭	areas
A. ceylanicum	Cats, dogs	Asia, S. America
Agriostomum vryburgei	Cattle, buffalo	S. Asia, S. America, Africa
Bunostomum phlebotomum	Cattle ⎫	Worldwide, especially
B. trigonocephalum	Sheep, goats ⎭	in the tropics
Gaigeria pachyscelis	Sheep, goats	S. Asia, Africa, S. America
Uncinaria stenocephala	Dogs, cats	Mainly in temperate areas

Transmission

The first-stage larvae hatch out of the egg and develop into the sheathed, infective third-stage larvae. *Ancylostoma*, *Gaigeria* and *Bunostomum* are favoured by higher temperatures than *Uncinaria*, but all require a moist environment. The infective larvae can penetrate the skin, but oral infection also occurs. *A. caninum* larvae can also infect their host prenatally, via the transmammary route or through suitable mammalian transport hosts, e.g. mice. *A. braziliense* larvae do not use the transmammary or prenatal routes. However, skin penetration is probably the most frequent route of infection for all these species.

Permanently moist sites such as water holes, which are regularly visited by the hosts, favour transmission.

Clinical features

All hookworms cause hypoalbuminaemia. However, in dogs, severe anaemia, often with bloody diarrhoea, is characteristic of *A. caninum* infection. Sudden death may occur, especially in young puppies where massive infections may prove fatal within 1–3 days. Skin reactions caused by the penetrating larvae range from a moist eczema to ulceration. Self-inflicted injuries may occur on irritated paws. Chronically infected animals show ill-thrift.

In ruminants, there may be anaemia and oedema. Poor growth rates or wasting and even deaths may occur. The disease may be exacerbated by fasciolosis, haemonchosis or other gastroenteric nematode infections.

Pathology

A. caninum infection is associated with haemorrhagic intestinal contents. Haemorrhagic pulmonary lesions may also be found, especially in hyperacute cases in young puppies. Several hundred worms will be present in severe cases.

Severe bunostomosis causes anaemia, oedema and erythrocytic hyperplasia similar to those seen in haemonchosis, but there will also be large numbers of punctate haemorrhages (2–3 mm in diameter) in the small intestine. These are usually visible from both the mucosal and serosal surfaces. The relatively large worms are readily seen and recovered in numbers which usually range up to 500.

Diagnosis

Clinical signs occur in animals exposed to infection, especially in humid tropical areas or when they are kept in groups in unhygienic, damp conditions. Confirmation is by detection of eggs in faeces, *post-mortem* examination, the demonstration of hypoalbuminaemia, eosinophilia and, in *A. caninum* infection, anaemia. *A. caninum* eggs (56–65 μm long) are smaller than *A. braziliense* eggs (75–95 μm long), without a significant overlap. As the eggs will usually be embryonated when examined in tropical areas, they may need to be distinguished from *Strongyloides* eggs, which are much smaller. Differential diagnosis from other causes of ill-thrift, anaemia, diarrhoea and skin lesions.

Treatment

The anthelmintics of choice in dogs are fenbendazole, mebendazole or dichlorvos incorporated in resin pellets. Most modern nematocides are effective against hook-worms in ruminants. Simultaneous measures should be taken to limit reinfection. In dogs, parenteral iron may be given and, in young puppies, a blood transfusion should be considered.

Immunology

Strong acquired resistance to reinfection with *A. caninum* develops in dogs and there is also some non-specific age resistance. However, adult bitches still transmit *A. caninum* via their colostrum. Resistant animals may carry small burdens but these lay relatively few eggs per worm.

Resistance is known to develop against *Bunostomum* infections but there has been no attempt to utilize this knowledge prophylactically.

Control

Measures for controlling other gastroenteric nematode infections will usually reduce the prevalence of hookworm disease. Avoid crowding animals together, indoors, at watering points or on pastures under warm, moist conditions. In tropical areas, it may be difficult to prevent dogs acquiring infection but the provision of hygienic, dry living quarters will be beneficial. Routine anthelmintic treatment may also be necessary at regular intervals. Pregnant bitches should be dosed at least once and puppies at 2 and 4 weeks of age. A course of fenbendazole at 50 mg/kg per day for 2–3 weeks before and after whelping will prevent prenatal and transmammary transmission of *A. caninum*.

ANOPLOCEPHALIDOSIS

Anoplocephalid tapeworms are very common in herbivores. *Moniezia* is up to 6 m long, while *Avitellina* and *Thysaniezia* are often over 1 m long. In contrast, *Anoplocephala perfoliata* is not more than 12 mm in length. No rostellum or hooks are present on the scolex of these tapeworms and the proglottides, which may be poorly demarcated, are usually much wider than they are long.

Aetiology

The adult tapeworms are usually found in the small intestine, but *Stilesia hepatica* and *Thysanosoma actinioides* occur in the bile ducts, while *A. perfoliata* is found in both the small and large intestines. These parasites are of very low pathogenicity except perhaps in heavy infections in undernourished animals, when their use of the available nutrients may be harmful.

Species affected

The common species and their final hosts are shown in Table 2.

Table 2 Final hosts and distribution of anoplocephalid tapeworms

Species	Main hosts	Range
Moniezia expansa *M. benedini*	Sheep and goats Cattle	Worldwide
Avitellina centripunctata (and other species)	Ruminants	Old World: Tropics and subtropics
Stilesia globipunctata *S. hepatica*	Ruminants	Old World: Tropics and subtropics
Thysaniezia giardi	Ruminants	Worldwide
Thysanosoma actinioides	Ruminants	Americas
Anoplocephala magna *A. perfoliata*	Equids	Worldwide
Paranoplocephala mamillana	Equids	Worldwide
Mesocestoides lineatus	Carnivores	Old World

Transmission

Transmission is indirect, via oribatid mites, which contain the cysticercoid larvae. These infect the final host when it ingests the mites. *Mesocestoides* has a vertebrate second intermediate host.

Clinical features

Possible ill-thrift in animals on marginal nutrition.

Pathology

Minimal enteritis. Large numbers of these cestodes may be found in apparently normal hosts.

Diagnosis

Demonstration of characteristic eggs in faeces. Definitive diagnosis only at post-mortem examination.

Treatment

If treatment is indicated or requested, albendazole is a safe and effective drug, although older and/or cheaper remedies such as niclosamide, copper sulphate or lead arsenate may be considered.

Immunology

Infections in ruminants are more common and heavier in young animals.

Control

Almost impossible in grazing animals because of the ubiquity of the vectors.

ASCARIOSIS

Infection with large ascarid roundworms. *Parascaris* is up to 500 mm and *Ascaris* up to 400 mm long, while *Toxocara vitulorum*, which used to have the generic name *Neoascaris*, is also a large ascarid, being up to 300 mm long. The ascarids found in carnivores are smaller. Thus *Toxocara canis* is up to 180 mm long and *Toxocara cati* and *Toxascaris leonina* up to 100 mm long. These latter are the arrow-headed worms, having large cervical alae, which are striated and particularly broad in *T. cati*. *T. canis* eggs are readily distinguishable from *Toxascaris* eggs, as the former have markedly pitted shells, whereas the external surface of *Toxascaris* eggs is relatively smooth.

Aetiology

The adult worms are normally found in the small intestine, but occasionally in aberrant sites such as the bile ducts. They usually only cause a low-grade enteritis but may cause obstruction. Larvae migrating through the lungs may cause pneumonia and/or bronchitis. The larvae of *Toxocara canis* readily undergo somatic migration in man. This condition – called *visceral larva migrans* – occasionally results in disease.

Occurrence

Most ascarid species occur worldwide, especially in unhygienic, moist environments. *T. vitulorum* is only prevalent in warm climates, where it is of particular importance in buffalo calves.

Species affected

The common species and their domestic hosts are shown in Table 3.

Table 3 Domestic hosts of ascarids

Species	Hosts
Ascaris suum	Pigs
Parascaris equorum	Equidae
Toxocara vitulorum	Cattle and buffalo
Toxocara canis	Dogs
Toxocara cati	Cats
Toxascaris leonina	Dogs and cats

Transmission

The infective larvae do not hatch out of the egg until ingested by a host and are therefore very resistant to adverse environmental conditions except heat and prolonged desiccation. Direct oral infection with a liver-lung-tracheal somatic migration is the only route of infection for *Ascaris* and *Parascaris*. Such direct infections also occur in dogs and cats but are only successful following very light infections in dogs over 3–4 months of age. *Toxocara* species also use the transmammary route for infection, while *T. canis* may also infect puppies transplacentally and both *T. cati* and *T. canis* use rodents or birds as paratenic hosts, in which they undergo their somatic migration. *Toxascaris* also uses mice as paratenic hosts. Following transmammary infection or infection via a paratenic host, there is no migratory phase in the final host. Nursing bitches commonly become infected by eating puppies' faeces containing expelled larvae. The prepatent period is 3–12 weeks depending on the species and the route of infection.

Clinical features

Acute ascariosis is usually only seen in young animals. Larvae migrating through the lungs cause pneumonic signs such as dyspnoea and coughing, particularly in heavy infections. Chronic infections may cause ill-thrift, pot-belly, occasional diarrhoea and vomiting. Adult worms occasionally cause intestinal or biliary obstruction. *Visceral larva migrans* has been associated with fever and hepatomegaly, as well as with central nervous and ocular disturbances in children and may be involved in some cases of epilepsy. Similar signs, including ocular lesions, have been described in dogs and cats.

Pathology

White spot liver in pigs. Foci of alveolar collapse, haemorrhage and infiltration in the lungs of susceptible animals with more widespread reactions including oedema and emphysema in older, resistant animals. The large adult worms usually only cause a mild, catarrhal enteritis.

Diagnosis

Clinical signs and ill-thrift, especially in animals kept in warm, moist unhygienic environments or in pigs or horses grazing pastures used repeatedly for these hosts. Confirmation by faecal and post-mortem examination. Very large numbers of eggs are found in the faeces of heavily infected animals (> 10,000 eggs/g), but the pneumonic condition may occur during the prepatent phase or in resistant animals in which the worms will not mature. Differential diagnosis from viral and other pneumonias and from other causes of ill-thrift and diarrhoea.

Treatment

Piperazine, the benzimidazoles and other modern nematocides are very effective against adult ascarids. A course of fenbendazole at 50 g/kg/day for 2–3 weeks before and after whelping will prevent prenatal and transmammary infection with *T. canis*.

Immunology

Pigs and horses rapidly develop resistance to ascarids, becoming refractory to reinfection and losing their existing burden. Puppies over 3 months of age and calves of over 6 months of age are resistant to direct infection. Neonatally acquired burdens are largely lost in both puppies and calves by about 6 months of age. Thus infections are usually low in adult animals. However, adult animals can acquire burdens of *T. cati*, *T. canis* or *Toxascaris* from paratenic hosts.

Control

Hygiene, including the provision of a clean, dry environment. This is impossible to achieve with grazing animals, and therefore routine anthelmintic treatment and prolonged alternate use of pastures may be essential, at least in areas without an extended dry season. In calves, a single treatment at about 3 weeks of age will suffice, but in puppies doses at 3, 6, 9 and 12 weeks of age may be needed. Pastures or earth-runs may remain a source of infection for the mothers – and hence of transmammary infection of neonates – for several years despite repeated chemotherapy. The use of paratenic hosts by the ascarids of dogs and cats makes control difficult if the final hosts have access to rodents.

CHABERTIIDOSIS

Infection with nematodes of the family Chabertiidae, including the genera *Oesophagostomum* and *Chabertia*, which have many similar features.

Oesophagostomes are bursate worms up to 25 mm long and are thicker and more rigid than the trichostrongyles. They have characteristic complex structures at the anterior end, including leaf crowns, head collar, cephalic vesicle and a ventral cervical groove. *Oesophagostomum columbianum* and *O. radiatum* also have lateral cervical alae and their cervical papillae are embedded in the alae, just posterior to the ventral cervical groove. *O. venulosum* has no cervical alae and the cervical papillae are behind the posterior end of the oesophagus.

C. *ovina* is superficially similar to the oesophagostomes but has a distinctive large buccal cavity, which can be seen with the naked eye.

Aetiology

The larvae of these parasites develop in the wall of the ileum and the large intestine, the adults being found in the colon and caecum. *O. columbianum* and *O. radiatum* are the most pathogenic oesophagostomes, heavy infections causing a protein-losing enteropathy and anaemia as the fourth-stage larvae emerge from nodules in the intestinal wall and from damage to the mucosa of the large intestine caused by the adults. Repeated infections of *O. columbianum*, *O. radiatum* or *O. quadrispiculatum* cause the formation of large nodules from which inhibited larvae emerge intermittently. These nodules may interfere with the motility and function of the intestine giving rise to chronic disease. Nodule formation does not occur with *O. venulosum*, while *O. dentatum* only causes the formation of small nodules.

The adults of C. *ovina* occur in the lumen of the colon where they browse on the mucosa. A few hundred of these worms will cause disease, although diarrhoea may result in many of the worms being lost before death.

Occurrence

Oesophagostomum spp. are found worldwide but are less common in cooler and drier areas. *O. columbianum* is common in tropical, subtropical and contiguous areas but is usually replaced in temperate areas by *O. venulosum*. C. *ovina* occurs most commonly in winter-rainfall subtropical climates and in temperate areas.

Species affected

O. columbianum occurs in sheep, goats and wild ruminants and these, together with camels, are also the hosts for *O. venulosum*. The common oesophagostome in cattle is *O. radiatum* and in pigs *O. dentatum* and *O. quadrispiculatum*. Other minor species of oesophagostomes occur locally in all these hosts. C. *ovina* also infects sheep, goats, cattle and other ruminants.

Transmission

There is a direct strongyle-type life-cycle in which the first-stage larvae hatch out of the eggs and the third-stage, sheathed infective larvae migrate from the faeces on to the herbage from where oral infection occurs.

The prepatent period in fully susceptible hosts is about 6–7 weeks, but in resistant animals the fourth-stage larvae may remain inhibited in the intestinal nodules for several months before emerging.

Clinical features

Acute oesophagostomosis is rare in pigs, but in heavy infections in young cattle and sheep (*O. columbianum*) there is severe diarrhoea, anorexia and wasting and there may be anaemia and oedema. Chronic infection is associated with ill-thrift and sometimes with intermittent diarrhoea and anaemia. *C. ovina* may cause severe diarrhoea in sheep and anaemia may develop. The diarrhoea is usually dark-coloured and may contain numbers of the easily recognized worms. Cattle rarely show clinical signs of chabertiosis.

Pathology

In acute oesophagostomosis, the large intestine contains large numbers of worms, which may be immature. However, large numbers of worms may be present in pigs and in *O. venulosum* infection in sheep without causing clinical disease, although there may be some reduction in growth rate. Large numbers of nodules in the intestinal wall ("pimply gut"), which may be up to 20 mm in diameter in sheep, are associated with chronic infections with *O. columbianum* or *O. radiatum*. In *C. ovina* infections, the wall of the colon is thickened and oedematous with congested areas containing many small haemorrhagic foci.

Diagnosis

Based on the clinical signs, known prevalence of pathogenic species, season, grazing history and post-mortem examination. Demonstration of hypo-albuminaemia and anaemia. In subtropical areas, *C. ovina* most often causes disease in lambs in the rainy winter season. Faecal egg counts may aid diagnosis but are often low as the disease may occur during the prepatent period. Diagnosis from other causes of diarrhoea, debility and anorexia may be necessary.

Treatment

Modern nematocides are effective against these parasites, including the inhibited larval stages of *Oesophagostomum* spp. in the mucosal nodules. Disease may recur without further infection in animals which have been treated with older anthelmintics.

Immunology

Cattle develop an effective resistance to reinfection with *Oesophagostomum* spp. but sheep do not. The intestinal wall of resistant animals may carry many nodules. Resistance to reinfection with *C. ovina* develops slowly.

Control

The methods used to control other gastrointestinal nematode infections are of value against both the oesophagostomes and against *C. ovina*.

DICROCOELIOSIS

Infection with liver lukes of the genus *Dicrocoelium*. *D. dendriticum* is the most common species, but *D. hospes* is found in several African countries. These are small flukes, about 10 × 2 mm, with a distinct dark-brown posterior end.

Aetiology

The adult flukes are found in the small bile ducts.

Occurrence

Worldwide, but less widespread in Africa, the New World and Australasia. The habitats cannot be clearly defined as none of the intermediate hosts require a water environment. Infections are more common in drier climates and where the soil is free draining.

Species affected

Primarily ruminants; occasionally other mammals.

Transmission

The life-cycle is indirect and two intermediate hosts are necessary. The first is a land snail and many different genera have been implicated. The second intermediate host is an ant of various genera including *Formica* or, in Africa, *Campanotus*.

The egg, which contains a miracidium when passed out of the mammalian host, hatches after ingestion by the snail. There are two generations of sporocysts before cercariae are produced. The cercariae collect in masses held together by slime ("slime balls"), in which they survive much longer in dry than in humid conditions. If they are eaten by suitable ants, the cercariae encyst to form metacercariae. Infection of the final host is by ingestion of the infected ant. The metacercariae excyst in the duodenum, migrate up the bile duct and distribute themselves in the lesser bile ducts throughout the liver. In contrast to fasciolosis, there is no parenchymal migration.

Clinical features

Most infections are subclinical but signs similar to those in chronic fasciolosis are seen in very heavy infections. Fatal epidemics have occasionally been reported in Europe.

Pathology

There is fibroblastic proliferation around the small bile ducts, the branches of the hepatic artery and the portal veins, with interlobular fibrosis. In heavy infections *post mortem*, the liver is cirrhotic and the smaller bile ducts are fibrosed.

Diagnosis

Very small, dark brown eggs are present in the faeces. The liver lesions are to be seen *post mortem* and confirmation may be obtained by recovering the small flukes.

Treatment

Albendazole is very effective at 15 mg/kg. Other benzimidazoles are also effective at high dose levels.

Immunology

There appears to be no immunity to reinfection and the heaviest burdens are found in older animals.

Control

Control is rarely called for. In any case, it would be very difficult, as it is impossible to define the breeding places of the snails because of the large reservoirs of adult flukes in many species of animals and because the eggs on the pastures are very resistant to adverse conditions.

DIROFILARIOSIS

Infection with filarial parasites of the genus *Dirofilaria*. Only the heartworm *D. immitis* is of major veterinary importance. This is a slender nematode up to 300 mm long.

Aetiology

The adult parasites of *D. immitis* are found in the right ventricle, pulmonary artery and venae cavae. They may cause mechanical obstruction or there may be allergic reactions.

Occurrence

Widespread in tropical, subtropical and many warm temperate zones. The prevalence is highest in humid regions where the mosquito intermediate hosts occur in the greatest numbers. Such conditions allow the mosquitoes to breed in sufficient numbers and also to live long enough after an infective feed for the third-stage larvae to develop and for transmission to occur.

Species affected

Dogs and, rarely, cats or man.

Transmission

There is an indirect life-cycle, the intermediate hosts being mosquitoes of several genera. The final host is infected when fed on by a mosquito in which microfilariae have developed to the infective stage.

Clinical features

Many cases are inapparent, sometimes in the presence of heavy infection. Signs may be present over a long period and are very variable and non-specific. The general signs are dyspnoea, chronic cough and anorexia, but may include debility, eczema, ataxia, anaemia and vomiting. Anaemia and other severe clinical signs may occur in afilaraemic dogs. In the terminal stages, ascites, subcutaneous oedema and hydrothorax may be present. If the worms obstruct the posterior vena cava, an acute hepatic syndrome, which may cause a sudden collapse, may be seen, especially in young dogs.

Pathology

There is loss of endothelial cells and smooth muscle proliferation in the pulmonary arteries, which cause substantial narrowing of the small branches. *Post mortem*, the adult worms are found in the right ventricle and pulmonary artery. In heavy infections, the anterior and posterior venae cavae may also be involved. There may be pulmonary infarcts from adult worms swept into the arterial branches and other lesions consequent on the chronic cardiovascular obstruction.

Diagnosis

Clinical signs and history, plus radiography to show the greatly dilated and tortuous pulmonary arteries. Most clinically infected dogs are over 2 years old. The presence of microfilariae in the blood may confirm the diagnosis, but up to 25% of infected dogs have no microfilariae in their blood. As there is some periodicity it may be necessary to examine blood samples taken at night if those taken during the day are negative. It may also be necessary to use a centrifugal concentration or a filtration method to demonstrate the microfilariae. The microfilariae must be differentiated from those of *D. repens*, *Brugia* and *Dipetalonema* spp. which are found in many tropical areas but which are of little clinical significance. The microfilariae of *D. immitis* are 286–349 μm long, with a mean of about 313 μm. Various serological tests have been described and kits based on an ELISA test are commercially available.

Treatment

Thiacetarsamide will kill the adult worms, albeit at some risk to the host from thromboembolism and toxic side-effects, especially in those with cardiopulmonary, liver or kidney disease. Acetylsalicylic acid (aspirin) at 7 mg/kg daily should be given to dogs for which arsenical treatment is contraindicated or not available as it slows the progression of the disease and may even permit resolution of the arteriosclerosis. Aspirin (10 mg/kg daily for 4 weeks) is also of value after arsenical treatment as it reduces the severity of the side-effects. Prednisolone (1 mg/kg daily for 4 weeks) may also be given to dogs that develop severe lung disease after treatment with thiacetarsamide.

The efficacy of adulticidal treatment may be monitored serologically by assaying the concentrations of circulating antigen. Surgical removal of the adult worms may also be considered.

Dithiazanine, levamisole and ivermectin are effective against microfilariae. Some dogs, notably collies, have suffered toxic reactions following treatment with ivermectin. There is a risk of anaphylactoid reactions to the dying microfilariae with all these microfilaricidal drugs.

Immunology

Circulating immune complexes, parasite-derived antigen and antibody have all been demonstrated. Microfilariae may be removed from the circulation by an immunological mechanism, but there seems to be no effective immune response against the adult parasites.

Control

Control of the mosquito vectors is not practical. Routine prophylaxis with thiacetarsamide at 6-monthly intervals, monthly ivermectin or daily diethylcarbamazine have been recommended. The dog must be free of all infection before diethylcarbamazine is given or a severe reaction may result.

ECHINOCOCCOSIS

Infection with adult tapeworms or the larval hydatid cyst of the genus *Echinococcus*. Two main species are recognized. The most widespread is *Echinococcus granulosus* and the other is *E. multilocularis*. The adult tapeworms are not more than 6 mm long with, usually, three proglottides in *E. granulosus* and five in *E. multilocularis*.

The larval hydatid cyst of *E. granulosus* is commonly up to 100 mm in diameter with a fibrous capsule, but it may be much larger, especially in horses and man. Multiple cysts occur and daughter cysts may develop within the original cyst. Fertile cysts are filled with fluid containing "hydatid sand", which consists mainly of brood capsules about 0.3 mm in diameter; these contain the protoscolices. Infertile cysts do not contain "sand".

E. multilocularis forms an alveolar cyst, with many interconnected vesicles, which are not encapsulated by the host and are locally invasive by budding. Metastatic spread may also occur.

Aetiology

The cysts act as space-occupying lesions. Clinical disease is rare in domestic livestock with either adult or larval infections but occurs in humans, partly because their long life-span allows the cysts to grow much larger.

Occurrence

E. granulosus occurs worldwide, especially in countries with large sheep populations. There are several subspecies of E. granulosus, one of which, *E.g. equinus* occurs in Europe and the Middle East and there may be another subspecies in camels in Africa. *E. multilocularis* is restricted to the northern hemisphere, from Europe across Asia to Alaska. However, it appears to be spreading south into the Indian subcontinent, the Middle East and Central Europe.

Species affected

Adult *E. granulosus* usually occurs in the dog with its hydatid cyst in sheep, camels, goats, pigs, cattle, buffalo, other ungulates and also in humans. A subspecies, *E. granulosus equinus* occurs in horses but is not infective for sheep and probably not for man. There is one strain in Africa for which man appears to be the main host.

Adult *E. multilocularis* is found mainly in the fox but also in dogs and cats. Its intermediate hosts are usually rodents but it may also infect man.

Transmission

The intermediate host acquires infection by ingesting the eggs from an environment which has been contaminated with infected canine faeces. The eggs are very resistant to chemical disinfectants, but much less so to desiccation. The dog's coat and muzzle are frequently contaminated. The oncosphere hatches in the small intestine and passes first to the liver via the blood. It may later be distributed more widely. The cysts of *E. granulosus* develop slowly, becoming infective in 6–12 months, whereas *E. multilocularis* takes 2–3 months. The cysts may remain viable for the life of the host and the protoscolices can survive for 1–2 weeks after the death of the host. The final host becomes infected by eating the cysts.

Clinical features

None in domestic animals, apart from enteritis in heavily infected dogs. In man, the cysts will ultimately cause the symptoms of a space-occupying lesion at the affected site.

Pathology

The characteristic cysts are found at post-mortem examination, usually in the liver or lungs. Rupture of the cyst may cause severe anaphylactic shock and even death.

Diagnosis

The eggs cannot be differentiated from other taenioid eggs; therefore, in the absence of any clinical signs, it is necessary to dose the dog with arecoline and then to examine the mucous which follows the faecal purge for the presence of the minute tapeworms. *Caution*: Operatives should wear protective clothing and the sample should be boiled for 5 minutes before removal to the laboratory. The worms may be isolated from the sample by sequentially washing in sieves or by salt flotation. The examination is best made under low magnification in a black tray.

Diagnosis of larval infection in domestic herbivores is usually made *post mortem*, but in man serodiagnosis, X-ray photography, computerized tomography (CT scan) and ultrasound imaging are widely used.

Treatment

The older taeniacidal anthelmintics are ineffective and their use may lead the owner into a false sense of security. Arecoline may be only 50% effective and should only be used for diagnosis. However, praziquantel and cantrodiphene are reported to be 100% effective.

Mebendazole, albendazole and praziquantel are at present under investigation for treatment of hydatid cyst infection in humans, with rather variable results. However, surgery is still the most common form of treatment.

Immunology

Despite much study and the demonstration of resistance to reinfection in the intermediate hosts and to a lesser extent in the final host, immunity plays little part in the epidemiology or control of this infection. There is a strong serological reaction in the intermediate hosts but cross-reactions with antigens from other parasites are common.

Control

Practical measures must include adequate meat inspection, with disposal of infected material by incineration or secure pit-burial. Dogs must be prevented from gaining access to potentially infected offal or carcases. Regular and compulsory testing of all dogs should be undertaken and infected animals should be slaughtered or isolated and repeatedly treated until testing shows them to be clear.

Public interest and support is essential for successful control, and therefore education and information services play a major role.

FASCIOLOSIS

Infection with liver flukes of the genus *Fasciola*. The most important species are *F. hepatica* and *F. gigantica*. Both are leaf-shaped trematodes, *F. hepatica* being up to 30 mm long, whereas *F. gigantica* reaches a maximum of 75 mm; there is evidence that intermediate strains exist in some countries. *F. gigantica* also differs from *F. hepatica* in having a shorter anterior cone, less perceptible "shoulders", more profusely branched caeca, more nearly parallel sides to the body and larger eggs. However, there is considerable overlap in size and shape of the worms and some of the differences may be obscured by poor fixation.

Aetiology

Immature flukes can cause sudden death from hepatic failure or from haemorrhage during the migratory phase in the liver parenchyma. In some areas, fasciolosis is a precipitating factor in infectious necrotic hepatitis (Black disease), an acute disease caused by the toxins released from the vegetative forms of *Clostridium novyi* type B as they multiply in the anoxic lesions caused by the migrating flukes. At the end of the migratory phase, the flukes enter the bile ducts. Chronic fasciolosis is caused by loss of red cells and plasma into the bile ducts.

Occurrence

F. gigantica is widely distributed in the tropical and subtropical areas of Africa and Asia, whereas *F. hepatica* is widespread in the cooler, highland areas of Africa and Asia, and in parts of Australia and North and South America. The disease is becoming of more importance in tropical and subtropical countries as water resources are developed.

Species affected

Primarily cattle, sheep, goats and other ruminants, but both species have a very wide range of hosts, which includes man.

Transmission

There is an indirect life-cycle involving snails. No development takes place until the eggs are free of faeces. Free-swimming miracidia hatch and infect suitable species of the genus *Lymnaea*, in which they develop to become sporocysts. These give rise successively to rediae, daughter rediae and cercariae. When the latter are shed from the snail, they soon encyst to become metacercariae, which are infective for the final host.

The intermediate host of *F. gigantica* is one of the larger lymnaeid snails of the *L. auricularia* type, e.g. *L. natalensis* in Africa, *L. rufescens* and *L. acuminata* in Indo-Pakistan and *L. rubiginosa* in Malaysia. These are all aquatic snails, which require a warm environment and well-oxygenated, unpolluted water. The sites at which transmission occurs are usually associated with permanent water. The metacercariae may survive for some time, especially under wet, cool conditions, and it is likely that most infections in savannah areas are acquired in the dry season, when the mammalian hosts graze around shrinking areas of permanent water. There is evidence that very young snails may aestivate for a period under suitable conditions, but that older ones are usually quickly killed by desiccation.

The intermediate host of *F. hepatica* is one of the smaller lymnaeid snails of the

L. truncatula type. These live in wet muddy habitats in cooler areas. However, the species which occur in the tropics or subtropics are able to tolerate much higher temperatures. *L. truncatula* can aestivate and survive more than a year in dry mud. In Kenya, it has also been shown to act as an intermediate host for *F. gigantica*.

Clinical features

Both acute fasciolosis and infectious necrotic hepatitis result in sudden death. Acute fasciolosis is common in *F. gigantica* infections in sheep and goats where even light infections may prove fatal. It is rare in other hosts.

Chronic fasciolosis is a persistent, wasting disease in sheep with anaemia, hypoalbuminaemia and oedema. In cattle, it is similar but often self-limiting, especially in *F. hepatica* infections. Animals on a high plane of nutrition are much more resistant to the effects of chronic infections and can tolerate a higher burden of flukes than those on a low plane. Conversely, the disease is exacerbated by inadequate nutrition, e.g. during a savannah dry season, or by anaemia resulting from intercurrent disease.

Pathology

In acute cases *post mortem*, the liver is enlarged, haemorrhagic and friable with numerous tracts caused by the migrating flukes. The gall bladder is enlarged and there is bloodstained fluid in the peritoneal cavity, a feature which is especially marked in *F. gigantica* infection in sheep and goats. Immature flukes may be squeezed from the cut liver. There may also be a moderate anaemia.

In chronic fasciolosis the cholangitis results in fibrosis of the bile ducts which may be very marked in longstanding infections and which later become calcified in cattle. The damaged parenchyma is replaced by fibrous tissue and the induration is palpable in areas where there have been many tracts. Biliary cirrhosis is less marked in sheep than in cattle and calcification is not seen. It is also less marked in cattle infected with *F. gigantica* than in those infected with *F. hepatica*. Anaemia is manifest except in lightly infected animals. Severely abnormal bile ducts, which contain few or no flukes, may be seen in longstanding cases in cattle.

Diagnosis

A provisional diagnosis may be based on the clinical signs, grazing history and season.

Acute fasciolosis should be suspected in cases of sudden death in sheep and goats exposed to an environment where infection is possible. Confirmation is by post-mortem examination, when the small flukes can be expressed from the liver parenchyma. In chronic fasciolosis, the characteristic eggs are found in the faeces but counts are often very low in cattle, especially in longer-standing cases. *Fasciola* eggs must be differentiated from paramphistome eggs, which are common in ruminant faeces in many countries. The diagnosis may be further supported by haematological examination and serum protein and enzyme assays.

Treatment

Most modern fasciolicidal anthelmintics such as brotianide, nitroxynil, oxyclozanide, rafoxanide, albendazole and triclabendazole are highly efficient against mature flukes. The choice will depend on economics and ease of use. Triclabendazole is also effective against the immature stages in the liver parenchyma. Diamphenethide is efficient against the parenchymal stages in sheep. Where the cost of the drug is likely to be of paramount importance, consideration might still be given to the use of carbon tetrachloride orally by capsule to sheep or intramuscularly in oil to cattle, although toxicity may be encountered. Hexachlorethane and hexachlorophene are still used in cattle in many countries.

Immunology

Some species, including cattle and pigs, have a moderate degree of natural resistance to infection with *F. hepatica*, whereas others, including sheep, have little resistance. The reason for such differences in host susceptibility is not clear. Furthermore, natural resistance within a species appears to be age-dependent, adults being more resistant than young animals.

There is a serological response to infection with *Fasciola* and substantial evidence of acquired resistance in cattle both to reinfection and against the survival of an existing burden. Such resistance does not arise in sheep under field conditions.

Control

Effective control of fasciolosis is always possible if sufficient funds are available. Drainage may be the best permanent solution, especially where *L. truncatula* is involved, but may be too expensive. Fencing off *Fasciola* transmission sites can be effective and the cost may not be prohibitive where the sites are small, especially if sisal or suitable thorny bushes are available locally. These can also be planted round watering places to make them inaccessible to livestock, except at points which are kept snail-free by providing a concrete or stone platform or by at least clearing away aquatic vegetation. The use of adequately maintained troughs fed by water pipes from dams, boreholes, deep wells or by hydraulic rams from rivers is also helpful, provided that other transmission sites are fenced off.

Under field conditions, molluscicides will rarely kill all the snails, even when applied by experienced staff and repopulation is usually very rapid. Hence repeated applications are necessary and considerable expense is involved. It may be more economic to use molluscicides strategically to kill infected snails shortly before those times of the year when most cercariae are shed. These times must be determined by surveys in each climatic area. There is evidence that shedding of cercariae is maximal by about the middle of the dry season in many African countries.

The use of molluscicides locally extracted from plants such as *Phytolacca dodecandra* may be considered, but these may also be toxic to mammals and fish. Many plants have molluscicidal properties, but problems associated with husbandry, harvesting and processing have restricted their use in effective control. One possibility might be to plant those *Eucalyptus* species with marked molluscicidal properties around the edges of *L. auricularia* habitats so that their leaves, which are shed intermittently throughout the year, will fall into the water.

Biological control of *Lymnaea* by certain species of fish and domestic ducks, sciomyzid larvae or the snail *Marisa cornuarietis* have shown promise experimentally but none have been used successfully under extensive field conditions.

One of the greatest problems in the control of fasciolosis is that grazing livestock in infested marshes in the dry season may be unavoidable. In such cases, it would be desirable to keep the animals away for as long as possible into the dry season, so that fewer viable metacercariae are present on the herbage. In any case, previously infected older cattle should be admitted first as they are much more resistant than the younger cattle, while the sheep and goats, in which the infection is most pathogenic, should be grazed in these areas last of all. Fasciolosis can often be materially reduced with minimal cost by such measures, coupled with the administration of fasciolicidal anthelmintics only to those groups of animals most seriously affected.

HABRONEMOSIS

Infection with spirurid nematodes of the genera *Habronema* and *Drascheia*. Three species are involved: *Habronema muscae*, *H. microstoma* and *Drascheia megastoma* (syn. *H. megastoma*). The adults are relatively rigid nematodes, *D. megastoma* being up to 13 mm long, while the others may reach 25 mm. The pharynx has a thick cuticular lining and, in *D. megastoma*, a characteristic funnel shape. The spicules are dissimilar.

Aetiology

Larvae that have been deposited on wounds or near the eyes migrate intradermally and may cause an exudative dermatitis termed "cutaneous habronemosis" or "orbital habronemosis". The adults occur in the stomach.

Occurrence

Worldwide, but particularly prevalent in the Far East, Australia and South and Central America. In areas with a distinct summer or warm wet season, the disease tends to be more prevalent at this time.

Species affected

Equids.

Transmission

The embryonated eggs laid by the adult worms hatch while still in the host. The larvae present in fresh faeces are ingested by maggots, *H. muscae* and *D. megastoma* developing in the house fly, *Musca domestica*, whereas *H. microstoma* uses the stable fly, *Stomoxys calcitrans*. The larvae reach the infective stage by the time the maggots pupate and are passed out via the mouth-parts on to the lips, nostrils or wounds of horses. Those which are swallowed by the horse develop to maturity in the stomach.

Clinical features

Pruritis and hard nodules or ulcerating, weeping granulomatous masses, especially around the head, legs and withers.

Gastric and pulmonary habronemosis rarely causes overt disease.

Pathology

Granulomatous reactions form around larvae in the skin and lungs. These may lead on to the formation of hard tumours or in more severe cases to large, granulomatous masses or "swamp cancer". *D. megastoma* may be associated with gastric tumours. The adults of *Habronema* spp. cause only a mild, chronic catarrhal gastritis.

Diagnosis

The seasonal incidence of the cutaneous lesions ("summer sores") in areas where this condition is known to occur. Characteristic larvae may be seen in biopsies from the granulomata. Larvae may also be recovered by gastric lavage or from flies which have developed from maggots allowed to feed on the horses' faeces.

Treatment

Modern broad-spectrum anthelmintics for treatment of adults in the stomach. Cutaneous habronemosis was difficult to treat but ivermectin and systemic organophosphates are reported to be effective. Surgical removal of suitable lesions may be indicated.

Immunology

Unknown.

Control

Difficult because of the mobility and ubiquity of the vectors. Consistent use of hygienic measures for disposal of manure, the use of insecticides and the prevention or protection of wounds are all of value.

MACRACANTHORHYNCHOSIS

Infection with the acanthocephalid (thorny-headed worm) *Macracanthorhynchus hirudinaceus*. This large, thick, pink worm looks rather like *Ascaris* but is more wrinkled and it is firmly attached by its proboscis, which has six rows of hooks. The female is up to 400 mm long and the male up to 100 mm long.

Aetiology

Large numbers of adult acanthocephalids may be found in the small intestine where they attach by burying their proboscides in the intestinal wall.

Occurrence

Worldwide, except for northern and western Europe. The highest prevalence occurs in parts of Central and South America and in the Far East.

Species affected

Pigs.

Transmission

The eggs may survive on pasture for several years and do not hatch until they have been ingested by a suitable arthropod intermediate host, usually the larval grub of a beetle. The larvae develop to the infective stage in 3–6 months, depending on the temperature. Pigs are infected when they eat the grubs.

Clinical features

These range from no overt disease to severe haemorrhagic diarrhoea, abdominal pain, emaciation and anaemia in heavy infections.

Pathology

The nodules around the proboscides are often visible from the serosal surface. Deep, necrotic and purulent lesions may form at the attachment sites, with haemorrhage and sometimes perforation and peritonitis.

Diagnosis

Clinical signs in pigs kept on pasture or free-ranging in endemic areas. Characteristic eggs in faeces.

Treatment

Ivermectin may be effective.

Immunology

Little is known, but there is some evidence of partial resistance to super-infection.

Control

Hygienic measures including housing and careful disposal of dung. Ring grazing pigs to discourage rooting. Pigs must be kept off heavily infected land for at least 3 years.

ONCHOCERCOSIS

Infection with nematodes of the genus *Onchocerca*. These are filariform nematodes up to 600 mm long with microfilariae 200–400 μm long.

Aetiology

O. gibsoni occurs in the brisket and subcutis of the lower limbs, *O. gutturosa* in the *ligamentum nuchae*, other ligaments and stifle joints, *O. lienalis* in the omentum, the splenic ligament and capsule, and *O. armillata* in the wall of the thoracic aorta of cattle. *O. reticulata* is found in the *ligamentum nuchae* and in the ligaments and subcutis of the lower limbs of equidae.

Occurrence

Worldwide, but more prevalent in the tropics and subtropics.

Species affected

Most species of veterinary importance occur in cattle, but *Onchocerca reticulata* is a parasite of equidae.

Transmission

There is an indirect life-cycle, the intermediate hosts usually being *Culicoides* or *Simulium* spp. The vector of *O. armillata* is unknown. The microfilariae are ingested from the cutaneous lymph vessels and spaces, develop to the infective stage and then infect the final host when the vector feeds.

The main requirement for breeding places of *Simulium* spp. is flowing water. This need not be near to the hosts, because simuliids are exceptionally strong fliers and may travel many miles from their breeding places. Conversely, the number of *Culicoides* spp. present is dependent on the local rainfall being sufficient to keep the breeding places moist, as they have a very limited range.

Clinical features

In *O. gibsoni* infection, there may be palpable nodules. There are very few external signs of the nodules caused by parasites in the *ligamentum nuchae*. In infection of the stifle joint, there is often local swelling. Disability may result if the main supporting ligaments of the limbs are involved. *O. reticulata* may cause soft painless swellings which later develop into small fibrous nodules in the lower limbs. No signs are associated with *O. armillata* infections.

Pathology

Granulomatous and fibrous nodules which contain the adult worms.

Diagnosis

The presence of infection, which has been suspected from the presence of nodules or swellings in the characteristic sites, may be confirmed by the examination of skin snips for microfilariae. Histological examination of the nodules shows the presence of nematodes.

Treatment

Ivermectin is effective against the microfilariae, but treatment may elicit an allergic response.

Immunology

No practical immunity to reinfection occurs.

Control

Control of the insect vectors is impracticable, but it may help to keep the hosts away from areas where there are large numbers of *Culicoides*.

PARAMPHISTOMOSIS

Infection with the conical flukes. A large number of species have been described in ruminants, most of which occur as adults attached to the mucosa of the rumen or reticulum. In many areas, a high proportion of ruminants is infected. One species, *Gastrodiscus aegyptiacus* is unusual as it occurs in the large intestine and sometimes in the small intestine of horses and pigs and has a conical anterior end and a disc-shaped posterior end.

Aetiology

Acute disease follows massive infections and is caused by the immature stages in the duodenum. Most reports have described infections with *Calicophoron* (previously *Paramphistomum*) *microbothrium*, *Cotylophoron*, *Gigantocotyle* or *Ceylonocotyle*. At least 50,000 infective metacercariae of *C. microbothrium* are needed to produce acute intestinal paramphistomosis in calves. An intake of this order over a short period requires an extremely dense aggregation of infected snails. A similar syndrome is seen in sheep and goats.

The disease may be exacerbated by intercurrent fasciolosis, schistosomosis or gastroenteric nematode infections.

Heavy infections of immature *G. aegyptiacus* cause severe colitis, but the adults only cause a mild enteritis.

Occurrence

As indicated in Table 4, *Calicophoron* spp. are mainly found in Asia and Australia, only one species being recorded from Africa. *Gigantocotyle explanatum* occurs in the bile ducts of buffalo in the Indian subcontinent and the Far East and *G. lerouxi* adults occur in the abomasum of cattle in Africa.

Species affected

The common species and their domestic hosts are shown in Table 4.

Table 4 Common paramphistomes of domestic animals

Species	Final host	Distribution
Paramphistomum spp. (*P. cervi*)	Ruminants	Worldwide
Cotylophoron spp. (*C. cotylophorum*)	Ruminants	Most parts of the world except the northern temperate region
Calicophoron spp. (*C. microbothrium*)	Ruminants	Tropical and subtropical regions excluding America
Carmyerius spp.	Ruminants	Tropical and subtropical regions
Gigantocotyle spp. (*G. explanatum*) (*G. lerouxi*)	Ruminants	Southern Asia, Middle East, Africa
Gastrothylax spp. (*G. crumenifer*)	Ruminants	Europe, Middle East, Asia
Fishoederius spp.	Ruminants	Southern and Eastern Asia
Ceylonocotyle spp.	Ruminants	Southern Asia, Australia, Africa
Gastrodiscus spp. (*G. aegyptiacus*)	Equids and pigs	Throughout the tropics
Homalogaster spp.	Ruminants	Southern and Eastern Asia
Gastrodiscoides spp. (*G. hominis*)	Pigs and humans	Most of Asia

Transmission

The life-cycle is indirect and closely resembles that of *Fasciola*. The main intermediate snail hosts of *C. microbothrium* are *Bulinus truncatus* in North Africa and *B. tropicus* south of the Sahara. These are aquatic snails which can aestivate for some time. Various other snails serve as intermediate hosts for other species of paramphistomes.

Clinical features

Acute intestinal paramphistomosis is often a seasonal problem and is usually only seen in calves and small ruminants. There is foetid diarrhoea, which does not contain blood or mucous and which may show remissions. Other signs include anorexia and marked loss of condition, while progressive weakness leads to recumbency. Death may occur within a few days of the first signs appearing but more often the disease extends over several weeks.

With most species, no clinical signs are seen with lesser infections or with prolonged low-level infections. However, heavy infections with adult *G. explanatum* may cause emaciation.

Pathology

The metacercariae excyst in the duodenum where they feed by ingesting plugs of mucosa before beginning their forward migration. They also penetrate the mucosa, sometimes as deeply as the *muscularis* layer. The duodenum and abomasum may show severe inflammation, with petechial haemorrhages. In less severe cases, the mucosa is corrugated with small erosions and petechiae. Serous effusions are present to varying degrees. There is also oligocythaemia and hypoalbuminaemia.

The adults of *G. lerouxi* may cause extensive chronic abomasal ulcerations. Adults of *G. explanatum* cause thickening and fibrosis of the walls of the bile ducts. The adult paramphistomes in the rumen and reticulum are not pathogenic except for *Carmyerius dollfusi*, which is haematophagous and has been reported to cause severe anaemia and death in heavy infections in cattle.

Diagnosis

In acute infections, clinical signs and grazing history; the small flukes may be observed in the diarrhoea. Duodenal and abomasal lesions may be seen *post mortem* and large numbers of the immature flukes may be found on and in the mucosa. In chronic infections, the eggs are present in the faeces. They resemble those of *Fasciola* but are clear rather than golden-yellow.

Treatment

Oxyclozanide and bithionol are effective against adults, while rafoxanide, niclosamide and niclofolan are effective against the immature forms. Resorantel is effective against all stages.

Immunology

There is field evidence of acquired resistance to reinfection in cattle.

Control

Similar to that for fasciolosis and schistosomosis. The most effective means of preventing acute infections is to keep calves and small ruminants away from places which are heavily infested with the intermediate snail hosts. Adult cattle can use these with far greater safety.

PARASITIC BRONCHITIS

Infection with lungworms of the genera *Dictyocaulus* or *Metastrongylus*, or of the family Protostrongylidae. *Dictyocaulus* and *Metastrongylus* are thread-like nematodes up to 100 mm long. The Protostrongylidae are smaller but are rarely seen because of their location.

Aetiology

Dictyocaulus and *Metastrongylus* inhabit the bronchi and bronchioles. *D. viviparus* may cause severe disease in calves, while *D. filaria*, *D. arnfieldi*, and *Metastrongylus* spp. are usually less pathogenic. *D. arnfieldi* adults are usually only found in donkeys and foals, but the larvae will cause bronchitis in adult horses. The Protostrongylidae occur in the alveoli and small bronchioles but are of little pathogenicity.

Occurrence

Dictyocaulosis occurs widely in calves in temperate areas and may also occur in tropical and subtropical highlands. *D. filaria* is common in sheep in winter-rainfall climates, such as the Middle East. The disease occurs primarily in young animals during their first summer or wet season.

Species affected

Dictyocaulus viviparus occurs in calves, *D. filaria* in goats and sheep and *D. arnfieldi* in donkeys and horses. *Metastrongylus apri* and *M. pudendotectus* occur in pigs and various protostrongyles are found in sheep. Wild ruminants and equidae may also be infected.

Transmission

First-stage larvae of *D. viviparus* and *D. filaria* hatch out of the eggs within the lungs and are found in fresh faeces. *D. arnfieldi* eggs hatch very soon after the faeces have been passed. Oral infection is by sheathed third-stage larvae. The prepatent periods within the host are 3 weeks for *D. viviparus*, 4 weeks for *D. filaria* and 5–6 weeks for *D. arnfieldi*. Light infections and inhibited larval stages in yearlings and older animals play a major role in maintaining the parasite species through an adverse climatic season. Very light infections of *D. filaria* will maintain a population of these parasites.

Clinical features

In the most severe cases of dictyocaulosis in calves, there is dyspnoea without coughing, anorexia and refusal to drink or move. These signs occur before the infection becomes patent and may recur after the calves have lost their lungworms. Frequent coughing is associated with less severe cases. Pyrexia indicates an intercurrent bacterial pneumonia. Coughing occurs in infected sheep and horses.

Pathology

At post-mortem examination of calves which die during the prepatent phase, the characteristic lesion is blockage of the bronchioles by a greenish, eosinophilic exudate, with collapse of the distal alveoli. At this stage, there may be no worms detectable or larvae may be found in the bronchial mucus. From about 3–8 weeks after infection, during the patent phase, extensive green pus consolidates the lobules and worms are present. The severe dyspnoea frequently results in interstitial emphysema and may cause cardiac dysfunction and hence pulmonary oedema. After the worms are lost, areas of pus-filled, secondarily infected bronchiectasis may still be found in animals which are not thriving. Red or fawn rubbery patches of proliferative alveolar epithelialization, which still contain air, are found in those calves which relapse at this time. The pathological changes in other hosts are generally similar but usually less severe.

Diagnosis

Clinical signs, age of animal, season, recent weather and grazing history usually afford a diagnosis, which may be confirmed by post-mortem examination. Demonstration of *Dictyocaulus* larvae in the faeces of the affected animals or of those which have grazed on the same pasture may confirm the diagnosis. Infected donkeys are often found grazing alongside affected horses. Differential diagnosis is from other causes of dyspnoea and coughing.

Treatment

Treatment with nematocides, including levamisole, most benzimidazoles and ivermectin is effective during the prepatent phase of dictyocaulosis, when the lung function recovers rapidly after removal of the worms. Ivermectin is the drug of choice against *D. arnfieldi*, while tiabendazole is not effective against *D. viviparus*. No chemotherapy is of much restorative value later in the disease. Removing affected animals from the infested pasture is an essential part of treatment, as is ensuring the maintenance of water intake. The administration of antibiotics is indicated if there is pyrexia.

Immunology

Resistance to reinfection develops relatively rapidly, but is more effective in sheep than in goats or cattle. Most of the adult worm burden is lost by 8–9 weeks after initial infection, but small numbers of worms may survive in resistant or susceptible animals for extended periods. Resistant animals will lose most developing larvae before patency. X-ray attenuated vaccines are available in Europe against *D. viviparus* and in Iraq against *D. filaria*.

Control

Although vaccination of young cattle before they are allowed to graze is a well-tried and effective control measure, supplies of vaccine are only readily available in Europe. The administration of three doses of ivermectin, 5 weeks apart, when the animals are first exposed to infection or three doses of levamisole, 3 weeks apart, when signs of infection are first observed are alternative control strategies. Otherwise, avoid exposing young animals to contaminated pasture at weaning. Control is rarely attempted in other hosts, except as part of a programme for controlling other strongyle infections or by avoiding grazing donkeys alongside horses.

SCHISTOSOMOSIS

Infection with trematodes of the genus *Schistosoma*. These parasites occur in many tropical and subtropical areas and are likely to become more important as water resources, irrigation schemes, etc., are developed. There is little detailed information on the economic importance of most of these infections, but it is likely that they have a considerable effect on productivity. Schistosomosis is one of the major endemic diseases of man in the tropics.

Besides the important species in domestic livestock, there are also several minor species, usually with a restricted geographical range. These flukes are not hermaphrodite, the longer, narrow female, up to 28 mm long being carried in the gynaecophoric canal of the male.

Aetiology

Except for *S. nasale*, which lives in the nasal veins, the adults of all these species live in the hepato-intestinal veins. *S. mattheei* is often also found in the veins of the urinary bladder.

Species affected

The common species and their domestic hosts are shown in Table 5.

Transmission

The life-cycle is indirect but differs from that of *Fasciola* (q.v.) in several respects. The egg already contains a miracidium when passed out of the host and hatches in water within a few minutes. The miracidia penetrate suitable snail hosts and develop as sporocysts and daughter sporocysts to the fork-tailed cercariae. There are no rediae.

Table 5 Hosts and distribution of schistosomes of domestic animals

Species	Final host	Intermediate host	Range
Schistosoma bovis	Ruminants	*Bulinus*	North and Central Africa Middle East, Southern Europe
S. mattheei	Ruminants, humans	*Bulinus*	Central and Southern Africa
S. japonicum	Domestic mammals, humans	*Oncomelania*	Far East
S. spindale	Ruminants, equids	*Indoplanorbis*	Indian subcontinent
S. indicum	Ruminants, equids	*Indoplanorbis*	Indian subcontinent
S. nasale	Ruminants	*Indoplanorbis*	Indian subcontinent
S. incognitum	Pigs and dogs	*Lymnaea*	Indian subcontinent
Orientobilharzia turkestanicum	Ruminants	*Lymnaea*	Asia

The intermediate snail hosts include several genera which are listed in Table 5. These are all aquatic snails except for *Oncomelania* which is amphibious. Many of them can aestivate for some time.

There is no metacercarial cyst. Infection of the final host occurs by skin penetration or by ingestion with the drinking water. The cercariae die in 1–2 days unless they infect a suitable host. After skin penetration, the young tail-less flukes (schistosomulae) travel via the lymphatics to the heart and then via the lungs into the systemic circulation and so to the liver. They mature in the portal vessels and then migrate to the mesenteric veins. After oral infection, the epithelium of the alimentary canal is penetrated and transport then takes place via the blood.

Clinical features

A high proportion of adult cattle in some parts of Africa are infected, but their burdens are often low and most infections are asymptomatic. However, infections in young animals may result in decreased growth rate, lowered resistance to other diseases and even death.

Heavy infections with the species found in the mesenteric veins cause diarrhoea, which may be intermittent, often with blood and mucus in the faeces, anorexia, anaemia, ascites, emaciation and death, especially in sheep, goats and calves. Sheep may die with severe anaemia after heavy infections with *S. mattheei*.

S. nasale causes a mucopurulent coryza followed by dyspnoea and, in chronic cases, the formation of characteristic nasal granulomata in cattle but is usually only mild or asymptomatic in buffalo, sheep or goats.

Animals which are exposed to infection with schistosomes may also be infected with *Fasciola*.

Pathology

The pathology associated with schistosomosis mainly results from the passage of the eggs through the tissues. Granulomata may be seen in the mucosa of the gastrointestinal tract. These are grey-white in colour, range in size from foci 1–2 mm in diameter up to areas 200 mm long in very heavy infections and are associated with petechiae and ecchymoses. Enlargement and haemorrhage of the ileo-caecal valve have also been reported in *S. mattheei* infections. There is a grey, sometimes almost black discolouration of the liver with white fibrous thickening of the portal vessels. White granulomata 1–2 mm in diameter may be scattered throughout the liver parenchyma. A grey discolouration of the lungs is also seen. In *S. mattheei* infection, granulomata are often present in the urinary bladder. Acute catarrhal inflammation of the small intestine has also been reported and serous effusions in the body cavities may be present to varying degrees.

In cattle severely affected by *S.nasale*, the nasal epithelium proliferates extensively, resulting in the granulomata. At post-mortem examination, the abscesses which form round the eggs in the nasal mucosal veins may be seen.

Diagnosis

Clinical signs, prevalence and grazing history. Immediately after death, the parasites can easily be seen if the mesenteric veins are stretched. However, they are not so easily seen after the blood has clotted. Serological tests have been extensively used in man and may be increasingly used in animals. The large, characteristically spined eggs may be found in the faeces or, in the case of *S. nasale* in the nasal discharge. However, the eggs hatch quickly in warm water, and therefore the faeces must be fixed in 10% formalin before using the standard sedimentation or sieving methods. The eggs are usually easily seen in squash preparations of blood clots or mucus from the faeces, although egg production falls to very low levels in the later stages of the infection. Similarly, a rapid diagnosis can be made from compressed tissue obtained as scrapings from intestinal lesions. It is probable that schistosomosis would be diagnosed more frequently if such preparations were examined routinely.

Treatment

The early drugs were mostly antimony compounds (tartar emetic and stibophen), but these are rather toxic and are being superseded by niridazole, lucanthone and metrifonate – an organophosphate given parenterally. Treatment needs to be given for several days. Praziquantel is very effective and would be the drug of choice but it may be too expensive to use in farm animals. Care must be taken with any form of chemotherapy as there is a risk of large numbers of dead schistosomes acting as emboli and so causing portal occlusion and focal hepatic infarction.

Immunology

A rather variable acquired resistance occurs against homologous species and an immune response which acts against the schistosomulae may have little effect on established adult worms. Recent work has demonstrated that irradiated schistosomulae of *S. bovis* are immunogenic in cattle following intramuscular injection and a vaccine based on this is undergoing field trials.

Control

Similar in principle to the measures adopted against *F. gigantica* (q.v.) but more difficult, because most of the snail intermediate hosts live in a wider, less well-defined range of habitats and may aestivate. In areas where *S. japonicum* or *S. mattheei* are prevalent, it is necessary to control the distribution of human faecal material as well as that from infected animals. Measures such as the use of molluscicides in the control of fasciolosis or human schistosomosis may also help in the control of animal schistosomosis.

SPIROCERCOSIS

Infection with the spirurid nematode *Spirocerca lupi*, a stout, pink, coiled worm up to 80 mm long.

Aetiology

S. lupi is found in nodules in the walls of the oesophagus, stomach or aorta.

Occurrence

Common in most tropical countries, especially in rural areas.

Species affected

Dogs and other Canidae.

Transmission

The eggs hatch after being ingested by a coprophagous beetle, and the larvae develop to the infective stage and encyst. They are released when the beetle is eaten and will develop directly if they are now in a suitable final host. If not, they will re-encyst within a variety of paratenic hosts including amphibia, reptiles, birds and mammals. In the final host, the larvae undergo a somatic migration via the arteries to the aorta and usually from there to the oesophagus.

Clinical features

Frequently none, but there may be persistent vomiting and emaciation. The nodules may be large enough to occlude the oesophagus. Associated signs include those of widespread metastatic neoplasia and thickening of the long bones. Sudden death will follow rupture of the aorta.

Pathology

Characteristic scarring caused by the migrating larvae is found on the intima of the aorta. The nodules in the oesophagus and stomach are hard and fibrous, up to 30–40 mm long and may be haemorrhagic. Highly invasive and metastasizing sarcomata may arise from the nodules.

Diagnosis

Clinical signs, X-ray and oesophagoscopy. Demonstration of the embryonated eggs in the faeces or vomit may be possible using flotation fluids of specific gravity of at least 1.36.

Treatment

Disophenol will kill the adult worms. Obstructive oesophageal nodules may be removed surgically.

Immunology

Not known.

Control

Difficult, especially in rural areas. Prevent dogs gaining access to the intermediate or transport hosts.

STEPHANOFILAROSIS

Infection of the skin with parasites of the genus *Stephanofilaria*. There are several species including *S. assamensis*, *S. dedoesi*, *S. kaeli* and *S. stilesi*. They are all small, filariform nematodes about 2–9 mm long.

Aetiology

The adult worms are found in the cutaneous lymphatics. *S. assamensis* causes "hump sore" in zebu cattle, while *S. dedoesi* causes "Cascado" and *S. kaeli* causes "Krian sore".

Occurrence

The distribution of *Stephanofilaria* is shown in Table 6.

Table 6 Distribution and lesions caused by *Stephanofilaria*

Species	Distribution	Lesions
S. dedoesi[a]	Indonesia	Head and neck
S. kaeli[a]	Malaysia	Legs, ears
S. zaheeri	India	Ears
S. assamensis[a]	Indian subcontinent Southern USSR	Hump
S. stilesi	Cosmopolitan	Ventral surface of body
S. okinawaensis[a]	India and Far East	Head, legs and teats

[a]May be synonomous.

Species affected

Cattle and buffalo.

Transmission

There is an indirect life-cycle, the intermediate hosts being anthomyid and other flies. The vector species has not yet been determined in some cases. The microfilariae are ingested from the open skin lesions and develop to the infective larval stage in the fly. Transmission to the final host occurs when the fly then feeds.

The highest prevalence of *S. stilesi* infections is seen where the faeces are kept moist by rain or irrigation and so remain attractive as breeding sites for the vectors. Similar considerations may apply to other species.

Clinical features

Lesions are localized and appear as a papular dermatitis. This later becomes exudative and even haemorrhagic, but resolution gradually takes place over many months, with the skin becoming dry and thickened.

Pathology

There are no internal lesions.

Diagnosis

Based on clinical signs and recent weather. Confirmation by skin snips or scrapings from the lesions, in which adult worms and microfilariae may be found.

Treatment

Topical application of 6% metrifonate in petroleum jelly or 2% coumaphos ointment have been shown to be effective, as has intramuscular levamisole or ivermectin.

Immunology

There is field evidence of acquired immunity in *S. stilesi* infections, where older animals, which have had repeated infections since calfhood, usually only have resolved lesions.

Control

Rarely feasible because the vectors are so numerous.

STEPHANUROSIS

Infection with the kidney worm, *Stephanurus dentatus*. A relatively stout nematode up to 45 mm long with a cup-shaped, thick walled, buccal cavity and a reduced bursa.

Aetiology

The adult worms are usually found in pairs in cysts in the peri-renal tissues, pelvis of the kidney and walls of the ureters, but usually cause little dysfunction.

The larvae cause considerable damage to the liver parenchyma during their migration and also thrombosis in abdominal vessels, which may prove fatal. In heavily infected pigs, there may be very little functional liver parenchyma and much cirrhosis, which results in ascites. Aberrant larvae or even small adults are commonly found encapsulated anywhere in the host's body, usually causing no overt disease, although they may be associated with paralytic conditions.

Occurrence

All tropical and subtropical countries where pigs are kept on free range or on pasture.

Species affected

Pigs. Calves may become infected, but adult worms do not usually develop in this host.

Transmission

The first-stage larvae hatch and develop to the infective third-stage larvae outwith the host. These larvae have little resistance to cold or desiccation. Infection of the host may occur prenatally, by skin-penetration or orally, including by ingestion of infected earthworms, which form an efficient transport host. The larvae migrate via the liver, in which they remain for about 3 months, and thence across the peritoneal cavity to the kidney. The prepatent period is at least 6 months. The adult worms in the peri-renal tissue and kidney may survive for up to 2 years.

Clinical features

Mainly ill-thrift, with anorexia and sometimes a mild anaemia and ascites. There may be paralysis in pigs and heavy infections may prove fatal. However, many infections are asymptomatic.

Pathology

This is mostly associated with the migrating larvae, which cause focal hepatic and pancreatic necrosis with leucocytic infiltration and cirrhosis, thrombosis in abdominal vessels and hypertrophy of mesenteric lymph nodes. Haemorrhagic areas and abscesses may be found in the lungs and white focal lesions on the surface of the kidneys. The adult worms are surrounded by greenish pus in cysts which communicate directly with the reduced lumen of the thickened ureter. Cystitis is common.

Diagnosis

Clinical signs, usually in pigs kept on pasture or on free range in areas where the parasite is known to occur. In patent infections, strongyle-type eggs are found in the urine. Many inapparent infections are diagnosed *post-mortem*. Immunodiffusion tests and ELISA have been developed but cross-reactions occur.

Differential diagnosis from other causes of ill-thrift, ascites, paralysis and sudden death.

Treatment

Modern benzimidazoles, levamisole and ivermectin are effective.

Immunology

Little is known although serological reactions have been demonstrated with antigens from *S. dentatus* and sera from infected pigs.

Control

The best method of control is to keep the pigs indoors or at least in clean, dry, concrete-floored pens to which earthworms do not have access. Avoid breeding from sows which may have been exposed to heavy infections and keep young stock away from paddocks grazed by older, possibly infected animals. Effective drainage of pig paddocks may also help. As patency is unusual in animals under 2 years of age, it has been suggested that using only gilts for breeding would provide a useful measure of control.

STRONGYLOSIS

Infection of Equidae with strongyle parasites. These are all relatively rigid, bursate nematodes. The most pathogenic species is *Strongylus* (syn. *Delafondia*) *vulgaris*. Other commonly occurring large strongyles include *Strongylus* (syn. *Alfortia*) *edentatus* and *Triodontophorus*. However, the most common strongyles are the small trichonemes, most of which belong to the genus *Trichonema*, in which there are many different species of varying size, ranging from 4 to 26 mm in length. There are several other genera and species which occur less commonly, including another large strongyle, *Strongylus equinus*.

S. *vulgaris* can be differentiated from the other large strongyles by its relatively small size, being 14–24 mm long compared with 23–44 mm for *S. edentatus*, and by its oval buccal cavity, which contains two ear-shaped dorsal teeth in contrast to *S. edentatus* which has no teeth, and *Triodontophorus*, which has a thick-walled, subglobular buccal capsule, with three pairs of teeth at the base.

Aetiology

The most serious disease associated with these parasites results from the thromboarteritis caused by the presence of *S. vulgaris* larvae in the anterio-mesenteric, ileo-caeco-colic and neighbouring arteries. The inflammatory thickening of the wall of these arteries forms the so-called "verminous aneurysm" although true aneurysms also occasionally occur proximal to the lesion. Intestinal infarction, which may cause colic or death, commonly results from emboli derived from the arterial thrombi. The animals will then only survive if an adequate collateral can be established sufficiently quickly.

S. *edentatus* larvae do not develop within the arteries but undergo an extensive migration via the liver to locate in the tissues beneath the parietal peritoneum in the flanks within 2–3 months of infection. Here they remain for a period of 1–2 months, after which they migrate back to the large intestine. Heavy infections may cause death from peritonitis or peritoneal haemorrhage, but this is relatively uncommon. Aberrant larvae may be found in widely distributed sites, e.g. kidney, spleen, testes.

Triodontophorus and *Trichonema* larvae do not undergo a somatic migration, but develop within the intestinal wall – mainly in the caecum and colon. *Trichonema* larvae are commonly found within nodules and secondary infection of these nodules may lead to ulceration. Ulcers may also form at the attachment sites. The adult large strongyles suck blood, as do immature trichonemes. There is leakage from ulcers and old attachment sites.

Occurrence

Although there are differences in species distribution, these parasites are of worldwide prevalence, being able to survive in most climates where horses are found.

Species affected

Equids.

Transmission

There is a direct life-cycle in which the first-stage larvae hatch and develop to the third-stage, sheathed infective larvae, which migrate from the faeces on to the herbage. Oral infection is followed by a prolonged period of development within the host. The prepatent periods are 3–4 months for *Trichonema*, about 6 months for *S. vulgaris* and 10 months for *S. edentatus*.

These prolonged development times and the inhibited development of *Trichonema* larvae in the nodules allow the parasite to survive within the host during prolonged periods of adverse climatic conditions.

Clinical features

The acute disease which follows infection of susceptible foals with *S. vulgaris* larvae is characterized by pyrexia, anorexia and severe colic, with death within 3 weeks of infection if a susceptible animal has ingested 800 or more larvae at one time. *S. edentatus* rarely causes clinical signs, although there may be peritonitis and peritoneal haemorrrhage. Chronic disease arising from mixed infections is associated with ill-thrift, poor performance and anaemia.

Pathology

Thromboarteritis with thickening of the wall and occlusion of the lumen of the anterio-mesenteric, ileo-caeco-colic and neighbouring arteries, with extension into the aorta, is the characteristic lesion associated with *S. vulgaris* infection. Evidence of such damage can be found in most horses, although the lesions regress in older, resistant animals. Embolism and infarction of the intestine, hind limb or testes may occur. *S. edentatus* larvae cause the formation or large haemorrhagic nodules in the sub-peritoneal tissue of the flanks and in the intestinal wall. Similar nodules are also caused by the *S. vulgaris* larvae when they break out of the arterioles after returning to the bowel wall. *Trichonema* larvae cause the widespread formation of nodules of varying size and colour in the large intestinal wall and in the ileum, while in heavy infections there may also be a generalized oedema and thickening of the wall. *Triodontophorus* causes the formation of large deep ulcers, while the attachment of the other large adult strongyles results in small haemorrhagic areas 2–3 mm in diameter, which may enlarge and coalesce to give shallow ulcers.

Diagnosis

Virtually all horses are infected with strongyles. As the most severe disease is associated with larval infections, the clinical signs, age, season and grazing history are of much greater significance than faecal egg counts. Confirmatory evidence may include a post-mortem examination and demonstration of anaemia, eosinophilia, hypoalbuminaemia and hyper-β-gammaglobulinaemia.

Treatment

Modern nematocides are very effective against equine strongyles but are of no curative value in the acute embolic disease caused by the immature large strongyles, and therefore symptomatic treatment should also be given. The modern benzimidazoles and ivermectin are effective against the larvae of the trichonemes and some of the migratory stages of the large strongyles. Removing only the adult trichonemes may stimulate the development of larvae already within the host. Some strains of strongyles have been reported to show resistance to the benzimidazoles.

Immunology

Young horses are usually more susceptible to strongyle infection than mature animals, and there is good evidence that an effective acquired resistance to reinfection with *S. vulgaris* may develop following a single previous infection.

Control

In climates where there is a prolonged dry season or winter, contamination of the pasture during the following favourable season for free-living larvae comes mainly from parasites which have survived within the hosts. Anthelmintic treatment of these older, infected animals can reduce the level of contamination, provided it is repeated at regular monthly or 6-weekly intervals with an anthelmintic which is effective against the larval stages. Otherwise, similar, regular anthelmintic treatment should concentrate on the younger animals, which should also have access only to the cleanest pastures. Alternate grazing by horses and ruminants is of value in reducing contamination levels. Unfortunately, occasional losses due to embolic infarction caused by immature *S. vulgaris* may occur in foals exposed to only light infections. With valuable horses or in climates where there is no unfavourable season for the free-living larvae, zero-grazing, constant medication and/or twice-weekly manual removal of fresh faeces from the pastures may be considered. When used consistently, this last procedure can provide better control than anthelmintics and can increase the grazing area by up to 50%.

STRONGYLOIDOSIS

Infection with parasites of the genus *Strongyloides*. There are many species including *S. stercoralis, S. fülleborni, S. papillosus, S. ransomi, S. westeri, S. cati* and others. The parasitic stages are all female. Their length varies from 2–9 mm and they have a relatively long filariform oesophagus, which distinguishes them from female trichostrongyles.

Aetiology

The parasitic adults are found in the small intestine. Large numbers of *Strongyloides* adults may cause enteritis with diarrhoea, which is often chronic. *S. stercoralis* and

S. ransomi are relatively pathogenic, but the other species are of little pathogenicity, except in massive infections. The skin-penetrating larvae may cause local pruritus and erythema or prolonged *cutaneous larva migrans* (creeping eruption) in man. Bronchopneumonia may occur as large numbers of larvae migrate through the lungs.

Occurrence

Worldwide, but more prevalent in humid, unhygienic environments.

Species affected

S. stercoralis occurs in man, apes, dog and cat, *S. fülleborni* in man and primates, *S. papillosus* in ruminants and rabbits, *S. ransomi* in pigs, *S. westeri* in equines and *S. cati* in cats.

Transmission

There are minor differences between the species, but both parasitic and free-living generations may occur in all species. Except for *S. fülleborni*, where the parasitic and free-living generations strictly alternate, the eggs derived from the parasitic females may give rise to either infective larvae or to a free-living generation of very small males and females. The free-living generation may itself also give rise to either a parasitic or a further free-living generation. The life-style tends to change to the parasitic type when the external environment becomes unfavourable. Infection is by skin-penetration, ingestion or transmammary in most, if not all, species. Auto-infection occurs and it has been suggested that a true endogenous egg-to-egg cycle may occur in man and carnivores. *S. stercoralis* infection of dogs can be acquired by man but tends to be self-limiting.

Clinical features

In puppies, there may be anorexia, coughing and bronchopneumonia, followed by diarrhoea. The diarrhoea may be blood stained and may lead to dehydration and even death. In piglets, the intestinal phase is relatively pathogenic, with signs ranging from ill-thrift with diarrhoea to continuous dysentery, anaemia, vomiting and sometimes up to 50% mortality. In other young domestic animals, the signs are similar to those in piglets but are rarely severe, and even heavy burdens may be asymptomatic.

Pathology

Haemorrhagic foci in the lungs and a severe catarrhal enteritis with fluid, sometimes haemorrhagic, small-intestinal contents. Large numbers of female *Strongyloides* are present on the mucosa.

Diagnosis

Except in humans, clinical enteritis usually only occurs in the very young. Skin lesions may be seen in older animals. Very large numbers of small embryonated eggs or, in the case of *S. stercoralis* and usually *S. ransomi*, larvae may be found in fresh faeces. In some tropical countries, other species of *Strongyloides* occur in domestic carnivores, which have embryonated eggs in fresh faeces and are not infectious for man. Light infections often occur together with trichostrongyle infections in ruminants.

Treatment

Most modern nematocides including the benzimidazoles, ivermectin and dichlorvos are effective. Topical thiabendazole is effective against creeping eruption.

Immunology

Except perhaps in man, resistance to reinfection develops rapidly even in very young animals and burdens tend to be small or absent in adults.

Control

Specific control measures are rarely necessary. Hygiene is the most important factor.

TAENIOSIS

Infection with the adult tapeworm or larval metacestode of the genus *Taenia*. The tapeworms, which in some species may be over 1 m long, occur in the small intestine. Except for *Taenia saginata*, which is unarmed, the scolex in both tapeworm and the larval metacestode bears a rostellum with hooks. Cysticerci are simple metacestode cysts which contain a single scolex. The cyst of *T. hydatigena* (syn. *Cysticercus tenuicollis*) may be up to 50 mm in diameter, that of *T. solium* (syn. *C. cellulosae*) 20 × 10 mm and those of *T. ovis* and *T. saginata* (syn. *C. bovis*) 10 × 5 mm. A coenurus is a metacestode which takes the form of a fluid filled cyst, up to 50 mm in diameter, with numerous scolices on its wall.

Aetiology

In domestic animals, neither the tapeworms nor cysticerci are commonly associated with disease, although the latter may act as space-occupying lesions. However, the coenurus of *T. multiceps* (syn. *Coenurus cerebralis*) causes central nervous dysfunction and the cysticerci of *T. solium* cause the severe disease neurocysticercosis when they occur in the brain of man.

Occurrence

These parasites are found worldwide with local variations in prevalence, which largely depend on the availability of the host species and on social factors where man is the final host. *T. solium* and hence human cysticercosis is relatively common in parts of Latin America and the Far East.

Species affected

The domestic hosts are shown in Table 7. The cysticerci found in wild ruminants are usually the larvae of tapeworms occurring in wild carnivores. The coenurus of *T. multiceps* has also occasionally been reported as occurring in the brain of other ruminants or man.

Table 7 Hosts and sites for *Taenia* parasites of domestic animals

Species	Final host	Intermediate host	Site for metacestodes
T. solium	Man	Pig, dog, man	Musculature
T. saginata	Man	Cattle	Musculature
T. hydatigena	Dog	Sheep	Peritoneal cavity
T. ovis	Dog	Sheep	Musculature
T. taeniaeformis	Cat	Rat, mouse	Liver
T. multiceps	Dog	Sheep	Brain[a]
T. serialis	Dog	Rabbit	Subcutaneous tissue[a]

[a]Coenurus – all the other metacestodes listed are cysticerci.

Transmission

Transmission is by oral infection of the intermediate host by unhatched eggs derived from proglottids in the faeces of the final host. These eggs are susceptible to desiccation but may be widely disseminated by flies. They hatch in the intestine and then migrate to the appropriate development sites where cysticerci develop over the next 10–12 weeks, while coenuri take 3–8 months. The final host becomes infected by eating viable infective cysts. Prenatal infection of calves with *T. saginata* is reputed to occur but is uncommon.

Clinical features

The adult tapeworms may cause various minor digestive disturbances in man and have been reputed to be associated with fits in young dogs. Cysticercosis rarely causes clinical signs in domestic animals, but neurocysticercosis in man may cause blindness, paralysis or epileptiform seizures and may be fatal. In cerebral coenurosis, there is slowly developing central nervous dysfunction, preceded by dullness, anorexia and ill-thrift. The signs vary with the site of the cyst but may include blindness and locomotor inco-ordination with ultimate recumbency and death.

Pathology

The only pathology associated with the adult tapeworms is the small area of enteritis at their attachment site. The metacestodes are mostly but not exclusively to be found in their characteristic development sites. Cysticerci may become necrotic, filled with greenish pus or calcified.

Diagnosis

The presence of the adult tapeworms may be detected by observing the gravid segments in the faeces of the host. This may be easy or, especially with *T. saginata*, it may be necessary to examine several faecal samples.

A diagnosis of cysticercosis in domestic animals is usually only made *post mortem* by direct observation of the cysts, although those of *T. solium* can often be seen beneath the surface of the tongue of the infected pig. The sites which are searched for the cysticerci of *T. saginata* are often dictated by commercial considerations, e.g. masseters, heart, diaphragm, etc. The heart and diaphragm may contain relatively large numbers of cysts in recent infections but fewer in older infections. Examination of the shoulder muscles has been shown to afford a significantly higher detection rate in African cattle but, even then, only a very small proportion of lightly infected carcases are detected by meat inspection. No reliable *ante mortem* serodiagnostic or other methods are at present generally available for use with domestic animals, although both serology and computerized tomography (CT scan) are useful in human cases.

Coenurosis may be diagnosed in sheep from the clinical signs and history and *post mortem*. An area of softening of the cranisal bones can sometimes be located by palpation over the site of the cyst.

Treatment

The adult tapeworms are susceptible to most cestocides but there is no effective, commercially available metacestocide, although high doses of praziquantel will kill cysticerci.

Extraction of a cerebral coenurus through a trephined hole in the skull may be possible.

Immunology

In calves infected shortly after birth, some metacestodes may survive for several years even in the face of constant reinfection. Such continuously infected calves become highly resistant to reinfection but may show little serological response. Cattle initially infected with *T. saginata* when over 6 months of age, develop a strong resistance to reinfection and also a demonstrable serological response. Such infections are usually self-limiting, the cysts dying within 10–12 months.

Relatively little is known about the immunology of the adult tapeworms or of the other metacestodes, apart from the fact that the latter all elicit a serologically demonstrable response.

Control

Treatment and hygienic measures may be applied to the final host, including man. The latter should include safe disposal of faeces and prevention of access by potentially infected final hosts to the intermediate hosts – notably by man to calves or pigs, or dogs to sheep. Dogs should not be allowed to feed on uncooked sheep meet or offal. Even the most careful meat inspection cannot be expected to ensure detection of lightly infected carcases, so thorough cooking of beef or pork for human consumption is advisable.

Deep freezing lightly infected carcases to at least $-10°C$ for 10 days or to a lower temperature for a shorter time will kill cysticerci.

THELAZIOSIS

Infection with spirurid nematodes of the genus *Thelazia*, including *T. rhodesii*, *T. lachrymalis*, *T. callipaeda*, *T. californiensis* and several other minor species. *Thelazia* spp. are white, thin nematodes up to 20 mm long and the cuticle usually carries clear transverse striations.

Aetiology

Disease is caused by the presence of the parasites in the eyes or lachrymal ducts.

Occurrence

Worldwide, although various species have restricted ranges. Thus *T. callipaeda* occurs in the Far East and *T. californiensis* in the southern USA. Often seasonal in incidence, varying with the prevalence of the vectors.

Species affected

T. rhodesii is relatively common in cattle and sheep, *T. lacrymalis* in horses, *T. callipaeda* in dogs and man and *T. californiensis* in sheep, dogs, man and other hosts.

Transmission

The worms are viviparous and the first-stage larvae are infective for various diptera, including *Musca* spp. They develop to the third stage in the fly and will then infect the eye of a further host as the fly feeds. No migration in the final host.

Clinical features

Marked unilateral or bilateral lachrymation, which is often purulent, and photophobia. The whole cornea may be opaque. May recover spontaneously in about 2 months.

Pathology

Conjunctivitis, keratitis, ulceration and sometimes perforation of the cornea. There may be residual corneal fibrosis.

Diagnosis

Clinical signs with a seasonal incidence and observation of the worms in the eye following local anaesthesia.

Treatment

Parenteral ivermectin or levamisole, which may also be given topically as a 1% aqueous solution. Alternatively, local anaesthesia and manual removal of *T. rhodesii* is usually possible but may be difficult with other species. Local antibiotic therapy.

Immunology

Unknown.

Control

Difficult because of the nature of the vectors. Treatment of symptomless possible carriers of the adult parasites during the season when the disease is not prevalent may help to reduce the incidence of new infections.

TRICHINELLOSIS

Infection with the nematode *Trichinella spiralis*. This is the only species in the genus, but strains in different geographical areas have different host specificities.

The adult worms are very small (<5 mm) and are rarely seen. The coiled larvae are found in spindle-shaped cysts (trichinae) about 0.5 mm long in muscular tissue.

Aetiology

Disease occurs as a result of the host's reaction to the presence of the larvae in the muscles.

Occurrence

Worldwide apart from Australasia, but more common in man in temperate countries.

Species affected

Most mammals. The strain found in Africa is infective for wild Suidae, wild carnivores and man, but not for domestic pigs or rats, in contrast to the wider infectivity of the strains in temperate areas.

Transmission

Direct from final host to final host when infected meat is eaten. The larvae develop to viviparous adults in the small intestine within 5 days but die within 2–16 weeks. The larvae they produce are distributed in the blood and those which reach the striated muscles are encysted within 7 weeks. They may remain alive for several years and survive in meat or carrion for 2–3 months after the death of the host.

Clinical features

Disease is seldom seen in naturally infected animals, but in man the reaction to the larvae encysting in the muscles causes widespread muscular pain. Myocarditis, meningitis and encephalitis may also occur and the infection may be fatal. The reaction subsides as encystment proceeds.

Pathology

Generalized myositis associated with recently established larvae in muscles. Well-encapsulated cysts, containing larvae, can later be seen at low magnification of suitable thin muscles, e.g. diaphragm. Many of the cysts eventually become calcified.

Diagnosis

Clinical signs in man, with a history of eating raw or lightly cooked meat. Muscle biopsy. Eosinophilia. Serodiagnosis by ELISA can provide valuable epidemiological information but should not be relied upon as a means of ensuring that pig meat is free from infection. Trichinoscopy and digestion techniques permit direct detection of the trichinae in meat.

Treatment

None in animals. High doses of benzimidazoles, corticosteroids and symptomatic treatment in man.

Control

Meat inspection and prolonged deep freezing or adequate cooking of potentially infected meat and of waste human food used to feed pigs. Hygiene in relation to cooking utensils.

TRICHOSTRONGYLIDOSIS

Gastric trichostrongylidosis

Infection of the stomach or abomasum with trichostrongylid nematodes. Often regarded as forming part of the parasitic gastroenteritis syndrome. The intestinal trichostrongylids are considered below under "Enteric trichostrongylidosis".

Haemonchus contortus and *H. placei* are the most widespread species of that genus. *H. similis*, *H. bispinosus* and *H. longistipes* having a more limited range, as does the superficially similar parasite, *Mecistocirrus digitatus*. The most common species of *Ostertagia* are *O. ostertagi*, *O. circumcincta* and *O. trifurcata*. The two latter species may be given the generic name *Teladorsagia*. *Grosspiculagia* is a very closely related genus of which the most common species is *G. lyrata*. Other related species include

Marshallagia marshalli, Camelostrongylus mentulatus and *Hyostrongylus rubidus.*
Trichostrongylus axei infection also occurs in the same site.

Haemonchus and *Mecistocirrus* are relatively large trichostrongyles, the former
being up to 30 mm long and the latter up to 45 mm long. *Haemonchus* has an
asymmetrically sited dorsal ray and the vulva is situated about two-thirds of the way
down the body, whereas *Mecistocirrus* has long slender spicules (4–7 mm long), a
small centrally placed dorsal ray and the vulva is very close to the posterior end of the
body. The different species of *Haemonchus* can be differentiated on spicule lengths,
which are < 340 μm for *H. similis*, 400–430 μm for *H. contortus*, 450–470 μm for *H.
placei* and >620 μm for *H. longistipes*.

Female *Marshallagia* may be up to 20 mm long, but *Ostertagia* and its related species
are all relatively small trichostrongyles not more than 12 mm long. They can all be
distinguished by differences in the shape of the spicules, while gravid female *Marshallagia* can easily be recognized because of the very large eggs in their uteri.

Aetiology

Only *Haemonchus* and *Mecistocirrus* are frank blood suckers, but all these parasites
impair the integrity and function of the gastric mucosa.

The acute disease can follow two epidemiological patterns:

Type I: Occurs within a few weeks of exposure to heavy infection and mostly in the
hosts' first grazing season. In sheep and pigs, the main source of this infection is the
post-parturient rise in the numbers of eggs in the faeces of the parturient females.
Heavy infections, especially with *Haemonchus*, usually occur at times when the recent
weather has been favourable for the development and survival of the larval stages on
the pasture. Because of the high fecundity and short generation interval, severe
outbreaks of disease may occur after only a short period of suitable weather.

Type II: Occurs only in areas where there is a prolonged unfavourable period for
larval development and survival outwith the host, when the climate is too cold, too hot
or too dry. This includes temperate areas with a cold winter, winter-rainfall subtropical
areas with a hot dry summer, and savannah areas with a long dry season. This form of
the disease occurs during the unfavourable season and mainly in yearlings but sometimes in older animals. It may occur in housed animals as it results from the delayed
maturation of larvae acquired during the latter part of the previous favourable season.
Type II haemonchosis has been described in cattle during a savannah dry season.

Occurrence

Haemonchosis is most prevalent in the permanently humid and in summer-rainfall
tropical and subtropical climates, but also occurs in many temperate areas. *M. digitatus*
predominates in parts of the Indian subcontinent and South East Asia and also occurs
in South America.

Ostertagosis occurs mainly in winter-rainfall subtropical areas and in temperate
areas. *Marshallagia* is mainly found in relatively arid tropical and subtropical regions.
T. axei occurs worldwide.

Species affected

Cattle, sheep, goats, camels and other ruminants.

H. placei, O. ostertagi and *G. lyrata* occur primarily in cattle, while *H. contortus, O. circumcincta, O. trifurcata* and *Marshallagia* occur mainly in sheep and goats. *H. longistipes* and *Camelostrongylus* occur in camels and sometimes in sheep and goats, whereas *Hyostrongylus* is found almost exclusively in the stomach of pigs. *T. axei* may occur in the abomasum or stomach of all these hosts and of equines.

Transmission

There is a direct life-cycle in which the first-stage larvae hatch out of the eggs and under suitable conditions of moisture and temperature the relatively resistant sheathed third-stage larvae migrate out of the faeces on to the herbage. *Haemonchus* larvae – and to an even greater extent *Mecistocirrus* larvae – are less able to survive and develop at low temperatures or to survive arid conditions than *Ostertagia* spp., which are characteristically able to survive and develop at relatively low temperatures. *Haemonchus* and *Ostertagia* infective larvae can also survive and develop for some time during a dry season in the crusted pats of bovine faeces but only for a much shorter time in ovine pellets. *Marshallagia marshalli* larvae remain within the egg until the second larval stage, which may aid their survival in arid areas. Infection occurs only by the oral route.

The inhibition of larval development late in the favourable season may be consequent upon either host resistance or a physiological change in the infective larvae. It is the main mechanism by which these parasites survive unfavourable seasons.

Clinical features

The most acute cases of haemonchosis or mecistocirrosis may present as sudden death, but otherwise anaemia, oedema, loss of wool and dark-coloured faeces, but no diarrhoea or pyrexia are characteristic signs. The animals are lethargic and milk yield is reduced. In chronic haemonchosis, there may be little anaemia or oedema and the poor growth rate or weight loss tends to be overlooked because all the animals in the group are affected or the nutrition is known to be poor.

Type I ostertagosis occurs mainly in young animals. There is a severe diarrhoea, which is green when the animals are grazing lush pastures, and also dehydration and wasting. No pyrexia or anaemia. The morbidity is usually high but mortality low.

Type II ostertagosis affects yearlings or older animals and is usually of low morbidity but may involve a high case mortality. There is an intermittent profuse diarrhoea and wasting. Oedema or anaemia may be present. The clinical signs of trichostrongylosis are similar but there may be an oligocythaemia.

Malnutrition or intercurrent disease such as fasciolosis may exacerbate the chronic or Type II conditions.

Pathology

At post-mortem examination of acute cases of haemonchosis or mecistocirrosis, there is evidence of anaemia and oedema with hyperplasia and extension of the red bone marrow. However, these features may not be evident in the most acute cases.

The abomasal mucosa is petechiated, eroded and/or hyperplastic and, even in less acute cases, there are usually over 1000 adult worms present, However, animals may lose their burden shortly before death.

In the chronic syndrome there is emaciation, a moderate anaemia, little oedema, hyperplastic thickening of the abomasal wall and extension of the bone marrow, with resorption of both cancellous and cortical bone, although in terminal cases the marrow may no longer be red because of exhaustion. A few as 100 adult worms may be present in such chronic cases.

At post-mortem examination in acute cases of infection with *Ostertagia* or the related species, the abomasum or stomach has a hyperplastic mucosa with epithelial lesions ranging from raised nodules of 2–3 mm diameter through confluent lesions to large areas of superficial necrosis and sloughing. There may be severe oedema or congestion of the abomasal wall and the contents are often foul smelling. Large numbers of parasites (10,000 +) can usually be observed with the naked eye, although many of these may not be mature in Type II.

Diagnosis

Should be based on the clinical signs, the age of the animal, the climatic region, the season and the grazing history, with confirmation from post-mortem examination and faecal egg counts in Type I disease. These counts are usually very high in acute cases of haemonchosis – over 10,000 epg in sheep, although disease may occur before the worms reach patency. In Type I ostertagosis, counts usually exceed 1000 epg. *Marshallagia* eggs are distinct, being nearly three times the size of most strongyle-type eggs. Plasma pepsinogen levels are usually elevated often to over 3 international units as compared with normal values of less than 1 i.u.

Differentiate haemonchosis and mecistocirrosis from other causes of anaemia and oedema or sudden death in several animals and ostertagosis from other causes of severe diarrhoea and wasting.

Treatment

Modern benzimidazoles and ivermectin are effective against all these parasites, but the older anthelmintics such as tiabendazole or levamisole are not effective against all inhibited larvae and may be of little value in Type II disease. Even after treatment, heavily infected animals may die and the growth rate of chronically infected animals may still be impaired. Removing the animals from the infected pasture forms an essential part of the treatment.

Immunology

Resistance develops relatively slowly and its efficacy in individual animals varies markedly. It is not effective in young animals and, although it may be sufficient to prevent deaths in adult animals, they will continue to contaminate the pastures. Resistance also tends to wane when the challenge is reduced, e.g. during a dry season. Pigs develop resistance against *Hyostrongylus* more quickly and effectively. In both sows and ewes, there is an apparent diminution in host resistance associated with lactation which results in a "post-parturient rise" in the numbers of eggs in their faeces. Ejection of a pre-existing burden of *Haemonchus* may follow reinfection but may also follow rainfall or the associated regrowth of the pasture.

Control

Type I ostertagosis or haemonchosis may be prevented by removing the young animals from their dams on to a clean pasture at weaning, perhaps with treatment at this time. Type II disease may be avoided by not returning the animals to pastures which had been contaminated earlier in the same grazing season. It is still probably better to risk an outbreak of the more readily treatable Type I disease than Type II. If clean pasture cannot be provided for young stock, repeated administration of anthelmintics may be necessary and economically advantageous. The numbers of infective larvae on a pasture will fall rapidly at the onset of a savannah dry season or of summer in a winter-rainfall climate, so that they may be considered to be free of infection before the onset of the next favourable season. However, some larvae may survive for an extended period within faecal material, especially that from cattle. Alternate grazing with cattle and sheep may help to reduce infection levels but is not consistently effective with *Haemonchus*, which becomes adapted to both hosts. Grazing by adult animals also tends to reduce the numbers of larvae on a pasture.

Prophylactic anthelmintic treatment may be considered necessary and cost-effective, especially against haemonchosis in sheep and young cattle, in valuable animals in areas where potentially dangerous weather conditions occur at predictable seasons, e.g. a well-spaced monthly rainfall in excess of 50 mm together with mean maximum temperatures over 20°C. Such treatment may include the administration of an anthelmintic at 3-weekly intervals. Disophenol may be given every 2–3 months against *Haemonchus* or hookworms. In cattle, consideration may be given to the use of sustained-release or pulse-release boluses or the administration of ivermectin at 5-weekly intervals. In other areas, tactical treatments in anticipation of an outbreak following short spells of suitable weather may be preferable.

Enteric trichostrongylidosis

Infection with small intestinal nematode parasites of the Family Trichostrongylidae. Often included with the trichostrongylids which occur in the abomasum or stomach (see "Gastric trichostrongylidosis") in a syndrome termed Parasitic Gastroenteritis.

Species of tropical and subtropical importance include *Trichostrongylus colubriformis*, *T. capricola*, *T. probolurus*, *Cooperia curticei*, *C. oncophora*, *C. punctata*, *C. pectinata* and *Impalaia nudicollis*. A number of other species have been described in the two former genera. Two other tropical species with many similarities to *Cooperia* are *Cooperioides kenyensis* and *Paracooperia nodulosa*. *Nematodirus* spp. and *Nematodirella* spp. occur in some areas.

These are small, thin, bursate nematodes. The largest are *Nematodirus* and *Nematodirella*, which are up to 25 mm long; none of the other species exceed 12 mm. *Trichostrongylus* has a simple anterior end and a small bursa, whereas *Cooperia* has a small cephalic dilation with a number of cross-striations and a larger bursa.

Aetiology

The adults of all these nematodes are mostly found in the proximal part of the small intestine, except in very heavy infections. Where disease occurs, it is usually later in the favourable season as their fecundity is rather less than that of *Haemonchus* or *Ostertagia*, and the numbers of infective larvae on the pasture need to have built up by repeated infection.

Occurrence

Several of these species are of worldwide prevalence. *Cooperioides kenyensis* occurs in Africa and *Paracooperia nodulosa* in Asia. *Nematodirus* and *Nematodirella* occur mainly in winter-rainfall or temperate areas, but *N. helvetianus* is found in some highland tropical regions.

Species affected

Domestic and wild ruminants. *Trichostrongylus colubriformis* may occur in all ruminants and occasionally in other hosts, *T. capricola* occurs in goats and sheep and *T. probolurus* occurs in camels and other ruminants. *Cooperia curticei* occurs mainly in small ruminants, while *C. oncophora*, *C. punctata* and *C. pectinata* occur mainly in cattle. *Cooperioides* spp. occur in wild ruminants while *Paracooperia nodulosa* is primarily a parasite of buffalo. *Impalaia nudicollis* is mostly found in wild ruminants but also occurs in camels and sheep. Various species of *Nematodirus* and *Nematodirella* occur in sheep, goats, camels and wild ruminants, while *Nematodirus helvetianus* is found in cattle.

Transmission

Direct strongyle-type life-cycles, with first-stage larvae which hatch out of the egg (except for *Nematodirus* where the larvae remain within the egg until the third stage) and oral infection by sheathed, third-stage larvae which have migrated from the faeces on to the herbage.

There is evidence to suggest that, except in the case of *Nematodirus* and probably *Nematodirella*, inhibited development is important for the survival of the species in the hosts during the dry season or winter.

Clinical features

General ill-thrift and anorexia, severe diarrhoea in more serious cases. The disease may be chronic or of sudden onset, with rapid loss of condition and death. However, large numbers of parasites may occur in the absence of severe clinical signs.

Pathology

The carcase is emaciated and often stunted, with heavy faecal contamination of the peri-anal region and very fluid intestinal contents. The duodenal and jejunal regions may contain very large numbers of the parasites (20,000 +).

Diagnosis

Based on clinical signs, season and grazing history taken together with *post mortem* findings. Plasma-pepsinogen levels will be normal except where there is concurrent trichostrongylid gastritis. Faecal egg counts may be in excess of 10,000 epg. *Nematodirus* eggs are characteristic, being large with relatively few large cells in the morula.

Treatment

Modern nematocides are effective against all these parasites but may not prevent death in severely affected animals. Removal to uncontaminated pasture is an essential part of treatment.

Immunology

Resistance to most of these parasites develops relatively slowly as with *Ostertagia* and *Haemonchus* (see "Parasitic gastritis"). They also appear to be involved in the post-parturient rise in ewes. In contrast, resistance to *Nematodirus* is relatively rapid in onset.

Control

The methods used in the control of other gastrointestinal nematode infections will be effective against these parasites.

TRICHUROSIS

Infection with nematodes of the genus *Trichuris* (syn. *Trichocephalus*). Many species have been described, some of which are of doubtful validity.

These are the whipworms which have a very characteristic appearance in that the very thin oesophageal region occupies at least two-thirds of the total length of the worms and the stouter end is markedly coiled in the male.

Aetiology

The adult parasites are found in the caecum, especially towards its blind end, where they attach by burying their narrow anterior end into the mucosa.

Occurrence

Particularly prevalent in unhygienic, moist, warm environments.

Species affected

The species of veterinary importance are listed in Table 8.

Table 8 Distribution and hosts of *Trichuris* in domestic animals

Species	Hosts	Distribution
T. ovis	Ruminants	Worldwide
T. globulosa	Ruminants	Africa
T. discolor	Ruminants	Europe, Asia, USA
T. suis	Suidae	Worldwide
T. vulpis	Dogs	Worldwide
T. campanula	Cats	North and South America, Caribbean
T. trichiura	Humans, simian primates	Worldwide

Transmission

The infective stage is the first larva, which does not hatch out of the egg, and is therefore resistant to adverse environmental circumstances except heat and desiccation. The eggs may survive in a cool, moist environment for up to 5 years. Oral infection. There is no somatic migration, the larvae developing in the caecum. Prepatent period 6–12 weeks depending on the species.

Clinical features

T. trichiura causes chronic diarrhoea in man and *T. suis* may be associated with a similar condition in pigs. Disease caused by *Trichuris* in ruminants is relatively uncommon, only occurring following massive infections. Clinical signs include diarrhoea, which may contain blood, anorexia, ill-thrift and anaemia, particularly in dogs, where trichurosis often occurs together with hookworm infection.

Pathology

T. vulpis is the most pathogenic species and heavy infections cause a severe inflammation of the caecal mucosa (typhlitis) as the parasites damage capillaries causing localized hae-morrhage. The caecal contents are fluid and bloodstained. There is evidence to suggest that *T. suis* only causes disease because a virtually ubiquitous spirochaete is also present.

Diagnosis

Clinical features in animals kept in an unhygienic, moist environment. Large numbers of characteristic eggs in the faeces. May be initially confused with ancylostomosis in dogs.

Treatment

Rarely necessary in ruminants, but the modern benzimidazoles, levamisole and inver-mectin are very effective against the adults. Dichlorvos in a resin base is also effective.

Immunology

Largely unknown, although sheep can develop an acquired resistance to *T. ovis*.

Control

Rarely necessary in ruminants. In dogs and pigs the provision of a dry, clean environment will prevent disease. However, a contaminated area may remain so for several years.

HELMINTH INFECTIONS OF LESSER IMPORTANCE

Nematodes

Ascarops strongylina occurs widely in the stomach of pigs. It is a spirurid nematode up to 22 mm long, with an embryonated, thick-shelled egg up to 40 μm long. A larger species, *A. dentata*, up to 55 mm long, occurs in South East Asia. A characteristic feature of this genus is the complex spiral thickening of the wall of the buccal cavity, which contrasts with the relatively simple spiral and ring-like thickenings in another spirurid, *Physocephalus sexalatus*, which is up to 23 mm long and occurs in the same host and site and also in camels, as does *Physocephalus cristatus*. Another related species, *Simondsia paradoxa* occurs in nodular cysts in the stomach wall of pigs in parts of Europe, Asia and Africa. All these parasites may cause ill-thrift but are otherwise of low pathogenicity. Their life-cycles involve coprophagous beetles as intermediate hosts and they may utilize transport hosts.

Gongylonema pulchrum is a long spirurid worm, up to 145 mm long, which occurs widely in the oesophagus and rumen of ruminants and occasionally in equidae and man. It has cervical alae and clearly demarcated cuticular thickenings at the anterior end. *G. verrucosum*, which occurs in the same sites, is up to 95 mm long. It has anterior cuticular plaques on the left side only and a single, festooned, left cervical ala. These nematodes, which use coprophagous beetles as intermediate hosts, are virtually non-pathogenic.

Dipetalonema spp. mostly occur in the subcutis of dogs and are not usually pathogenic. However, as they often occur in the same areas as *Dirofilaria immitis*, their blood-borne microfilariae should be differentiated. Adult *Dip. evansi* of camels live in the pulmonary and internal spermatic arteries and lymphatics and may cause orchitis or cardiac dysfunction. The microfilariae also occur in the blood, the vector being *Aedes*.

Elaeophora poeli is a filarial nematode which occurs in nodules of the aorta of cattle and buffalo. It is widely distributed in South East Asia and has also been recorded from Africa. It has no pathogenic significance.

Mammomonogamus laryngeus (syn *Syngamus laryngeus*) occurs in the trachea and *M. nasicola* in the upper trachea and nasal cavities of ruminants and occasionally in man in the tropics. A related species, *M. ierei*, occurs in cats in the West Indies and Sri Lanka and there are several species in elephants. These worms are permanently *in copulo*, the larger female being up to 22 mm long. Their eggs are of the strongyle type. They may cause coughing and loss of condition.

Micronema deletrix is a minute saprophytic nematode which is an occasional parasite of horses. It may cause granulomatous lesions around the face or nares. It has also been reported to invade the central nervous system, where it causes haemorrhagic necrosis and malacia, with signs similar to those of a viral encephalitis. The infection is usually diagnosed *post mortem*, the worms being seen in histological sections.

Parafilaria **spp**. occur in the subcutaneous tissues of equidae and cattle. *P. bovicola* occurs throughout the Old World. It is a slender, white worm up to 60 mm long. Mature females puncture the skin to lay eggs on the surface and there is a haemorrhagic exudate from the lesions. The inflammation and oedema at the sites of infection resemble subcutaneous bruising. Such areas have to be trimmed off at meat inspection and the hides downgraded. Ivermectin or nitroxynil may be used to treat non-lactating cattle; the less effective levamisole may be used in lactating cattle. *P. multipapillosa* is also of some importance as it causes nodular haemorrhagic skin lesions which may incapacitate horses for some months. These parasites have a wide distribution.

Rhabditis bovis is a soil-living nematode, about 1 mm long, which has become adapted to infecting the ears of cattle in East and Central Africa and Brazil. Clinical signs include a putrid discharge from the ear, chronic wasting and a severe drop in milk yield. Intercurrent bacterial infection is common. Central nervous signs and death may result. The infection is usually acquired from contaminated toxaphene in dip tanks but it has been reported that the nematodes are killed by adding nicotine to the dip at 2 p.p.m. Treatment of infected cattle with ivermectin is effective.

Setaria labiato-papillosa (syn. *S. cervi*). The white adults, which are up to 120 mm long in the peritoneal cavity of cattle, are non-pathogenic, but immatures may occur in the spinal canal of horses, sheep and goats, causing a severe disease (cerebrospinal nematodosis), which often results in paralysis or death. This parasite is widely distributed, especially in the Middle and Far East. The closely related but non-pathogenic *S. equina* is often found free in the peritoneal cavity of equids.

Trematodes

Artyfechinostomum malayanum is an echinostome which causes wasting and deaths in pigs and may also be found in dogs in the Indian subcontinent and South East Asia. The mammalian host becomes infected when it eats an infected molluscan host. There are no recommended drugs, but resorantel, bithionol or oxyclozanide would probably be effective.

Eurytrema pancreaticum is a fluke which occurs in the pancreatic ducts of ruminants in Eastern Asia and parts of South America. It measures up to 19 × 9 mm and has the brown, posterior uterus characteristic of the Dicrocoeliidae. It may cause ill-thrift, but is usually of little pathogenicity. The infection is usually diagnosed *post mortem* although the small, brown eggs may be found in the faeces. Land snails are the initial intermediate hosts and grasshoppers the second. Nitroxynil at 20–30 mg/kg/day for 3 days has been reported to be an effective treatment.

Fasciolopsis buski is a large, thick fluke up to 75 × 20 mm, which occurs in the small intestine of man and pigs in Eastern Asia. It may cause severe enteritis with diarrhoea, oedema and ascites. The eggs are brown and up to 140 × 90 μm. The intermediate hosts are water snails. The cercariae encyst on aquatic vegetation, often on the water chestnuts, *Trapa* spp. or *Eliorchis* spp. Praziquantel is the most effective drug.

Heterophyes heterophyes and *Metagonimus yokogawai* very small flukes up to 3 mm long with small brown eggs. They, and a number of related species, occur in the small intestine of dogs, cats and sometimes in man, mainly in Eastern Europe and Asia. They are of low pathogenicity but may cause some enteritis. The intermediate hosts are water snails followed by fish.

Opisthorchis tenuicollis occurs in the bile ducts of cats and less often of dogs, pigs and man in Eastern Europe and Asia. These flukes are up to 12 × 3 mm and do not have the prominent brown posterior uterus seen in the Dicrocoeliidae. The closely related, larger species *O.* (syn. *Clonorchis*) *sinensis*, which occurs in Eastern Asia, is more common in man than the other hosts. These flukes may cause jaundice, ascites and emaciation. Their intermediate hosts are water snails followed by fish. Praziquantel is probably the drug of choice.

Paragonimus **spp.** occur sporadically but widely in pulmonary cysts and aberrant sites in many carnivores and man. They are thick flukes, up to 16 × 8 mm, with large brown eggs up to 120 μm long. The flukes in the lungs cause coughing, while those in other sites may cause various signs including blindness, paralysis and death. Their intermediate hosts are water snails followed by crayfish or crabs. Praziquantel is probably the drug of choice.

Platynosomum fastosum are small flukes up to 8 mm long, which occur in the bile ducts of cats in many tropical areas. They have the posterior, brown uterus characteristic of the Dicrocoeliidae. Small brown eggs up to 50 μm long. May cause diarrhoea, vomiting and jaundice and may be fatal. The three successive intermediate hosts are a land snail, an isopod crustacean and a lizard. A related species, *P. arietis*, occurs in sheep in Brazil, but is probably non-pathogenic. Treatment with praziquantel or nitroscanate is effective.

Diseases caused by protozoa

C.G.D. Brown, A.G. Hunter and A.G. Luckins

BABESIOSIS

The babesioses are tick-borne diseases of domestic, wild and laboratory animals, and of man, caused by protozoa of the genus *Babesia*. These diseases are characterized by fever, haemolytic anaemia, haemoglobinuria, jaundice and, frequently, death. *Babesia* are even more strictly intraerythrocytic parasites than the closely related *Theileria*, organisms of the two genera being collectively known as "piroplasms". Of more than 70 known species of *Babesia*, 18 cause disease in domestic animals, notably in cattle, sheep, goats, horses, pigs, dogs and cats. These diseases occur worldwide, their distribution being dependent on a wide variety of vector ticks through which they are transmitted.

Some of the important *Babesia* spp. which cause disease in domestic animals and man are listed in Table 9. They are described collectively as "large" or "small" on the basis of their size (>3 or <3 μm). Size also serves as a crude indicator of their susceptibility to chemotherapy – the larger the *Babesia* the more susceptible it is to treatment.

Transmission of *Babesia* is by one-, two-or three-host ticks and may be either trans-stadial or transovarian. Most, the so-called "classical" *Babesia* spp., are transmitted transovarially. They are picked up by the engorging adult female and transmitted in the next generation by the larva, nymph or adult. Only the smallest of the *Babesia*, until recently classified as *Nuttallia*, are transmitted trans-stadially, from one stage to the next within one generation of the vector tick's life-cycle. Notable examples of *Babesia* which are transmitted trans-stadially are *Babesia equi* of the horse, mule and donkey and *Babesia microti* of rodents and man.

Babesia are rarely pathogenic to man, normally only affecting immunocompromised hosts, following splenectomy, immunosuppressive chemotherapy or concurrent infection with resultant immunosuppression. A rare epidemiological circumstance in the north-western USA has resulted in *B. microti*, usually a parasite of field rodents, infecting people across the spectrum of the resident human population, though generally only causing disease in the more elderly.

Treatment of babesiosis has been effected, with varying degrees of success, since the earliest days of chemotherapy. Trypan-blue was the first agent used and it is still effective, administered intravenously, against the large *Babesia* spp. Since then, a wide variety of acridine, quinoline and diamidine derivatives have been synthesized and shown to be chemotherapeutically active in the treatment of babesiosis. The choice of drug, route of administration and dose is dependent on a number of factors. These include: the size of the animal, with larger doses per unit weight for smaller species; the *Babesia* spp. to be

Table 9 The common *Babesia* spp. of domestic animals

Animal	*Babesia* spp.	"Large" or "Small"	Principal vectors	Distribution
Cow	*Babesia bigemina*	Large	*Boophilus microplus, Bo. decoloratus, Bo. annulatus, Bo. geigyi*	Central and South America, Africa, Australia, Asia, southern Europe
	B. bovis	Small	*Bo. microplus, Bo. annulata, Bo. geigyi, Ixodes ricinus*	As *B. bigemina*
	B. major	Large	*Haemaphysalis punctata*	Europe, North Africa
	B. divergens	Small	*I. ricinus*	Northern Europe
	B. jakimovi	Large	*I. ricinus*	Northern USSR
	B. ovata	Large	*H. longicornis*	Japan
	B. occultans	Large	*Hyalomma marginatum rufipes*	Southern Africa
Horse, mule, donkeys	*B. caballi*	Large	*Dermacentor (anocentor) nitens, Hyalomma* spp., *Rhicephalus* spp.	Worldwide
	B. equi	Small	As *B. cabilli*	As *B. caballi*
Sheep, goat	*B. motasi*	Large	*Haemaphysalis* spp., *Rhipicephalus* spp.	Asia, Africa, Europe
	B. ovis	Small	*Rhipicephalus* spp.	Africa, Middle East, southern Europe
Pig	*B. trautmanni*	Large	Not known	Africa, USSR, southern Europe
	B. perroncitoi	Small	Not known	Africa, southern Europe
Dog	*B. canis*	Large	*Rhipicephalus sanguineus, Rhipicephalus* spp., *Haemaphysalis* spp.	Africa, southern Europe, Asia, North America
	B. gibsoni	Small	*R. sanguineus, Haemaphysalis bispinosa*	South and East Asia, (southern Europe, North America)
Cat	*B. felis*	Small	Not known	Africa, southern Asia
	B. herpailuri	Large	Not known	Africa
Man	*B. microti*	Small	*Ixodes dammini*	North-west USA
	B. divergens	Small	*I. ricinus*	Europe

Table 10 Treatment of babesiosis

Group	Pharmacological name	Proprietory name	Manufacturer
Acridine derivatives	Acriflavine	Gonacrine	Rhone, Merieux, Baker (RMB) Dagenham, UK
	Flavine, euflavine, trypaflavine	–	–
Diamidine derivatives	Amicarbalide	Diampron	RMB
	Diminazene aceturate	Berenil	Fabwerke Hoechst, Frankfurt, West Germany
		Ganaseg	Squibb, Mexico City, Mexico
	Pentamidine isethionate	–	RMB
	Phenamidine isethionate	Lomadine	RMB
	Propamidine	–	RMB
	Stilbamidine	–	RMB
Quinoline derivatives	Quinuronium sulphate	Acaprine (Ludabal)	Farbenfabriken Bayer, Leverkusen, West Germany
		Babesan	ICI, Wilmslow, UK
		Pirevan, Akron, Baburon	–
		Pyroplasmin	
Others	Imidocarb	Imizol	Coopers Animal Health, Crewe, UK
	Trypan blue, haemosporidin, novoplasmin	–	–

treated, as the "small" *Babesia* may be retractory or may need a larger dose of the same drug than the more sensitive "large" species; the host animal to be treated, as dogs and cats experience toxic side-effects more readily than other species, while horses often exhibit severe local reactions. The babesicides commonly used in the treatment of babesiosis in domestic animals are listed in Table 10.

Of these drugs, the most widely used and effective are diminazene, imidocarb, amicarbalide, quinuronium and phenamidine. The aim of treatment is normally to promote recovery from clinical disease while allowing some organisms to persist in order to allow the animal to develop an immunity to the disease. Too rapid a cure, when treatment is administered early, can result in the subject being susceptible to reinfection. Thus, while early diagnosis is important, particularly in peracute, fulminating disease such as can be seen in canine babesiosis in young puppies or bovine babesiosis in adult cattle, treatment which immediately sterilizes the infection should, if possible, be avoided. Selection of drug and dosage is therefore most important. Chemotherapy can also be used prophylactically, in the face of an anticipated challenge, and also for legal or public health requirements, to sterilize infections, particularly in animals to be moved from one country to another. This is mainly done with horses – show jumpers, polo ponies and racehorses.

Bovine babesiosis

Aetiology

Bovine babesiosis is caused by one of four species of *Babesia*. In temperate zones, *Babesia divergens* is usually the causative organism, but *B. major* is sometimes implicated. In tropical areas, the parasite is either *B. bigemina* or *B. bovis*. The babesias appear within red blood cells as non-pigmented, pear-shaped organisms which reproduce by binary fission. Two organisms are thereby commonly seen together, with their narrow ends in apposition. Irregularly shaped amoeboid forms are also seen. "Large" species may be nearly as long as the parasitized cell (6 μm), whereas "small" species may be only 1.5 μm in length.

Occurrence

Bovine babesiosis has a worldwide distribution related largely to the distribution of the vector ticks. The incidence of the infection can be seasonally dependent on the occurrence and activity of the vectors.

B. divergens occurs in temperate climates in Northern, Western and Central Europe. *B. major* occurs in Europe, the USSR and North America. *B. bovis* (syn. *Babesia argentina*) occurs in South and Central America, Europe, the USSR, Africa and Australia. It has recently also been reported from the southern states of the USA. *B. bigemina* occurs in North, Central and South America, parts of Europe, the Middle East, North, Central and South Africa and Australia. These last two organisms are the important causes of babesiosis of cattle in the tropics and subtropical regions of the world, where some 600 million cattle are at risk.

Transmission

B. bovis and *B. bigemina* are primarily transmitted by one-host ticks of the genus *Boophilus*, which are distributed worldwide between latitudes 32°S and 40°N. The principal species of tick involved are:

1. *Boophilus microplus* (Cattle tick): Asia, Australia, Mexico, Central and South America (not Chile), West Indies, Indonesia, Malaysia, the Philippines, Southern and Eastern Africa and Malagasy. It is not native to Africa where its distribution is irregular.
2. *Boophilus decoloratus* (Blue tick): Africa south of the Sahara.
3. *Boophilus annulatus* (Texas fever tick): Mexico, Central America, Egypt, Sudan, Asia Minor, the Mediterranean Basin and North Yemen.

    B. bovis and *B. bigemina* are both transmitted by *Bo. microplus* and *Bo. annulatus* and, in parts of the world where both *Babesia* parasites exist, *B. bovis* is generally the more pathogenic. *Bo. decoloratus* can only transmit *B. bigemina* and thus in Africa, where this is the most common *Boophilus* species present, *B. bigemina* assumes greater importance than *B. bovis*.

    Transmission through these one-host ticks is transovarial. Following detachment, the infected, engorged, adult female *Boophilus* ticks pass the *Babesia* to the larvae of the next generation through the eggs. Following attachment to a new host, infection is transmitted by the larval stages (*B. bovis*) or by the nymph and adult stages (*B. bovis* and *B. bigemina*).

Clinical features

The clinical signs of infection with *B. bovis* and *B. bigemina* are similar except that *B. bovis* is generally more pathogenic. However, although *B. bigemina* is itself less pathogenic, it frequently occurs with other infections and may exert a synergistic pathogenicity. Notably in Africa, it may give rise to a peracute, fulminating disease with very a high parasitaemia. *B. bovis* infections, other than in splenectomized calves, normally exhibit low parasitaemias ($<1\%$).

    Adult cattle are more susceptible to infection than calves. Clinical signs can be acute and severe, or mild with parasitaemic episodes lasting 1–3 weeks.

    Following infection, the parasites multiply within the host's erythrocytes. Escaping parasites destroy the infected erythrocytes and invade new erythrocytes. The released parasite and host constituents from destroyed erythrocytes are toxic, resulting in various physiological disturbances and shock. The destruction of erythrocytes causes anaemia and tissue anoxia and the release of excessive amounts of haemoglobin results in icterus (jaundice) and haemoglobinuria (red water). This last is regarded as pathognomonic and has given rise to the descriptive term for the disease, i.e. "redwater".

    Although the incubation period of *B. bovis* (the time from tick attachment to the appearance of parasites in the erythrocytes) is variable, depending on such factors as the weight of infection, it is normally in the range 8–16 days. The incubation period for *B. bigemina* is at least 9 days longer, because infection is not transmitted until the nymph stage of the tick begins to feed. The first sign is pyrexia, which may be sudden in onset, due to the parasites multiplying. Animals become listless, anorexic, anaemic and jaundiced. Other signs are haemoglobinuria, dehydration and general weakness. Severe cases of *B. bovis* infection may end terminally with CNS signs (ataxia, paddling of limbs, coma) associated with sludging of parasitized red blood cells in brain capillaries.

Animals that survive acute early disease may have diarrhoea due to alimentary disturbances; later, animals may become constipated.

Diagnosis

A fever, associated with haemoglobinuria, anaemia and jaundice with the demonstration of *Babesia* spp. in the red blood cells is considered diagnostic.

Smears made from peripheral blood, fixed and stained with Giemsa or another Romanowsky stain, reveal the maximum numbers of parasitized red cells during the thermal reaction. With remission, the numbers of parasites diminish and can be so sparse as to be difficult to detect in blood smears. This is particularly so with *B. bovis*, which shows a marked tendency to accumulate in capillaries, especially those of the brain. In animals examined *post mortem*, it is useful to make brain crush preparations which often reveal, in *B. bovis* infection, capillaries packed with red cells, many of them parasitized. In chronic infections, finding parasites is sometimes facilitated by using direct acridine orange staining and scanning on the microscope with ultra-violet illumination.

The *post mortem* changes are those of a haemolytic anaemia. Apart from the cerebral form of the disease caused by blockage of the brain capillaries, the pathological changes are concurrent with destruction of the red blood cells. Anaemia of the carcase is marked. There is degeneration of the kidneys and liver; the gall bladder is enlarged and distended with dark green bile; the spleen is enlarged and friable and the pulp is very fluid in consistency. The lungs are often oedematous and bloodstained fluid sometimes occurs in the pericardium. Petechiation is seen in many tissues and the kidneys are often congested. Haemorrhagic areas and streaks are found in the mucous membranes of the gastrointestinal tract. The carcase is often jaundiced and the urine stained pink or red with haemoglobin.

In addition to the appearance of the parasites as seen under the microscope, differentiation from infections such as anaplasmosis and theileriosis can be assisted by checking the response to babesicidal drugs, which will provoke a rapid recovery where *Babesia* is the primary pathogen. Other aids to clinical diagnosis are the detection of haemoglobin in the urine, an increased bleeding time, reduced red cell count, packed cell volume and haemoglobin concentration and accelerated red blood cell sedimentation.

If there is anaemia and jaundice with no haemoglobinuria, anaplasmosis must be considered. Cases of cerebral babesiosis are easily confused with heartwater, but examining the capillaries microscopically in brain crush preparations readily facilitates the differentiation of these two diseases in the dead animal. In the living animal, reliance is usually placed on clinical differences and the detection of babesial parasites in capillary blood.

Epidemiology

The distribution of bovine babesiosis caused by *B. bovis* and *B. bigemina* is confined strictly to the distribution of their vector ticks. This is particularly marked in Africa, to which the tick *Boophilus microplus* was introduced at the end of the last century. *Babesia bovis* is only present in those areas of Africa to which *Bo. microplus* has spread, because the indigenous African "blue tick" (*Bo. decoloratus*) only transmits *B. bigemina*.

Ticks other than *Boophilus* spp. have been cited as vectors but they are relatively unimportant. Similarly, mechanical transmission by biting flies, surgical instruments, etc., although theoretically possible, is unimportant.

On recovery from initial infection, cattle are immune but harbour the parasite (premune), and may remain carriers for up to 2 years. In enzootic areas, constant reinfection ensures that such cattle remain carriers permanently, although the premunity may break down due to other factors such as stress or intercurrent disease, resulting in clinical babesiosis. Calves are less susceptible than adults and, if cattle are infected in calfhood, clinical signs may be minimal. Thus in enzootic areas, two epidemiological states are recognized:

1. *Enzootic stability*: The continuous presence of *Babesia* in both cattle and ticks with frequent acquisition of the parasite from active infective ticks ensures that cattle are infected in calfhood and remain carriers due to constant reinfection. Under these conditions, clinical babesiosis is minimal.
2. *Enzootic instability*: The infection rate of *Babesia* is such that not all cattle are infected as calves, and therefore some animals remain susceptible. If these are infected as adults, they may suffer severe clinical reactions. Such conditions arise when the numbers of infected ticks fluctuate due to factors such as seasonal variation, drought, dipping and pasture spelling.

Serology

A number of excellent serological procedures are available which can be applied to the serodiagnosis of bovine babesiosis. Chronologically, the procedures were developed and applied in the following order:

1. Complement fixation test (CFT)
2. Indirect fluorescent antibody test (IFAT)
3. Indirect haemagglutination test (IHA)
4. Other agglutination tests (latex, slide, card, capillary)
5. Radioimmunoassay (RIA)
6. Enzyme-linked immunosorbent assay (ELISA)

The most widely used procedures have been the CFT, IFAT and, most recently, ELISA. ELISA has, perhaps, the most potential. It is a highly sensitive test which is not subject to operator interpretation. The assay at present needs some technically sophisticated equipment and good laboratory facilities for preparation of the antigen and for reading the test. With present antigens, it is less specific than CFT or IFAT, giving limited discrimination between the different pathogenic species of *Babesia*. However, there are immediate prospects of defined antigens prepared by fractionation of the whole organism or by genetic engineering with cloned recombinant material. Such antigens should provide a durable test of high sensitivity and specificity.

Serodiagnosis is an invaluable tool in epidemiological studies of bovine babesiosis. Cattle which have been infected may have antibodies which are detectable for many years after infection and for some time (months, years) after the parasite has been eliminated. Thus the presence of antibodies will show that an animal has been infected and, probably, that it is immune, though not necessarily that it is carrying the infection. Seroepidemiological surveys, which give a prevalence rate in cattle across age cohorts, can help define the epidemiological balance in the population and determine strategies for controlling the disease.

Further anticipated progress in diagnostic technology includes the development of an antigen detection ELISA, using monoclonal antibodies to detect circulating antigen in infected cattle, and of DNA probes to detect miniscule amounts of parasite DNA in an infected animal.

Treatment

Large species of *Babesia* are more sensitive, and hence more responsive, to chemotherapy than small species. Thus *B. bigemina* and *B. major* require lower doses for both clinical cure and elimination of the parasite than do *B. bovis* and *B. divergens*. Selection of drug and dose rate are important, as most babesicides are quite toxic (see Table 10).

In the tropics, two drugs – diminazene aceturate and imidocarb diproprionate – are perhaps the drugs of choice. However, quinuronium sulphate, phenamidine and many other agents have been widely used. Diminazene is highly effective against *B. bigemina* at levels as low as 2 mg/kg, but needs to be used at 5 mg/kg to treat *B. bovis* infections, at which level it will probably not sterilize the infection. Imidocarb is very active and effective against both organisms, curative doses of 0.5–1.0 mg/kg being used.

Both diminazene and imidocarb are prophylactic if used at high doses – diminazene giving some protection for 2–3 weeks and imidocarb for 6–8 weeks. Care must thus be taken, particularly with imidocarb, if it is being used in conjunction with vaccination with living organisms.

The efficacy of treatment of clinical bovine babesiosis depends greatly on early diagnosis and the prompt administration of appropriate drugs. Because, in acute infections, anaemia will be severe, supportive therapy and management are important. Fluid replacement and even blood transfusion may be indicated in extreme cases. If so, a single early administration of a large volume of blood will avoid the problems of blood matching.

Immunology

Calves possess an innate resistance enhanced by maternal antibodies, but susceptibility to the disease increases with age. *Bos taurus* cattle appear more susceptible to the disease than *Bos indicus*. Recovery is followed by a period of immunity, variously reported as lasting for months or years, and is associated for most of this time with the persistence of the organism in the peripheral blood (co-infectious immunity or premunity). This carrier state, however, can be broken down by stress factors such as calving, or concurrent disease, and clinical signs may reappear. Reinfection at the time of declining immunity has been reported to produce an occult infection and to raise the level of residual parasitaemia.

The occasional phenomenon of a recently recovered animal succumbing to a second and fatal attack after being moved to new but possibly nearby grazing, may be due to the existence of different antigenic types within a species of *Babesia*. Animals which have recovered from *B. bigemina* infection may show some resistance to *B. bovis* but the converse is not the case.

Immunity to babesiosis is both humoral and cellular. It can be transferred passively with serum and adoptively with spleen cells to a syngeneic recipient. It is normally induced by infection of the animal with live organisms, with recovery of the animal being a consequence of one or more of chemotherapy, innate resistance (e.g. by infecting calves rather than adult cattle), or the use of attenuated organisms. It has been shown that crude, killed antigens can be used to immunize cattle, but they require adjuvants such as Freund's complete adjuvant to be effective and so are presently unacceptable for field use.

At present, vaccination of cattle against babesiosis is widely practised, particularly against *B. bovis* infection. A "blood" vaccine is used, based on traditional methods used since the turn of the century, whereby calves are "premunized" by deliberate infection with blood from a cow known to have had, and hence to be carrying, the infection. The system has been refined in Australia to use defined numbers of infected erythrocytes containing parasites attenuated by specific methods of passage. For *B. bovis*, the method is rapid passage in splenectomized calves; for *B. bigemina*, it is slow passage in intact calves followed by splenectomy to induce relapse. Such "attenuated" parasite stocks are obtained in bulk by bleeding out the infected splenectomized calves by carotid cannulation, counting the infected RBCs and diluting the blood with a buffered isotonic diluent containing bovine serum to give the number of parasites needed to get the required, reliable infectivity, yet with the minimal number of red cells present as undesirable antigen. This "vaccine" may be kept in wet ice or at 4–10°C for 5–7 days, or indefinitely stabilized at −196°C in liquid nitrogen, using DMSO or glycerol as cryopreservatives. In this frozen state, the vaccine can be shipped around the world.

Such vaccines are very effective in inducing immunity and promoting or maintaining enzootic stability in a population, as the organisms, although attenuated, are generally still infective for ticks. However, great care must be taken in the production to ensure that no diseases are transmitted with the vaccine. Scrupulous care must be taken with each of the components, particularly to ensure the disease-free status of the infected donor and of the cattle used to provide serum for diluent.

Recent developments in Australia and the USA give hope for defined *Babesia* antigens, particularly of *B. bovis*, which have been engineered by recombinant DNA technology and may provide a subunit or peptide vaccine against bovine babesiosis. Until such a vaccine is produced, however, the live vaccines presently available are invaluable tools for controlling the disease.

Control

Control measures which are currently applied to bovine babesiosis are immunization of susceptible stock, treatment of infected animals, control of ticks by use of acaricides or cattle resistant to ticks, and control of stock movement.

In areas of endemic infection, where all indigenous cattle are infected as calves, no control is usually necessary, but babesiosis is an important barrier to livestock improvement as imported, improved breeds are usually very susceptible. Such importations should only be carried out with animals immunized prior to importation, immunized immediately after arrival or brought into a locally tick-free environment. Reliance on drugs to control infection is possible only in situations where the animals can be frequently and individually examined.

The most difficult control situation occurs when the vector distribution in a country is very localized. Infected areas must then be defined and stock movements controlled both in and out.

The decision in relation to control of bovine babesiosis, with which anaplasmosis due to the nature of its transmission is nearly always inextricably associated, is whether to go for a "disease-free" situation or to aim for "enzootic stability". This decision is usually quite clear-cut and, where this is not so, can be made with the help of controlled seroepidemiological studies to define the prevalence rate of infection in cattle. This, coupled with some assessment of the incidence of the disease as a clinical entity, the numbers of ticks on cattle and hence the transmission rate of the infection, will provide the information needed to define the threat posed by the disease.

In simple terms, where the disease is a continual threat, the creation and maintenance of a state of enzootic stability should be the target. It is then a question of balancing the damage caused by the ticks, which in Australia and South America are in the main *Bo. microplus*, but in Africa include many tick species, against the dangers posed by babesiosis and other tick-borne diseases to a susceptible cattle population. It is, for example, safer to reduce the dipping frequency if the cattle are potentially tick-resistant *Bos indicus*. Some form of protection against ticks must be provided for taurine cattle. At present, this is afforded by strategic dipping, aiming to control the ticks but not the disease they transmit. In future, there is the potential of tick vaccines. Cattle otherwise susceptible to babesiosis must be protected against the disease. Vaccination can achieve this. Subsequent maintenance of the enzootically stable state is then dependent on maternal antibodies, inherent calfhood resistance and ensuring that calves are exposed to the infection while they are most resistant. If the challenge is still sporadic, continual vaccination of the calf crop from year to year may be necessary.

It is important to place control of bovine babesiosis within the overall disease control strategy, particularly within the strategy for control of tick-borne disease. The use of acaricides to control other ticks transmitting other diseases may have an unexpected effect on babesiosis transmission. For example, short-interval dipping for two-or three-host ticks will dramatically alter the population of one-host *Boophilus* spp. However, *Boophilus* is normally the first tick to develop resistance to novel acaricides. The consequences may then be catastrophic.

Equine babesiosis

Aetiology

Equine babesiosis is caused by *Babesia caballi* and *B. equi*. *B. caballi* resembles *B. bigemina*, the large species which affects cattle, but *B. equi* is only 2 μm long, and exhibits rounded, amoeboid or pear-shaped forms. These last can be found in a group joined by their pointed ends indicating that binary division has occurred twice ("Maltese cross" forms). These small *Babesia*, which apparently divide into four in this manner, have, until recently, been classified as *Nuttallia*. A further distinction from most *Babesia* spp. is that *B. equi*, like *B. microti*, is transmitted trans-stadially and not transovarially. Yet another, most significant, recent finding has been that *B. equi* has, like *Theileria*, an exoerythrocytic cycle in lymphoid mononuclear cells. Such small *Babesia* may thus prove indeed to be members of another genus, perhaps intermediate between *Babesia* and *Theileria*.

Occurrence

Equine babesiosis is present throughout the world wherever the tick vectors of *B. caballi* and *B. equi* exist. The disease is reported from North, Central and South Africa, South and Central America and the USA, Southern and Eastern Europe including the USSR, Asia Minor, the Middle East and India. *B. equi* appears to be somewhat more widespread than *B. caballi*.

Species affected

Horses, mules and donkeys are susceptible to infection with either of the two *Babesia* species. Other equines are likely to be infected by these *Babesia* spp. For example, both are said to be capable of infecting Burchell's zebra (*Equus burchelli*), which can act as a carrier of these parasities.

Transmission

Ticks of the genera *Dermacentor*, *Hyalomma* and *Rhipicephalus* are directly responsible for the transmission of both these *Babesia* spp. It would appear that, while *B. caballi* is transmitted transovarially from one generation of the tick to the next, *B. equi* is transmitted trans-stadially, most commonly from nymph to adult within a generation.

Both organisms can be transmitted mechanically, but there is little evidence for the role of this method in the field.

Clinical features

B. equi is the more pathogenic of the two species and can cause acute disease involving fever, anaemia, haemoglobinuria and jaundice. *B. caballi* causes a persistent fever and anaemia. However, clinical infections with both species can easily be overlooked, particularly where a concurrent infection with another disease has caused a breakdown of premunity.

Pathology

Parasitaemia and other changes in the blood are similar to those seen in bovine babesiosis. *Post mortem* features are also similar, but jaundice is more common and haemoglobinuria occurs less frequently – hence the synonym "biliary fever".

Diagnosis

As with other *Babesia* infections of domestic animals, a fever associated with anaemia, jaundice and haemoglobinuria and the demonstration of *Babesia*-infected red blood cells is diagnostic. However, chronic cases are difficult to diagnose because the signs may be obscure, with haemoglobinuria absent and parasitaemias low. Confusion with infectious equine anaemia easily occurs where this disease is also endemic. Useful techniques in addition to Giemsa staining of blood films include: concentration by centrifugation of the blood, as red blood cells infected with *B. caballi* are less dense and concentrate under the buffy coat, and examination of blood films stained with acridine orange under ultra-violet light. Estimation of bilirubin can also be used as an aid to diagnosis.

Epizootiology

The disease is maintained in the tick by the transovarial transmission of the organism (*B. caballi*) and recovered carrier equine animals remain a source of infection to the tick population. Prenatal infection of horses has been reported more often than with canine or bovine babesiosis, but is exceptional.

Immunology

Young animals are the least susceptible to infection. Recovered animals have an immunity lasting 12–24 months with an associated persistence of the organism in the blood. However, this premunity is easily broken down by physical stress or concurrent disease leading to a chronic infection.

Serology

Few serological tests are available for the routine assessment of disease prevalence. They are presently most important in the diagnosis of infection in individual horses being moved from one country to the next, such as 3-day eventers to the Olympic Games, racehorses and show jumpers around Europe, polo ponies between North, Central and South America.

The most commonly used procedures are the complement fixation test (CFT) and indirect fluorescent antibody tests (IFAT). Neither are appropriate for detecting the infection in its early stages but are reliable, though perhaps subjective, in picking up carrier animals in which it is difficult to detect the parasite in the blood.

Treatment

The horse is a particularly difficult subject for treatment, showing severe reactions to many babesicides, particularly if they are used at levels high enough to sterilize infections. *B. equi* is much more resistant than *B. caballi* to chemotherapy and requires high doses of drugs, which are often irritant, to eliminate the infection. Sterilization of carrier animals is most frequently required in the most valuable and hence most highly bred and sensitive horses; this compounds the problem.

While diminazene (5 mg/kg) and amicarbalide (8 mg/kg) are both highly effective, when administered with care, against *B. caballi*, and other babesicides are also active against this parasite, only imidocarb can sterilize *B. equi* infections. Even this cannot be achieved with certainty. Imidocarb may be used to treat clinical *B. equi* infection at dose levels around 2 mg/kg, but repeated doses as high as 5 mg/kg are used in attempts to sterilize *B. equi* infections. These are dangerously close to the toxic limit.

Control

The general principles of control are the same as those for bovine babesiosis, namely either to eliminate the disease and break the tick – horse contact or to induce and maintain infections deliberately. There is no commercial vaccine yet available, but infection of the young horse, carefully monitored, is a pragmatic approach in situations where it will be infected in any event.

Ovine and caprine babesiosis

Aetiology

Two species of *Babesia* are mainly responsible for babesiosis in sheep and goats. These are *B. motasi*, a large form, and *B. ovis*, a small form.

Occurrence

Babesiosis of sheep and goats is widespread in Europe, the Middle East and most tropical and subtropical regions.

Transmission

Ticks of the genera *Rhipicephalus*, *Haemaphysalis*, *Dermacentor* and *Ixodes* transmit these parasites and, depending on the vector involved, the parasites can pass through the egg or from stage to stage.

Clinical features

The diseases caused by *B. motasi* and *B. ovis* correspond in most characteristics with those caused in cattle by *B. bigemina* and *B. bovis*, respectively.

Diagnosis

The acute form has characteristic clinical signs and can be confirmed by microscopic examination. Cases which die suddenly may be confused with anthrax, particularly in view of the splenic enlargement, but jaundice and haemoglobinuria are characteristic of *Babesia* infection. Milder forms can only be diagnosed with certainty by demonstration of the parasite in the blood.

Immunology

As with *Babesia* in cattle, indigenous sheep in enzootic areas usually acquire a mild infection and are immune thereafter. Severe infections usually occur in adult sheep. Immunization can be effected by inoculation of infected blood and treatment of any severe reaction which results.

Serology

Serological tests are being developed, with prospects for an ELISA which will help considerably in understanding the epidemiology of the disease.

Treatment

This is approached as for bovine babesiosis. The same drugs are applicable for treatment, though quinuronium sulphate has perhaps been most widely used.

Control

Dipping is not regularly practised with sheep, other than one or two seasonal immersions in acaricide. The approach should be to establish a stable situation and to eliminate the opportunity for sporadic or, particularly, for epidemic infection in a flock.

Porcine babesiosis

The vectors of the two porcine babesias, *B. trautmanni* (large) and *B. perroncitoi* (small), have not been determined. *B. trautmanni* infection has been recorded in the USSR, Southern Europe and Africa and is supposedly more widespread than *B. perroncitoi*, which has only been recorded in Sudan, Sardinia and Italy. Transovarial transmission of *B. trautmanni* by *Rhipicephalus sanguineus* has been recorded.

Clinical signs of both infections are indistinguishable and typical of babesiosis, with fever, anaemia, jaundice and haemoglobinuria. The organisms' susceptibility to drugs is, respectively, similar to that of the large and small babesias of other domestic hosts.

Canine babesiosis

Aetiology

B. canis and *B. gibsoni* are responsible for the infection in dogs. They correspond in most characteristics to *B. bigemina* and *B. bovis* in cattle. *B. canis* is a large species, typically pear-shaped and approximately 5 μm in length. Multiple infection of the erythrocytes often occurs. *B. gibsoni* is a small species, most often appearing as annular or oval bodies but, occasionally, larger oval or elongate forms half the width of the host cell are found.

Occurrence

B. canis is reported from Africa, Asia, Southern Europe, the USSR, Central and South America and limited areas of the USA. *B. gibsoni* has a more limited distribution in India, Ceylon and the Far East, including Japan and parts of China.

Species affected

Domestic dogs of all breeds are susceptible to both species of *Babesia*, as are jackals (*Canis mesomelas*) and the wolf (*Canis lupus*). In addition, the fox (*Vulpes* spp.) is susceptible to *B. gibsoni*.

Transmission

B. canis is transmitted by ticks of the genera *Rhipicephalus*, *Dermacentor*, *Hyalomma* and *Haemaphysalis*, and *B. gibsoni* by ticks of the genera *Haemaphysalis* and *Rhipicephalus*. Transovarian transmission occurs in some species of tick and stage to stage transmission in others. Thus the organisms can survive in the tick population by transovarian infection from one generation to another. A carrier state occurs in recovered dogs and can be assumed to occur in wild carnivores, so providing a reservoir of infection in the mammalian part of the cycle.

Clinical features

Signs can vary from a mild fever lasting several days before the onset of anaemia to an acute disease involving a sudden high fever, marked anaemia and haemoglobinuria, with a later development of jaundice. Susceptible dogs imported into an area where *B. canis* infection is endemic, may die within a day of the signs first being noticed, but *B. gibsoni* usually produces a more chronic disease. Cerebral forms of babesiosis causing hyperexcitability can occur. Other clinical forms of canine babesiosis are common, depending on the individual animals, their degree of resistance and the nature of the infecting organism. They include episodes in which the alimentary tract appears to be involved, producing stomatitis, gastritis and enteritis; a predominantly respiratory form; a circulatory form which is marked by oedema; a form in which keratitis and iritis are noticeable; and a muscular form in which the signs give the impression that the animal is suffering from rheumatism.

Pathology

The pathology of canine babesiosis is that of anaemia varying from a very marked and rapidly developing type in highly susceptible dogs to a more chronic manifestation, with jaundice, in dogs reared in an endemic area. Except where adult dogs are introduced into an area where the parasites occur, the disease tends to manifest itself primarily in young pups, which are the susceptible population. There appears to be no equivalent of the "calfhood immunity" of bovine babesiosis. Puppies may get a series of infections or relapse infections in the first year of life, with a gradual development of immunity, as in malaria in man.

Diagnosis

Diagnosis in uncomplicated cases is based on the presence of a fever, haemoglobinuria and anaemia, together with the demonstration of *Babesia* spp. in a blood smear.

If facilities for examining a blood smear are not immediately available, treatment is desirable even without microscopic confirmation, as in acute cases delay may result in death of the patient. Diagnosis may be complicated by a concurrent infection with canine rickettsiosis. The presence of rickettsial bodies as clusters of cocci in monocytes and neutrophils, with some signs similar to those of babesiosis but with erosions of mucosa and skin and evidence of oedema, suggests infection with *Ehrlichia canis*. This pathogen is transmitted by the same species of ticks as those which transmit *B. canis*. If the cerebral form of canine babesiosis occurs, it is always wise to keep in mind the possibility of rabies infection. In cerebral babesiosis, examination of smears or sections of the brain should show the smaller capillaries packed with infected erythrocytes.

Treatment

Phenamidine isethionate, diminazene aceturate and imidocarb diproprionate are the most effective babesicides against *B. canis*. *B. gibsoni* is less amenable to treatment but large doses of diminazene aceturate (5–10 mg/kg) or imidocarb appear to be the most promising treatments. Care must be taken with high doses of certain drugs, notably the diamidines (e.g. diminazene, phenamidine), in dogs, because they may induce severe, sometimes fatal, toxicity.

Immunology

Recovered dogs have an immunity coincidental with, but not necessarily dependent on, the continued presence of the organism in the peripheral blood. Immunity lasts up to 2 years in the absence of reinfection. Where clinical infection occurs more than once, the phenomenon can be explained as a breakdown of the premunity under stress, by the occurrence of different antigenic types, or by the dog having been kept out of contact with the vector.

The resistance of young animals to *Babesia* infections does not apply to dogs, as acute babesiosis due to *B. canis* can occur in puppies under 6 months of age.

Control

Dog owners have a choice of either attempting to keep their animals free of ticks and seeking early diagnosis and treatment if infection is suspected, or attempting to immunize their animals by exposure to the natural disease, with careful observation so that treatment can be administered at the first signs of clinical infection. The removal of ticks by hand, together with frequent application of suitable acaricides, is important in the prevention of infection.

A recent, exciting development has been the release of an inactivated vaccine against *B. canis* based on an antigen harvested from the supernatants of cultures of that organism in canine red cells. This vaccine, presently released in the south of France and in South Africa, will perhaps change the approach to control of canine babesiosis. However, the epidemiological impact of the use of such a vaccine will need to be studied carefully.

C.G.D.B.

BESNOITIOSIS

Besnoitiosis is a disease of cattle and Equidae caused by *Besnoitia* parasites which are obligatory two-host coccidial parasites. The disease is characterized by the formation of cysts in connective and cutaneous tissues of the bovine and equine intermediate hosts.

Aetiology

There are two species of veterinary importance. *Besnoitia besnoiti* is a parasite of cattle and various African wild ruminants; the final host is a felid. *B. bennetti* is a parasite of horses, asses and burros, but the final host is unknown.

In the final host, *B. besnoiti* has typical coccidial stages of development in the intestine leading to faecal excretion of oocysts. In the intermediate host, *Besnoitia* parasites are crescent-shaped organisms up to 9 μm in length, slightly pointed at one end and rounded at the other. Following initial infection of the intermediate host, the parasite multiplies in mononuclear cells in various parts of the body, but, as infection proceeds, the parasites develop in dermal cysts up to 0.6 mm in diameter containing the parasites.

Occurrence

B. besnoiti infection has been recorded most frequently in southern Africa (South Africa, Botswana, Mozambique, Angola), but also in Central and East Africa, Israel, France, the Iberian peninsula and the USSR and it may have a worldwide distribution. *B. bennetti* infection has been recorded in Africa, Europe, Mexico and the USA.

Species affected

B. besnoiti infection occurs in cattle and various wild ruminants. In cattle, it can cause severe disease. *B. bennetti* is a similar parasite of Equidae.

Transmission

Until recently, the transmission of these parasites was not known. It has now been shown that cats can be the final host of *B. besnoiti* but the final host of *B. bennetti* is unknown. Intermediate hosts are infected by ingestion of sporulated oocysts from faeces of infected cats. It is probable, however, that other forms of transmission take place. Infection can be transmitted mechanically under experimental conditions by injections of blood of infected animals in the early febrile stage of the disease, or by inoculation of parasites from ruptured cysts, and it is suspected that infection can be transmitted mechanically by biting flies (experimental infection has been transmitted mechanically to rabbits by *Glossina* sp.).

Clinical features

Cattle over the age of 6 months are susceptible and the course of clinical besnoitiosis is divided into two stages:

1. *Acute febrile stage*: Following an incubation period of 6–10 days, cattle become febrile due to the multiplication of the parasites in mononuclear cells. Cattle may have fever up to 107°F, photophobia, anasarca, diarrhoea and enlargement of the lymph nodes. Orchitis and sterility may occur in bulls. Warm painful swellings occur on the ventral abdomen; lacrimation and nasal discharge may occur. The febrile stage lasts 2–10 days, and mortality rates may reach 10%. Oedema of the eye-lids and conjunctivitis has been observed in acute cases in cattle in the USSR. The febrile stage may be mild with little clinical change and recovery, but more severe cases may progress to the second stage.

2. *Chronic seborrheic stage*: In association with multiplication of the parasites in cysts in cutaneous tissues, the skin becomes thickened and wrinkled (scleroderma) and hair may fall out (alopecia). Denuded areas of skin become scurfy, cracked, secondary infected and fly-blown. Death occurs in severe cases. Recovered animals remain permanent carriers of cysts which contain numerous parasites. Cysts may also develop in the conjunctival selera. Chronic orchitis and epididymitis with calcification of the testicles may occur in bulls.

Besnoitiosis in horses caused by *B. bennetti* is similar to the disease in cattle, but is less severe and protracted.

Pathology

Early in the infection of the intermediate host the parasites multiply extracellularly or in blood monocytes. As infection progresses, parasites invade the dermis, subcutaneous tissues, mucosae of the upper respiratory tract, eye-lids and elsewhere. As the parasites multiply in the tissues, the intermediate host reacts by forming cysts (pseudocysts) to contain the parasites. Pseudocysts packed with thousands of the parasites can reach 600 μm in diameter.

Diagnosis

The early stages of clinical bovine besnoitiosis could be confused with bovine malignant catarrh. The later stages of the disease must be differentiated from other skin conditions, e.g. lumpy skin disease, photosensitization, streptothricosis and sweating sickness. Diagnosis is based on clinical signs and demonstration of subcutaneous cysts containing the typical banana-shaped parasites (bradyzoites). Conjunctival cyst formation is regarded as diagnostic in South Africa.

Treatment

There is no specific therapy but symptomatic treatment may be applied. Experimentally, sulphadiazine and pyrimethamine are effective against murine besnoitiosis.

Immunology

Infected intermediate hosts may become permanent carriers of the parasites in cysts. Antibodies can be detected by a complement fixation test.

Control

Clinical cases should be segregated. Fly control may be indicated.

A live tissue culture vaccine prepared from a strain of *B. besnoiti* isolated from blue wildebeest has been developed in South Africa and is reported to give good results in cattle, although it does not prevent subclinical infection.

Further reading

Bigalke, R.D. *et al.* (1974). Studies in cattle on the development of a live vaccine against bovine besnoitiosis. *Journal of South African Veterinary Medical Association*, **45**, 207–209.
Soulsby, E.J.L. (1986). Besnoitia. In *Helminths, arthropods and protozoa of domesticated animals*, pp. 686–687. Baillière Tindall, London.

A.G.H.

CANINE LEISHMANIOSIS

Leishmaniosis is an infectious disease of man and other mammals that manifests itself in various forms, and which can be classified into two main groups, the visceral and the cutaneous. Asymptomatic infections in a wide range of wild animals commonly occur.

Aetiology

Leishmaniosis is caused by several species of *Leishmania*, the taxonomy of which is very complex, but it is generally accepted that there are four main groups of the parasite, namely the *L. donovani*, *L. tropica*, *L. mexicana* and *L. braziliensis* groups. The various species and subspecies are morphologically identical and closely related anti-genically. The parasites occur as rounded oval amastigotes, 2–3 μm in diameter in the vertebrate host, and as promastigotes in the arthropod vector. In the vertebrate host, the parasite inhabits macrophages and other reticulo-endothelial cells, in which it multiplies by binary fission until the host cell ruptures and other cells are infected by the released parasites. In the invertebrate hosts, which are various species of sandfly, the parasites develop extracellularly either in the mid-gut or in the oesophagus and pharynx. Here they are found as the motile flagellated promastigote form.

Occurrence

Leishmaniosis is widely distributed in its various forms. It is prevalent in the countries of the Mediterranean basin including North Africa and the countries of Southern Europe from Spain to Greece. It is found in Central and South America, India, Central Asia, China, the southern USSR, Sudan, Ethiopia, East and West Africa. Climatically, it is associated with those areas and periods in which sandflies are common, although because of the variable and sometimes long periods of incubation it is difficult to define seasonal incidence.

Species affected

Leishmaniosis is primarily a disease of man and dog, but lizards and many species of wild mammals are the principal hosts, many acting as asymptomatic reservoirs of infection to dogs and man. The distribution and hosts of the important species are shown in Table 11.

Transmission

The disease is transmitted by species of sandfly – *Phlebotomus* spp. in the Old World and *Lutzomyia* spp. in the New World. On commencing to feed, the vector ejects the parasites into the vertebrate host. In some species of sandflies, the parasite remains in the mid-gut and is then believed to be transmitted to the vertebrate host when the sandfly is crushed on the skin.

Sandflies are principally active at night and this together with their very short life makes the part played by reservoir hosts of great importance. All infected vertebrates can act as reservoirs, but those of most importance in the epidemiology of the disease in man are dogs in some areas and wild mammals – probably rodents – in others. While the dog can be infected in any area where *Leishmania* occurs, it appears to act as a reservoir host principally in the Mediterranean, southern USSR, Chinese, Sudanese and South American areas. In other areas, the dog appears to play little or no part in the maintenance of human infection, and in India human visceral leishmaniosis (kala azar) is believed to be an anthroponotic disease.

Clinical features

Most of the information available refers to the various syndromes recognized in man and, although very little is published on the natural disease in dogs, the clinical features are essentially similar.

Table 11 Species, distribution, hosts and disease patterns of leishmaniosis

Species	Geographical distribution	Natural host	Disease[a]
L. donovani complex			
L. donovani	India,[b] Far East, Africa north of the equator	Man, wildcats and rodents in Africa	VL in man (kala azar or Dum Dum fever)
L. infantum	Mediterranean littoral, S.E. Europe, USSR, Middle East, North Africa	Dog, jackal, fox, wolf, rock, hyrax	VL in children VL in dogs
L. chagasi	South and Central America	Fox, dog, cat	VL in man and dogs
L. tropica complex			
L. tropica	Mediterranean littoral, USSR, Middle East, North Africa	Man, rodents, dog	Chronic urban oriental sores in man; CL in dogs
L. major	Middle East, USSR, North and West Africa	Burrowing rodents	Wet rural CL in man
L. aethiopica	Ethiopia, Kenya and South Yemen	Rock hyrax	Chronic dry oriental sores in man
L. mexicana complex			
Several spp.	Central America, Brazil	Forest rodents	Various forms of CL in man
L. braziliensis complex			
Several spp.	Central and South America	Forest rodents, sloths, porcupine	Various forms of CL in man including mucocutaneous form
L. b. guyanensis	The Guyanas and Brazil	Natural hosts unknown. Dogs?	CL in man

[a]VL, Visceral leishmaniosis; CL, cutaneous leishmaniosis.
[b]Studies indicate that kala azar in India exists as an anthroponotic disease.

Visceral leishmaniosis in dogs is particularly attributed to *L. infantum* infection in the Old World and *L. chagasi* in the New World. Infection commences as a cutaneous lesion from the vector bite, and spreads through various organs, especially spleen, liver and bone marrow. The disease is normally chronic, causing diarrhoea, emaciation, abdominal distension and eventual death, although acute forms of visceral leishmaniosis sometimes occur. Cutaneous lesions often occur in the dog, especially in the more chronic form of the disease. These can vary from eczematous eruptions to ulcerations of the skin, especially around the nose, lips and eye-lids, tip of the ears, tail, back and feet. There is sometimes alopecia in patches, and adenopathy may be evident, particularly hypertrophy of the prescapular and popliteal lymph nodes.

Cutaneous leishmaniosis in the dog attributed to *L. tropica* usually occurs as small focal lesions, and generalized skin disease is more commonly associated with visceral leishmaniosis. The mucocutaneous form of cutaneous leishmaniosis associated with

L. braziliensis infection can occur in the dog; metastases spread to the mucous membranes of the nose and mouth and produce a more recalcitrant form of the disease. Recovery in such cases is uncommon.

Pathology

In both forms of the disease, the basic lesion comprises infection of macrophages by the parasites accompanied by lymphocyte and plasma cell infiltration. Lesions range in severity from small localized cutaneous granulomas to widespread infection resulting in enlargement of spleen, liver and lymph nodes associated with hyperplasia of the reticulo-endothelial system.

Diagnosis

The most reliable means of diagnosis is the demonstration of the parasite in smears made from skin and ulcer scrapings, lymph node biopsies and, where necessary, bone marrow biopsy smears. At post-mortem examination of visceral leishmaniosis, large numbers of amastigotes in macrophages in spleen and other viscera in histological sections are a feature. Flourescent antibody tests to detect serum antibodies have been used in epidemiological surveys of dogs, but the results must be interpreted with care as cross-reactions between species of leishmania and trypanosomes can occur.

In man, the leishmanin intradermal skin test is used extensively for the diagnosis of all forms of leishmaniosis.

Parasites can be isolated either by inoculation of clinical material into laboratory hamsters or by culture.

Treatment

Most forms of cutaneous leishmaniosis recover spontaneously and require no treatment. Visceral and mucocutaneous leishmanioses require treatment. In man, certain pentavalent organic antimonial compounds, such as neostibosan, and aromatic diamidines are effective. In the dog, treatment is less effective, but if necessary canine leishmaniosis may be stabilized by repeated courses of intramuscular injections of meglumine antimonate (glucantine).

Immunology

Recovery from the visceral form of the disease is rare and does not appear to leave the dog immune, although recovered human beings are believed to have some immunity. Recovery from the skin form of the disease confers an immunity in both man and dog.

Control

The main step to be taken in the prevention and control of leishmaniosis is the breaking of the cycle, vertebrate reservoir – sandfly – vertebrate host. This is best effected by the elimination of the insect vector and the reduction of reservoir hosts. Phlebotomine sandflies usually fly near to the ground and residual insecticide strategically applied can have a marked effect in reducing the incidence of the disease.

The insects are very susceptible to adverse climatic conditions and have adapted themselves to the environment provided by rodent burrows and termite mounds, and in some areas rodents are probably significant reservoir hosts. Insecticidal treatment of such areas of breeding and resting can be of value in control of the disease.

In areas where the dog is an important reservoir host, treatment can be tried, but destruction of the infected animals is probably the wisest course.

Immunization against cutaneous leishmaniosis caused by *L. tropica* spp. has been extensively and successfully used in man in the Middle East, either by crude vaccination using clinical material from cutaneous lesions or more recently by inoculation of cultured promastigotes. These practices have been confined to man.

Further reading

Cahill, K.M. and Cox, K.B. (1975). Leishmaniasis. In *Diseases transmitted from animals to man*, 6th edn (W.T. Hubbert, W.F. McClulloch and P.R. Schnurrenberger, eds). Charles C. Thomas, Illinois.

Kirmse, P., Mahlin, L. and Lahrech, T.M. (1987). Canine leishmaniasis in Morocco with special reference to infantile kala-azar. *Transactions of the Royal Society of Tropical Medicine and Hygiene*, **81**, 212–213.

Losos, G.J. (1986). Leishmaniasis. In *Infectious tropical diseases of domestic animals*, pp. 319–345. Longman, London.

A.G.H.

THEILERIOSIS

Theileriosis of domestic animals comprises a group of tick-borne protozoan diseases of cattle, sheep and goats caused by pathogenic species of *Theileria*. These organisms are transmitted trans-stadially but not transovarially by two-and three-host ixodid ticks. In the vertebrate host, *Theileria* proliferate as schizonts in lymphoid mononuclear cells, releasing merozoites which invade erythrocytes to become piroplasms. The diseases produced by these parasites are thus lymphoproliferative disorders which may be associated with leucopenia and/or anaemia.

In a tick (larva or nymph) which feeds on piroplasm-infected blood, gametocytes are formed and, after syngamy, a zygote develops in the tick gut. Coincidental with the tick moult, motile kinetes migrate to the salivary gland of the next stage in the tick's life cycle (nymph or adult). Here sporogony occurs to give rise to sporozoites, the forms infective for the vertebrate host. This last developmental process in the tick is usually triggered by feeding, but it is also affected by the environmental temperature.

Pathogenic *Theileria* of cattle, sheep and goats are found worldwide, but the important pathogens are in East and Central Africa (the *T. parva* complex) and across the northern Mediterranean and subtropical regions of the Old World (*T. annulata* and *T. hirci*) (Table 12). *Theileria spp.* may also infect wild or feral ungulates in all continents, but are rarely associated with disease in these animals, except those reared in captivity or translocated to zoos.

Table 12 Pathogenic *Theileria* of cattle, sheep and goats

Species	Host	Vector	Disease/distribution	Serotype	Schizonts	Piroplasms
*Theileria parva parva***	Domestic cattle (African buffalo)	*Rhipicephalus appendiculatus*	East Coast fever (ECF)/East and Central Africa	*T. parva*	+++	+++
*T. parva bovis***	Cattle	*R. appendiculatus*	January disease/Central Africa	*T. parva*	+	+
*T. parva lawrencei***	Buffalo, cattle	*R. appendiculatus*, *R. zambeziensis*	Buffalo disease, Corridor disease/East and Central Africa	*T. parva*	+	±
T. taurotragi	Eland, cattle	*R. appendiculatus*	Benign theileriosis/East and Central Africa (? turning sickness)	*T. taurotragi*	+	+
*T. mutans**	Cattle	*Amblyomma* spp.	Benign theileriosis, turning sickness/Africa, south of Sahara	*T. mutans*	+ (morphology distinct)	+++
T. velifera	Cattle, buffalo	*Amblyomma* spp.	Theileriosis/Africa, south of Sahara	?	?	+ (distinct veil)
*T. annulata***	Cattle, (swamp buffalo)	*Hyalomma* spp.	Mediterranean Coast fever, tropical theileriosis/Morocco to China	*T. annulata*	+++	+++
*T. orientalis***	Cattle	*Haemaphysalis longicornis*, *Haemaphysalis* spp.	Oriental theileriosis/Japan, Korea: pathogenic; elsewhere: mild	*T. sergenti*	+ (very rare)	+++
*T. hirci***	Sheep and goats	*Hyalomma* spp.	Malignant ovine theileriosis/North Africa, Middle East to India	*T. hirci*	+++	+++
T. ovis	Sheep and goats	*R. bursa*	Benign ovine theileriosis/worldwide	*T. ovis*	?	++
Others: *T. spp.* *T. separata*	Sheep and deer	?	Germany, USA/East and South Africa	?	?	+ (may be characteristic)

Note: The asterisks refer to grades of importance as pathogens.

East Coast fever

A non-contagious, febrile disease of cattle, East Coast fever (ECF) is characterized by high fever, leucopenia and severe damage to the lymphoid system.

Aetiology and occurrence

Theileria are piroplasms, apicomplexan parasites closely related to *Babesia*. *T. parva parva* is the major pathogen in ECF, a disease complex of cattle in East and Central Africa. *T. p. parva* causes "classical" ECF and is transmitted from cattle to cattle in East Africa by *Rhipicephalus appendiculatus*, the brown ear tick. Other *T. parva* subspp. also contribute to the disease complex. *T. p. lawrencei* causes corridor disease carried by African buffalo, *Syncerus caffer*, and transmitted to cattle by *R. appendiculatus* and *Rhipicephalus zambeziensis*. *T. p. bovis* is primarily a pathogen of cattle in the high veldt of Central Africa, where it may be the only component of the ECF complex remaining after eradication of *T. p. parva* by a dipping campaign and of *T. p. lawrencei* by elimination of the buffalo.

ECF caused by *T. p. parva* is of particular importance in East Africa – Kenya, Uganda, Tanzania, Rwanda, Burindi and Malawi. It also extends into Zaire, Zambia, southern Sudan and Mozambique. *T. p. bovis* has a wider distribution, extending into East Central Africa, notably Zimbabwe. *T. p. lawrencei* extends further south and west, where it is carried in buffalo and transmitted to cattle wherever there is buffalo – cattle contact and the vector tick. There may thus be sporadic or epidemic disease caused by this parasite from East Africa down to the low veldt of Zimbabwe, areas of the Republic of South Africa adjacent to game reserves and into Angola.

Transmission

The disease is transmitted trans-stadially by ixodid ticks. Nine species of the genus *Rhipicephalus* and three *Hyalomma* spp. have been shown to transmit the disease experimentally. However, in the field, the distribution of the disease is confined within the known distribution of *R. appendiculatus* except where, in the low veldt of Central Africa, *R. zambeziensis* has been shown to be responsible for transmitting *T. p. lawrencei*.

Piroplasms in the blood of an infected animal are picked up by engorging immature stages of the vector. These complete feeding, drop off and moult and then, at the next stage in their life-cycle, attempt to feed. If picked up by a susceptible bovid, the parasites in their salivary glands complete their development over the first 3 days after attaching and, between the third and fifth days of feeding, the tick secretes infective sporozoites into its new host. On rare occasions, the tick is able to transmit the infection in less than 3 days. This is normally after exposure to temperatures approaching 37°C, stimulating premature sporogony of the parasite in the salivary glands of the questing tick.

Mechanical transmission is of no significance, being difficult to achieve even in laboratory conditions.

Clinical features

The severity of the disease is quantum-dependent, but one tick will transmit sufficient sporozoites to kill a susceptible cow. Both *Bos taurus* and *Bos indicus*, from areas where the disease is not endemic, are susceptible, though *Bos indicus* is comparatively more resistant at end-point dilutions of sporozoite suspensions. This, coupled with their relative resistance to ticks, makes *Bos indicus* significantly more resistant than *Bos taurus* to ECF. Despite this, mortality figures of 97% have been recorded in Boran (East African shorthorn Zebu) cattle introduced to ECF enzootic areas.

Following inoculation of sporozoites into a cow, schizonts appear 4–12 days later (i.e. 8–16 days after the ticks attached) in the lymph node draining the site of their attachment. With *R. appendiculatus*, the brown ear tick, this is most commonly the parotid lymph node. This node becomes hyperplastic and enlarges at this time. Then, 1–3 days later, the animal becomes febrile and other clinical signs ensue, thus giving an apparent incubation period of 9–18 days, most commonly 14–16. Other superficial lymph nodes enlarge, the body temperature rises to 41–42°C and there is a fall in milk yield. Early in disease, there is little decline in condition or inappetence, but these develop late in the disease, when there is a rapid deterioration in condition. It is at this point that the disease is most frequently recognized for the first time, by which time prognosis is poor. By day 16, the first piroplasms appear in the blood. From this day on the animal is infective to ticks.

Signs other than hyperthermia and lymphadenopathy are irregular. Respiratory distress, with evident developing pulmonary oedema and pneumonia, is the most common sign. There may be violent and even blood-tinged diarrhoea, or posterior paresis and wasting of muscles with occasional CNS involvement ("turning sickness"). Mucosal petechiation of the lower gum, under the tongue and of the vulva may be evident. Photophobia, ophthalmia and a milky infiltration of the eye is not uncommon. The animal collapses and dies, most commonly, between 18 and 26 days after infective ticks first attach.

Clinical pathology

During the disease the parasites are evident as macro-and microschizonts in lymphoid cells in biopsy smears of the enlarged lymph nodes, stained with Giemsa. Similar smears of blood may show piroplasms in the erythrocytes from day 16, increasing in number to death. Schizonts may also be seen in the circulating lymphocytes in blood smears. The haematological picture is pathognomic – a panleucopenia and thrombocytopenia, with little anaemia, developing late.

Pathology

At death there is most commonly evidence of pneumonia and pulmonary oedema, with froth in the trachea, bronchi and nares. The lungs may be full of fluid with extensive pleural transudate. Other "classical" lesions include punched erosions of the abomasum, white or red "infarcts" of the kidney (lymphoproliferative foci in the renal cortex), epicardial blood splashing, serosal petechiae and ecchymoses – on the peritoneum over the rumen, spleen and gall bladder – and, frequently, haemorrhages in the muscles, subcutaneous tissue and myelin sheaths of nerves.

The involvement and state of the lymphoid organ may vary between infection caused by different parasite stocks and is dependent on the length of disease reaction. There may be generalized hyperplasia of lymph nodes, spleen, and lymphoid tissue in liver, kidneys and gut. Alternatively, despite aberrant proliferation, the lymph nodes and spleen may be "exhausted"; the spleen dry and aplastic, the lymph nodes oedematous.

Diagnosis

In essence, diagnosis is dependent on identifying the parasite in the animal. This is achieved using Giemsa-stained thin blood smears for piroplasms and lymph node biopsy or organ smears for schizonts.

In an area where ECF is a possibility, it must be a prime suspect. A blood smear is an essential early step. If there is any evidence of lymph node enlargement, then lymph node biopsy is necessary. Between these two it is then necessary to find schizonts to make a definite diagnosis. In clinical disease, these should be common for *T. p. parva* but less so for *T. p. bovis* and perhaps rare for *T. p. lawrencei*. Piroplasms will be rare or absent in *T. p. lawrencei* infections but, late in disease, will be numerous in *T. p. parva* and *T. p. bovis* cases.

Differential diagnosis from other tick-borne diseases and trypanosomiasis which cause anaemia may be helped by haematological examination, which should indicate a leucopenia and thrombocytopenia but no anaemia. Identification of the parasite will confirm the diagnosis and will also discriminate from other lymphoproliferative disorders such as malignant catarrh.

A knowledge of the disease history will also help. As with all tick-borne diseases, cattle movement within or on to the farm or a change of management conditions 2–3 weeks earlier, may be the first lead to a diagnosis. A broken fence, intrusion of buffalo, grazing in thick bush or against forest edges must be viewed with suspicion. On a broader, epidemic scale, movement of cattle to new pasture, increased rainfall or improved ground cover to help tick survival may all be inducing or exacerbating factors.

Epizootiology

The epizootiology of classical ECF caused by *T. p. parva* in East Africa is relatively straightforward and is defined by a number of simple factors. However, once *T. p. lawrencei* or *T. p. bovis* are considered as components of the syndrome, the situation is much more complex.

The disease, caused by *T. p. parva*, is tick-borne, transmitted in the field by *R. appendiculatus*, trans-stadially but not transovarially. Thus larvae are *not* infective; nymphs and adults may be.

The distribution of ECF is geographically confined by the distribution of the tick and by whether the tick can undergo more than one life-cycle in a year. This really confines it to East Africa, in areas of rainfall of more than 750 mm per annum and where it is not too cold or high. There are large areas of Africa where the tick is present but not the disease. There are no areas where the disease is present without the tick.

After an infected tick attaches there is a delay of 3–5 days before it becomes infective and inoculates sporozoites. This gives additional leeway to acaricidal control but there are exceptional circumstances in which this pre-infective period may be as short as 24 hours.

Infected or clean ticks do not move, although they may be carried by animals or man. Infected ticks may live for 1–2 years, but normally they lose the infection in about 11 months. Only exceptionally may the parasite survive in the tick for up to 2 years.

Clinically infected cattle, exhibiting piroplasms, are the chief (and in most cases the exclusive) source of infection for the tick. In classical *T. p. parva* infection, cattle do not remain as carriers, though exceptions are now reported with increasing frequency. Effective disease control programmes have been based on this premise.

A very large proportion of cattle infected with the disease die. This itself limits maintenance of the parasite.

Corridor disease, caused by *T. p. lawrencei*, is classically transmitted from buffalo to cattle and is not normally maintained in cattle. Epidemiologically, it requires close contact between these species, usually at the forest edge or on uncleared land with dense bush. Buffalo are difficult to restrict and may break fences. Buffalo are carriers of *T. p. lawrencei* and cattle may become carriers, though normally exhibiting very low parasitaemias. Other wild ungulates also carry *R. appendiculatus*, but not *T. p. lawrencei*.

T. p. bovis causes theileriosis (January disease) which is maintained in cattle in the high veldt of Central Africa without the presence of buffalo. Cattle are carriers and mortality is lower than from infection with *T. p. parva*, but may be as high as 30% in epizootics.

The carrier status of cattle and buffalo infected with these two parasites of the *T. parva* complex and their potential to transform into a form indistinguishable from *T. parva* makes control measures based on a sterile immunity open to question.

Theileria taurotragi, a parasite of low pathogenicity for cattle transmitted from eland, for which it is pathogenic, is an example of a group of parasites of wild ungulates which may complicate the epizootiology of ECF.

Theileria mutans, transmitted by *Amblyomma* ticks, was until recently considered to be benign; it has now been shown to be significantly pathogenic for cattle. Both cattle and buffalo are known to be carriers and the organism and the anaemia it induces may complicate clinical theileriosis caused by more pathogenic species.

Serology

There are a number of serodiagnostic techniques using antigens prepared from the two major stages of the vertebrate cycle, namely schizonts from infected lymphoblastoid cell lines grown *in vitro*, and piroplasms from infected blood. The tests most widely used are the indirect fluorescent antibody (IFA) test, using cultured schizonts or intra-erythrocytic piroplasms as antigen, and the indirect haemagglutination (IHA) test, using a piroplasm antigen.

Other tests which have been developed but which are not widely used are the complement fixation test (CFT), the capillary agglutination (CA) test and the enzyme-linked immunosorbent assay (ELISA). This last test, with increased specifity, holds most promise for future seroepidemiological studies.

A strong antibody response is almost invariably recorded with both IFA and IHA tests 21–28 days following infection, but these antibodies do not persist for the duration of the immune state of the animal, declining to insignificant levels 6 weeks to 9 months after a single infection. Antibodies are usually absent during a clinical reaction, almost invariably so in fatal cases. Repeated challenge of immune cattle with a homologous strain of *T. p. parva* does not induce an anamnestic response unless the schizonts become established. High antibody levels may be induced in susceptible cattle by inoculation of killed antigen but these cattle are not immune to ECF.

Serological tests are of restricted value in disease surveys because of the above limitations. Moreover, in none of these tests can immunologically distinct strains of *Theileria* be distinguished. Indeed, *T. p. parva* cannot be distinguished serologically from *T. p. lawrencei* or *T. p. bovis*.

There are indications that cell-mediated immune techniques, monoclonal antibodies, isoenzyme electrophoresis and DNA probe technology may help in the identification of *T. parva* strains or subspecies. However, to date this still depends on very expensive cross-immunity trials with immunization and challenge of cattle.

Treatment

Two specific series of compounds have recently been shown to exhibit chemotherapeutic activity against the macroschizont stage of *T. parva*, and thus are effective in treating the clinical disease. These are the naphthoquinones and the febrifugines, a number of which also show activity against malaria and coccidiosis. Of the former, two analogues have been developed and released in countries where theileriosis is a problem, i.e. parvaquone and buparvaquone. Halofuginone is the coccidiostatic febrifugine which has also been shown to be highly effective in treating clinical theileriosis.

The regimens used for treatment of patent disease are:

1. Parvaquone[a] 1 × 20 mg/kg or 2 × 10 mg/kg i.m. at 48-hour intervals.
2. Buparvaquone[b] 1 × 5 mg/kg or 2 × 2.5 mg/kg i.m. at 48-hour intervals.
3. Halofuginone[c] 1 × 1 mg/kg by mouth.

[a]Clexon (Coopers Animal Health); [b]Butalex (Coopers Animal Health); [c]Terit (Hoechst/Roussel).

Chemotherapeutic agents can also be used prophylactically in the control of theileriosis. In this context, the tetracycline antibiotics can be added to the above three drugs. These are most widely used in the infection-and-treatment method of immunization against ECF to block parasite and disease development after inoculation of a cryopreserved stabilate of sporozoites prepared from ground-up infected ticks. Regimens which can be used for this purpose are:

1. A long-acting oxytetracycline[d] 20 mg/kg i.m. on day 0.*
2. Short-acting oxytetracyclines 5–10 mg/kg i.m. on days 0 and 4.
3. Buparvaquone 2.5–5 mg/kg i.m. on day 0.
4. Parvaquone 10–20 mg/kg i.m. on day 8.

[d]Terra LA (Pfizer); *day 0 being the day on which sporozoites are inoculated.

These recent developments in chemotherapy and chemoprophylaxis of theileriosis have opened new avenues in the approach to control ECF. In an outbreak of disease, however, specific chemotherapy must be complemented by early and efficient diagnosis and elimination of the infective challenge. This will require strict quarantine, movement control and intensive application of acaricides to prevent pick up and further transmission of the infection by ticks.

Immunology

In ECF enzootic areas, a high proportion of cattle naturally acquire immunity to the disease when first exposed as young calves of immune dams. This immunity effectively protects them against an otherwise lethal challenge and is classically accepted as being a sterile immunity. Recently, however, it has been shown that cattle which have recovered from field infection with *T. parva* may be carriers infective for ticks.

Experimentally, cattle immunized with *T. p. parva* have been shown to be solidly immune to challenge with the homologous strain of the parasite for more than 3 years. There is, however, laboratory and field evidence that antigenic differences exist between different strains or stocks of the parasite. These differences cannot be detected serologically, but only by cross-immunity trials, cattle immunized with one stock being partially or fully susceptible when challenged with another.

At present, immunity can only be induced by establishing the parasite within the cells of the host. Thus immunity is cellular and, being genetically restricted, may be adoptively transferred with lymphocytes from an immune twin. Cytotoxic lymphocytes in an immune animal have been shown to kill autologous lymphocytes infected with *T. parva* schizonts. Other mechanisms, such as antibodies which block sporozoites entering target lymphocytes, may also have a role, but these have not yet been shown to be protective on their own.

Susceptible cattle can thus be immunized against ECF but, at present, only following recovery from a deliberate infection. This is achieved by the infection-and-treatment method using sporozoites to infect and a chemoprophylactic or chemotherapeutic drug to block the clinical reaction. At present, this is implemented by preparing sporozoite stabilates, cryopreserved in liquid nitrogen, from ground-up, partially fed, infected ticks (GUTS), and using aliquots of these stabilates to produce infections with one or more parasite stocks. The infection is then blocked by treatment as indicated above, most commonly with a long-acting oxytetracycline.

Such procedures, using selected individual *T. p. parva* stocks or "cocktails" of *T. p. parva*, *T. p. bovis* and *T. p. lawrencei* stocks, are presently being evaluated and are showing much promise in large-scale field trials throughout East and Central Africa.

Control

Since the first recognition at the turn of the century of the disastrous impact of ECF on susceptible cattle in East, Central and southern Africa, control has depended primarily on breaking the transmission cycle between the cattle and the tick. This has depended on short-interval application of acaricides to cattle using immersion baths or dip tanks, or sprays and spray races. In restricted conditions, using effective acaricides to provide assidious control of the vector tick, *R. appendiculatus*, coupled with stringent movement control and quarantine, the disease could be and has been eradicated from farms, districts and even countries. Such control has, however, only been achieved at great cost. The capital expenditure on fencing and construction of dip tanks and the recurrent costs of acaricide for weekly, or even more frequent, application are now generally considered to be unacceptably high. Nevertheless, until recently this was the only way to control the disease and was essential if highly productive yet highly suscept-ible stock were to be reared in endemic areas or if the disease was to be eradicated from marginal areas. Widespread success was achieved only in regions where the climate for transmission of the pathogens was borderline, such as South Africa and Zimbabwe. However, very effective local control was achieved on farms and in districts of high endemicity in East and Central Africa.

The resistance to acaricides by the tick vector, the drain on foreign currency resources and political problems have meant that control of ECF can no longer rely solely on the use of strict acaricidal regimens of short-interval dipping. However, two recent developments – the discovery of specific chemotherapeutic agents with which clinical ECF can be cured, and the development of the infection-and-treatment method of immunization – have meant that it is now possible to reduce the impact of ECF using integrated control measures. These also involve the strategic application of acaricides timed to coincide with periods of greatest tick challenge, coupled with the deliberate choice of cattle with higher potential for tick resistance. At present, these are cattle with a significant Zebu component in their genetic make-up, rather than pure *Bos taurus*. Such measures are only possible now that the availability of vaccines and therapy, at a cost, have abrogated the previously unacceptably high morbidity and mortality levels of ECF.

Tropical theileriosis

Tropical theileriosis or Mediterranean Coast fever is a non-contagious disease of cattle characterized by fever, enlargement of the peripheral lymph nodes, wasting, progres-sive anaemia and jaundice.

Aetiology

Tropical theileriosis is caused by *Theileria annulata* (syn. *T. dispar*, *T. sergenti*, *T. turkestanica*), the schizonts of which are found in the lymphoid tissue and are morphologically similar to those of *T. parva*. However, in *T. annulata* infection the erythrocytic stages of the parasite are predominantly round (annular) or oval forms, whereas with *T. parva* rod-and comma-shaped types are more common. The piroplasms appear in the erythrocytes shortly after the schizonts are first detected and, in fatal cases, may be present in very large numbers. In chronic or subacute infections, they persist in the blood for years. In such established infections, the few piroplasms which can be seen in blood films are also infective for ticks. There is evidence that a schizont carrier state also persists, recrudescence of schizonts being detectable on splenectomy of recovered animals.

Occurrence

The disease occurs across a wide zone of Africa, Europe and Asia, predominantly north of latitude 10°N. The area affected stretches from Morocco to China, thus covering much of the Mediterranean littoral of Europe and Africa, the Near and Middle East, and parts of the Indian subcontinent, the USSR and China. Its distribution is dependent on the presence of susceptible animals and vector ticks (*Hyalomma* spp.) in sufficient numbers to ensure contact from year to year. In the east, this distribution probably overlaps that of *Theileria orientalis*, transmitted by *Haemaphysalis* spp., whereas in the south, but probably only in southern Sudan, it may co-exist with *T. parva*, transmitted by *R. appendiculatus*.

Transmission

T. annulata has a life-cycle similar to that of *T. parva* and is transmitted trans-stadially but not transovarially by three-, two-and one-host ixodid ticks of the genus *Hyalomma*. All species of *Hyalomma* can probably transmit the disease, at least in the laboratory, but in the field transmission is dependent on tick – cow contact and, in particular, on immature stages of the tick feeding on infected animals. For many *Hyalomma* spp., the preferential host of the larva and nymph is a small animal and thus these species do not transmit *T. annulata* in the field. Effectively, *H. detritum* (syn. *H. mauritanicum, H. scupense* in USSR) and *H. anatolicum anatolicum* are the most common vectors.

An unusual feature about this arthropod – vertebrate host relationship is that the tick actively seeks its host. Larvae or nymphs engorge on infected, frequently carrier, cattle in late summer and autumn, over-winter in crevices in walls, moult in the spring and, as adult ticks, cause a marked seasonal incidence of the disease in the summer. The length of the season is dependent on tick activity and hence on the climatic zone, being very short at high altitudes or high latitudes but occurring almost all year round in much of India, for example.

Where the vector is, or behaves on cattle as, a three-host tick, the nymph or adult can transmit the disease which it picked up when feeding as a larva or nymph, respectively. However, many of the vectors, notably *H. detritum*, are two-host ticks, the disease being picked up by the engorging larva/nymph and thus only transmitted by the adult tick. As with *T. parva*, the infected tick normally needs to feed for some time (2–3 days) before the parasite matures in its salivary glands and infective sporozoites are injected. However, again as with *T. parva*, this process of maturation can be abbreviated if the tick has been exposed to high temperatures while questing for a host.

Mechanical transmission can be effected by the inoculation of schizonts as schizont-infected lymphoid cells from infected to susceptible cattle. However, though rare instances of intra-uterine transmission have been recorded, mechanical transmission by biting flies does not seem to occur.

Clinical features

Calfhood infection in areas where the disease is endemic takes the form of a mild fever but mortality as high as 25% has been reported. The acute form of the disease, most commonly observed in adult susceptible animals, shows an initial fever which can persist for several days and is accompanied by inappetence, rumenal stasis, nasal and ocular discharge and swelling of the superficial lymph nodes.

After a few days, marked anaemia develops, causing pale mucous membranes, which may later become icteric. Constipation is common in the early febrile period, but diarrhoea and blood stained faeces are common in the later stages. The disease runs a course of 8–15 days with rapid loss of condition. Mortality following the acute disease is up to 90%, and peracute cases with death after 3–4 days sometimes occur. Subacute and chronic forms of the disease are seen in which an intermittent fever can persist for 15–28 days and anaemia, icterus and general malaise may be observed during this period. In such cases, recovery can occur but convalescence is protracted. The subacute or chronic form of the disease sometimes develops into an acute episode and the animal dies.

Clinical pathology

Lymph node biopsy smears may show schizonts but these tend to be more common in the liver than in the peripheral lymph nodes, of which only the node draining the site of attachment of the infected tick may exhibit a high level of infection.

The schizonts, which exert the principal pathogenic effect in *T. p. parva* and *T. p. lawrencei* infections, are also actively pathogenic in *T. annulata* infection but, in addition, the piroplasms in the erythrocytes cause destruction of the cells leading to anaemia. A panleucopenia and thrombocytopenia, similar to but less severe than that recorded in ECF, are common features of the acute and peracute disease syndromes.

Pathology

The chief pathological features of tropical theileriosis, which are broadly similar to those of ECF, are associated with the dysfunction of the lympho-reticuloendothelial system and the haematological features of the disease. *Post mortem*, the mucous and serous membranes are pale and often show numerous petechiae; the liver is enlarged, pale brown or yellow, and friable; the spleen is enlarged and soft and the malpighian corpuscles prominent; the lymph nodes are enlarged, oedematous, frequently hyperplastic and hyperaemic; the kidneys are pale and sometimes show lymphoproliferative foci manifested as "pseudoinfarcts"; haemorrhagic ulceration of the abomasum is common, and the lungs are oedematous and congested. The heart has petechiae and ecchymoses of the epi-and endocardium and the adrenal cortex may be severely infiltrated and haemorrhagic.

Diagnosis

It is essential to identify the causative organism to confirm the diagnosis. This is done with blood smears to detect the intraerythrocytic piroplasms and with lymph node or liver biopsy smears to demonstrate the intralymphocytic schizonts. Liver biopsy is performed with a 4-inch (100-mm) needle in the right, penultimate intercostal space, a hand's-breadth from the spine, directing the needle towards the sternum. Air-dried smears are fixed with methanol and stained with a Romanowsky stain, such as Giemsa, May-Grunwald/Giemsa, Leishman/Giemsa, Wright's, etc., to demonstrate the parasites. *Post mortem* smears can be prepared from any organ, including the lung, liver, kidney, spleen, adrenal gland, or draining lymph node, which is showing evidence of pathological disturbance.

In the live animal, the haematological features of anaemia and leucopenia help in directing the diagnosis towards haemoparasites, but detection and recognition of both the schizont and the piroplasm is conclusive evidence. These provide differential diagnosis from babesiosis and anaplasmosis, which both cause anaemia, from *T. orientalis* in the East (where only the piroplasm is evident) and *T. parva* in southern Sudan, which does not cause anaemia.

Epizootiology

In enzootic areas, tropical theileriosis can go almost unnoticed. In India, it was only detected in the 1920s after the introduction of exotic cattle. There can be a balance between cattle, tick and parasite in which all the cattle are infected and carriers, and the majority of ticks that feed on cattle are also infected. In this respect, the disease is similar to babesiosis or anaplasmosis rather than to ECF, with the normal state being one of enzootic stability.

However, when susceptible cattle are present, the disease is seasonal, dependent on tick activity. Thus, except in the tropical zones such as southern India, where ticks are active throughout the year, there is no theileriosis in the winter months. The length of this "winter" relates to both latitude and altitude.

Cattle throughout much of this area are "zero grazed" and the ticks have adapted to living on or off cattle in houses or yards. This is usually associated with environmental pressures, to avoid arid desert or semi-desert conditions or extremes of heat and cold. *H. scupense*, for example, may behave as a one-host tick, overwintering on the cattle. In such situations, the disease may occur early in the year, at times when there is negligible tick activity in the field.

Recovered cattle are carriers, for at least 9–12 months, probably longer. Immunity lasts for more than 1 year, probably for many years. Infection with a single parasite stock protects against most other stocks.

In an enzootic situation almost all the *Hyalomma* ticks that feed on cattle in their immature stages will be infected. Swamp or water buffalo (*Bubalus bubalis*) may be infected and be carriers, but show little evidence of clinical disease. It is possible that sheep and goats may also carry *T. annulata*. Ovine and caprine theileriosis may interfere with the transmission, control and interpretation of bovine theileriosis.

The parasite overwinters in carrier cattle but also in engorged immature ticks (e.g. engorged nymphs of *H. detritum*) which only moult to become infective adults in the spring. Ticks may remain infective for 6–18 months. As with *T. parva* and *R. appendiculatus*, ticks are not usually immediately infective but the time required after starting to feed before ticks infected with *T. annulata* will secrete sporozoites is less (normally 2–3 days) than with *T. parva*. Because heat also stimulates maturation of the parasite in the salivary glands of infected ticks, some ticks may be infective immediately they attach to a susceptible host.

Serology

Serological tests similar to those used for *T. parva* are available. Little is known about the relationship between serological reactions and disease or carrier status. Such evidence as is available points to long-term persistence of antibodies, associated with the presence of piroplasms. However, immunity may be of shorter duration, and therefore antibodies, detectable on serological tests, may indicate carrier status but not necessarily immunity. Complete serological cross-reactivity exists between all the strains presently identified.

Current serological tests (IFAT, ELISA) exhibit significant levels of cross-reaction between *T. annulata* and *T. parva*. The piroplasm is presently of more general use as an antigen in these tests than the schizont.

Treatment

As for East Coast fever, the naphthoquinones – parvaquone and buparvaquone – and the febrifugine, halofuginone, are effective in the treatment of clinical *T. annulata* infections but perhaps less effective than against *T. parva*. Similarly, while the tetracyclines may be used chemoprophylactically to block deliberate infections, they appear to be less reliable than in ECF.

Buparvaquone is the most effective chemotherapeutic agent presently available for the treatment of tropical theileriosis.

Immunology

The immune mechanisms involved in tropical theileriosis appear to be similar to those shown to operate in ECF.

Effective immunity against tropical theileriosis may develop naturally or be induced by immunization with living material, i.e. by infection and recovery. This immunity may be accompanied by carrier status and will last for at least 1 year and probably much longer.

Different antigenic strains of *T. annulata* exist, there being evidence for a broad geographic spectrum of strains. Much cross-reactivity and cross-protection is observed, however, and a single stock may, if used as a "vaccine", protect against other stocks from the same area and also against stocks from other areas and different countries.

Infective material from ticks, i.e. sporozoites, appears to induce better protection against homologous and heterologous challenge than infective material in the form of schizont-infected lymphoid cells from blood or cell culture. However, schizont-infected cells can be used to infect cattle, and cattle recovered from such infections are resistant to both homologous and heterologous challenge. Only infected ticks or sporozoites harvested from them provide a valid challenge when evaluating immunity.

Tropical theileriosis can thus be controlled by vaccination. Two forms of vaccine exist, one of which has been widely used:

1. *A schizont vaccine*: This may be either blood from a cow infected with a mild strain of the parasite (e.g. the Kouba strain of *T. annulata* used in Algeria and elsewhere since 1932) or a cell culture vaccine, containing a parasite that has been attenuated by passage *in vitro*, in an infected lymphoid cell line. Such a vaccine has been used in Israel since 1965, and subsequently in Iran, the USSR, China, India, Tunisia, Turkey, Iraq and elsewhere. The cell culture vaccine is practicable as only 10^2 cultured cells are needed, although 10^6 or more cells in 1–2 ml of culture are normally used, to give a mild reaction and subsequent immunity. This living vaccine has been extensively used in the field with most encouraging results in all the countries in which it has been tested.

2. *A sporozoite vaccine*, as for *T. parva*: The infection and treatment method is being developed. The indications at present are that it may be useful to boost the immunity provided by the schizont vaccines, as it may give better protection against heterologous challenge. This approach is as yet untried in the field and suffers from the same limitations as the culture vaccine in that, as it is a live vaccine, its immunogenicity is dependent on its infectivity. The strain used is also not attenuated and so is potentially dangerous. Hence particular care needs to be taken to ensure that the dose of tetracycline is sufficient to block the sporozoite dose administered.

Control

Control of tropical theileriosis depends on establishing or maintaining a stable situation. In endemic areas, indigenous cattle live with the tick and infection. It is only when valuable, highly susceptible *Bos taurus* are introduced in cross-breeding programmes initiated to improve the genetic potential of indigenous cattle that specific control of tropical theileriosis needs to be considered. Dependent on the system of management, the environmental conditions and the type of cattle, the decision then lies between living with the disease and creating a state of enzootic stability, or eradicating the disease.

In extreme conditions pertaining to the maintenance of pure-bred exotic taurine cattle in an environment where tropical theileriosis is endemic – as in a dairy herd or on a stud farm – it may prove worthwhile to take costly and extensive precautions. These might include zero-grazing, bringing in feed from tick-free lots, and the strict movement control of cattle; construction and maintenance of stalls and pens which are tick-free though not necessarily tick-proof, with a facility for washing them down with acaricides so as to kill any ticks and avoid creating a resident vector population; dipping or spraying the cattle, should there be a risk of exposure to ticks or, strategically, in spring and autumn.

These steps should keep susceptible cattle free from tropical theileriosis but, given the success with vaccination in recent years, it would be recommended that, where possible, such cattle should be vaccinated with living, cell culture vaccine. Such a step would not necessarily create carrier cattle, as the vaccine should have been sufficiently passaged *in vitro* to ensure that it does not produce piroplasms infective for ticks in the cattle immunized in this way.

Where the cattle under consideration are indigenous, control of tropical theileriosis must be part of an integrated programme for the control of ticks and tick-borne diseases. Almost invariably the aim will be to maintain the disease so that young calves are infected and a stable situation persists. This means not dipping the cattle too assiduously and not upgrading the stock too radically without providing supplementary control of the disease. Using vaccination offers such a method of disease control, complemented by the use of novel methods of treatment.

The most difficult situation in which to control the disease is on a ranch, using improved or selected cattle, or on a dairy farm where cattle are grazed out. Here, unless they are protected, the cattle will experience a morbidity and mortality rate which is too high to be acceptable. Vaccination and strategic control of the ticks together with an enlightened and pragmatic breeding programme is the most realistic approach. This should be integrated with the activities on adjacent farms and coupled with judicious movement control to prevent the introduction of susceptible or carrier cattle.

Benign bovine theileriosis

Benign theileriosis, caused by *Theileria mutans*, is a tick-borne disease of cattle characterized by pyrexia, malaise, variable but sometimes severe anaemia and slight swelling of lymph nodes.

The parasite *T. mutans* is transmitted by ticks of the genus *Amblyomma* in Africa south of the Sahara and potentially elsewhere within the distribution of the vector ticks. *Amblyomma variegatum* in East and West Africa, and *A. hebraeum* in Central and South Africa, are incriminated as the likely vectors. Other *Amblyomma* spp. have, however, been shown to transmit *T. mutans*.

The parasite is of comparatively low pathogenicity in cattle, rarely causing death even in susceptible, exotic animals. Schizonts are rare and characteristically different from those of *T. parva*, appearing 12–18 days after inoculation of sporozoites by the vector. Piroplasms are more easily found, from about the same time after infection, and are the pathogenic form of the parasite, the main disease feature being a haemolytic anaemia, as with anaplasmosis or babesiosis. In splenectomized calves, the disease is highly pathogenic and frequently fatal. Carrier status follows infection and splenectomy will induce relapse in carrier cattle, though only of the piroplasm form.

Other bovids may be infected and be carriers, and therefore wild ungulates act as a potential reservoir of the disease. African buffalo are proven carriers and *T. mutans* has been transmitted from buffalo to cattle by *A. cohaerens*.

With the distribution of the vector ticks closely paralleling that of *R. appendiculatus* in Africa, this disease is perhaps most important as a complication of ECF. Inter-relating immunosuppression may exacerbate its virulence and the anaemia may contribute significantly to the pathogenesis of the disease complex even in partially resistant or immune cattle.

This parasite is antigenically distinct from those of the *T. parva* complex. There is no cross-immunity and the parasite can be distinguished in serological tests and assays.

T. mutans can be treated effectively with the antimalarial 8-amino-quinolines (primaquin and pamaquin) and most probably with parvaquone and buparvaquone.

Control is by controlling the vector, as for *R. appendiculatus*, though this is not necessarily wholly desirable, because the vector may also be involved in transmitting *Cowdria ruminantium*, the causative agent of heartwater. Such action might therefore have an effect on the enzootic status of that disease. Immunization and production of the carrier state might be indicated. It is potentially possible to immunize cattle simply by inoculating infected blood.

Oriental theileriosis

Oriental theileriosis of cattle is caused by *Theileria orientalis* (syn. *T. sergenti*, *T. buffeli*, *T. mutans*), which is transmitted by ticks of the genus *Haemaphysalis*.

This is a relatively benign theileriosis only recognized as a disease of significance in imported cattle in the Far East, i.e. Japan and Korea. It is believed, however, that the organism is present throughout Asia, Europe, Africa and Australia and probably in the Americas.

T. orientalis is transmitted by ticks of the genus *Haemaphysalis* – *H. longicornis*,

H. japonica in the Far East, *H. truncatum* in Britain and north-western Europe. In many instances, the organism transmitted by these ticks has been called *T. mutans* because of its lack of pathogenicity, but recent serological studies have shown that the Japanese, Korean, Australian and British parasites are antigenically indistinguishable from each other, yet distinct from African *T. mutans* transmitted by *Amblyomma* spp. It is not understood why the organism should be pathogenic in Korea and Japan yet completely avirulent in Europe, Australia and Africa.

In the Far East, where *T. orientalis* causes disease and occasional deaths in exotic cattle, there is evidence that a high percentage of ticks are infected in the field, resulting in epizootics characterized by high morbidity but low mortality. Anaemia is the most significant clinical manifestation of the disease, being associated with the presence of intraerythrocytic piroplasms. Schizonts of *T. orientalis* are rarely found.

T. orientalis can be treated with the 8-amino-quinoline antimalarials primaquin and pamaquin, usually administered intramuscularly at 1.0–2.5 mg/kg of the phosphate. These drugs have been used both therapeutically and prophylactically. It is common practice in both Korea and Japan to immunize cattle by deliberately exposing them to tick infestation and then treating them prophylactically. The babesicide imidocarb (Imizol: Coopers Animal Health) has recently been used to treat *T. orientalis* infections in Korea, with apparent success. The dose used was 1–3 mg/kg. It is probable that parvaquone and buparvaquone will also prove to be effective in the treatment of oriental theileriosis.

IFAT and ELISA, using piroplasm antigens, are serological tests described for the diagnosis of *T. orientalis* infections and used in surveys of the disease.

The disease can be controlled by the use of acaricides applied to the cattle to prevent tick attachment during spring to autumn. As the only means of control for highly susceptible cattle, this would seem unnecessarily risky. The creation of a state of enzootic stability by immunization, with deliberate maintenance of the infected state, would seem to be a better option.

Malignant ovine theileriosis

This disease of sheep and goats is caused by *Theileria hirci*. It is of much importance in Iraq, Syria, Jordan and Iran and is probably endemic from North Africa to India, where it is possibly distributed over the same area as *T. annulata*. In susceptible sheep, the disease may be highly pathogenic. In Iraq, for example, losses of up to 40% have been attributed to theileriosis in indigenous Awassi sheep moved from one area to another. Losses in imported sheep may be higher. Although the parasite is apparently widely distributed, losses of the magnitude of those described in Iraq have not been reported elsewhere.

Diagnosis is confused by the widespread presence of the benign species *T. ovis*. Without a recognized serological test or significant knowledge of the epizootiology of the two organisms, this confusion will persist. To date, the only valid transmission studies show that the virulent *T. hirci* may be transmitted by *Hyalomma anatolicum anatolicum*. If this is so, other ticks of the genus *Hyalomma* will probably transmit this pathogen, transmission being dependent on the feeding of larvae and/or nymphs on infected sheep. *Rhipicephalus bursa*, a vector of *T. ovis*, has also been incriminated as a vector of *T. hirci*.

It is important that these two parasites are distinguished from each other and, because they probably co-exist with *T. annulata*, also from that organism. Epizootiological, transmission and cross-immunity studies are necessary before clear-cut recommendations on control and diagnosis can be made.

The disease caused by *T. hirci* in sheep may be considered to be equivalent to that caused by *T. annulata* in cattle. Both schizonts and piroplasms are incriminated in the pathogenesis, though the disease, in fatal cases at least, is almost invariably associated with anaemia.

There are early indications that parvaquone and its analogue buparvaquone are effective in treating the disease.

The schizonts can be cultured *in vitro* in ovine lymphoid cell lines. This gives hope for a vaccine and has also provided antigenic material for the development of an IFA test.

C.G.D.B.

TOXOPLASMOSIS

Toxoplasmosis is a disease of animals and man, caused by a protozoan parasite *Toxoplasma gondii*, which is an intracellular parasite capable of infecting a wide variety of tissues in a wide range of mammals and birds. Infection is probably extremely common, but clinical toxoplasmosis is relatively rare. It is important as a human disease and as a cause of ovine abortion.

Aetiology

The causal organism *Toxoplasma gondii* is an intracellular protozoan parasite found in many types of nucleated cells. The life-cycle is very complicated, but the parasite has a simple coccidian life-cycle in the final host – the cat – in which it is very common. The cat is the only known host in which *T. gondii* completes its life-cycle and produces oocysts. Infective sporulated oocysts ingested by the intermediate host, which can be from a wide range of other mammals and birds, result in the rapid multiplication of the parasite (tachyzoites) in a variety of tissues. A few weeks later, the parasites localize in certain tissues (brain, muscle, lungs, placenta) and their multiplication slows down (bradyzoites) as they become contained in a cyst and the infection becomes chronic.

The proliferative stages or trophozoites in the intermediate hosts are crescentic in shape, 4–6 μm long, one end being more rounded than the other and the nucleus is centrally placed. In fixed and stained preparations, the parasite appears more rounded. Movement is by flexion of the body and gliding.

Occurrence

Toxoplasmosis occurs widely throughout the world in all types of climate. Human infections appear to be associated with the presence of cats, and the consumption of inadequately cooked meat.

Species affected

This ubiquitous parasite has a wide range of approximately 200 species of mammalian and avian intermediate hosts including all domestic animals and man. Cats are the only known final host.

Transmission

Oocycts shed in the faeces of the final host sporulate within 2–3 days and become infectious to other cats and all intermediate hosts. Ingestion of sporulated oocysts by cats results in a typical direct coccidial-type life-cycle in the intestine, resulting in further faecal excretion of large numbers of oocysts. Ingestion of sporulated oocysts by intermediate hosts results in initial rapid multiplication of tachyzoites in a wide range of tissues. During this stage, the parasite can be transmitted to other intermediate hosts and cats by various routes, namely congenitally via the placenta in pregnant animals, in excretions and secretions including milk, and by carnivorism. Later, when infection is chronic and the parasites are contained as bradyzoites in host-tissue cysts, transmission by ingestion of infected tissues is possible.

Clinical features and pathology

Although infection appears to be common and widespread, most are symptomless or mild. Clinical signs depend on the tissues infected and the stage of the parasites, e.g. acute disease results from rapid multiplication of tachyzoites. Symptoms are exceedingly varied and include pneumonia, endocarditis, febrile exanthema (rash) and neonatal mortality.

Clinical toxoplasmosis tends to be sporadic and, because of the wide variation of possible clinical symptoms, it is usually undiagnosed.

Toxoplasmosis as an important cause of abortion in sheep is recognized in Australia, New Zealand, Canada and the UK, and probably occurs worldwide. The pattern of abortion depends on the stage of pregnancy when animals are infected. Infection early in pregnancy (45–55 days gestation) results in foetal death and apparent barrenness or abortion of a mummified foetus. Infection later in pregnancy causes placentitis and abortion of a relatively fresh, well-developed foetus. The cotyledons have small multi-focal necrotic lesions (white spot abortion). Some lambs congenitally infected may be born alive but are weak and die within a few days. Infection of sheep outside pregnancy is asymptomatic but results in immunity.

Outbreaks of porcine toxoplasmosis have been reported in the Far East, particularly in Japan. Young pigs appear to be more susceptible than adults. Clinical symptoms are very variable, ranging from latent to severe, and include pneumonitis, encephalitis and abortion.

In cattle, *T. gondii* does not appear to be very pathogenic, and clinical toxoplasmosis is rarely recorded. The parasite is quickly eliminated from infected tissues, and the milk of infected cows is of negligible importance in transmission.

Diagnosis

Diagnosis cannot, with confidence, be based on clinical features. The parasite can be isolated from infected animals by various means, the most sensitive being the intraperitoneal inoculation of suspect material into mice which are highly susceptible to infection. Parasite cysts can also be isolated direct from infected tissues by centrifugation on a discontinuous density gradient of a colloidal silica solution.

Various serological tests for detection of *Toxoplasma* antibodies are in use; namely, the complement fixation test, the indirect fluorescent antibody test, the latex agglutination test and the indirect haemagglutination test, all of which to a certain extent have superseded the dye test. These tests can be used to detect *Toxoplasma* antibodies in foetal fluids from ovine abortion material.

Treatment

Treatment is rarely applied to the toxoplasmosis of animals but, if used in the early stages, sulphadiazine combined with pyrimethamine has proved efficacious in man. Under experimental conditions, monensin given in the feed of sheep can significantly reduce the abortion rate in an infected flock.

Control

No vaccines are available commercially, although animals can be immunized by exposure to controlled infection. On known infected farms, susceptible female sheep should be exposed to *Toxoplasma*-contaminated areas several months before breeding in order to infect and immunize them before pregnancy. In uninfected flocks, contamination of supplementary feed with cat faeces should be prevented.

Further reading

Blewett, D.A. and Trees, A.J. (1987). The epidemiology of ovine toxoplasmosis with especial respect to control. *British Veterinary Journal*, **143**, 128–135

Dubey, J.P. (1986a). A review of toxoplasmosis in pigs. *Veterinary Parasitology*, **19**, 181–223.

Dubey, J.P. (1986b). A review of toxoplasmosis in cattle. *Veterinary Parasitology*, **22**, 177–202.

Fayer, R. (1980). Epidemiology of protozoan infections: The coccidia. *Veterinary Parasitology*, **22**, 75–103.

Soulsby, E.J.L. (1982). *Toxoplasma*. In *Helminths, arthropods and protozoa of domesticated animals*, pp. 670–682. Baillière Tindall, London.

A.G.H.

TRICHOMONOSIS

Trichomonosis is a non-febrile, contagious disease confined to the reproductive tract of the cow and the preputial sac of the bull, which gives rise to irregular returns to service, early abortions and some cases of pyometra.

Aetiology

The causal organism is *Tritrichomonas foetus*, a pear-shaped protozoan about three times the size of a red blood cell, with three terminal flagellae and a characteristic motility. It can be grown readily in the laboratory. Three antigenic types have been described, namely Belfast, Manley and Brisbane. All three are equally pathogenic, although they have both unique and shared antigens. The Belfast strain shares antigens with an apparently identical trichomonad found as a normal commensal in the intestine of the pig. Infections with more than one serotype is uncommon.

Occurrence

Bovine trichomonosis has a worldwide distribution and has been diagnosed in all the major cattle producing countries.

Species affected

Cattle, and possibly pigs, horses and roe deer, are natural hosts of the parasite, but only cattle are affected clinically.

Transmission

Trichomonosis is primarily a venereal disease, but the infection can also be transmitted by artificial insemination using semen from infected bulls, or mechanically via insemination instruments, vaginal palpation, etc.

Clinical features

T. foetus infection is confined to the reproductive tract. The parasite can invade most parts of the female genital tract and infection normally persists for about 3 months, although infections of a longer duration have been reported. A mild vaginitis may be evident soon after the infective coitus, but significant pathological changes do not normally occur until about 50–60 days after infection, and the resulting symptoms commonly include vaginitis, cervicitis, endometritis, pyometra and early abortion.

Abortions are often undetected and the main feature observed is often the failure of cows to hold to service.

Infection in the male is usually confined to the surface of the prepuce and penis, and although it may cause a mild inflammatory response, it is inapparent clinically.

Pathology

Although *T. foetus* can colonize all parts of the female reproductive tract within 15 days of infection, there is little pathological change until about the 50th day when mild inflammation characterized by accumulation of neutrophils, macrophages and lymphocytes may occur throughout the tract. Pathological lesions become severe on about the 60th day of infection or later, causing the clinical features mentioned above. Cows eventually clear themselves of infection and the uterus is usually restored to normal 2–6 months after infection.

Infection in the male produces little histopathological change, but once infected bulls tend to remain permanent carriers.

Diagnosis

Trichomonosis can be suspected in any breeding cattle if there is a history of reproductive failure characterized by a lower than expected pregnancy rate, a wide range of gestational ages and cases of early abortion and pyometra. The disease must be differentiated from campylobacteriosis which it resembles clinically and epidemiologically.

Diagnosis can be confirmed by demonstrating the trichomonad organism in vaginal or prepucial secretions, either directly under the microscope or in culture. Various similar methods are used to obtain suitable samples for examination. Bulls are sampled by scraping the preputial mucosa, preferably after a period of at least 1 week's sexual rest to allow the trichomonads to increase to detectable levels. Bulls should be tested in three consecutive occasions 1 week apart before they can be regarded as free of infection. Cows can be sampled by aspirating vaginal mucus. Other material containing large numbers of trichomonad organisms and suitable for examination are foetal and placental fluids from abortions, and the uterine contents of culled pyometra cases.

Motile trichomonad organisms may be detected in fresh samples by direct examination under the microscope using 100–400 × magnification. More sensitive is the isolation of the organism in culture, usually in a tube of nutrient medium containing trypticase peptone, yeast extract and maltose (Diamond's medium) modified by addition of a small quantity of agar. The culture is incubated aerobically at 37°C and the motile trichomonad organisms migrate downwards and multiply in the anaerobic conditions at the bottom of the tube.

Samples should be cultured as soon as possible but, if delayed, suitable transport media are available which are effective for up to 4 days.

Less sensitive than culture is the vaginal mucus agglutination test. Mucus samples become positive for antibody about 6 weeks after initial exposure, but it is essentially a herd test because it only detects approximately 60% of naturally infected cows. Mucus samples for this test should be kept cool but delays in transport are less important.

Treatment

As the majority of infected cows or heifers recover completely and clear the infection, they are not normally treated. In bulls, acriflavine douches of the prepuce and penis used to be popular but this approach has been superseded by parenteral or oral administration of various imidazole preparations. Dimetridazole has proved useful using a 5-day course by mouth at a dose of 50 mg/kg/day. Others have used metronidazole as a single dose intravenously, but this must be done with some care to avoid systemic side-effects. Drug resistance has been reported. More recently, ipronidazole hydrochloride (Ipropran) administered by intramuscular injection has been used successfully without any side-effects; before treatment, bulls should receive a course of broad-spectrum antibiotic therapy to reduce preputial commensal bacteria which might inactivate the ipronidazole.

Immunology

Circulating antibody is produced, but a natural agglutinin in bovine sera interferes with a blood test. Local antibody is produced in the cervicovaginal mucus but individual levels of immunity are variable and often transient.

After vaginal infection and multiplication, uterine invasion occurs only when an active corpus luteum is in the ovary, i.e. during mid-cycle, pregnancy or pyometra. When the corpus luteum regresses, the organisms leave the uterus and may be destroyed by the presence of vaginal antibody.

Like the females, infected bulls show circulating antibody and frequently a positive skin test with an extract of trichomonads. Neither of these reactions has proved useful as a diagnostic test.

Attempts to immunize cattle have largely been ineffective. Cows that recover are mostly susceptible to reinfection, and to date vaccination has not proved practicable.

Control

Trichomonosis can be controlled by breeding only from cattle known to be free of infection, or using artificial insemination with the semen of known non-infected bulls. The measures required are readily applied to closed intensive herds and, in general, where intensive cattle husbandry is practised, trichomonosis is a disease of the past.

In extensive conditions where it may be impossible to segregate herds or isolate infected animals, however, it is more difficult, and trichomonosis is still an important reproductive disease. The segregation of an infected herd from a clean herd with unexposed females and clean young bulls, is most difficult to maintain for more than a short time. A compromise is to allow clean bulls to serve previously infected cows after they have completed a 60-to 90-day rest after a normal parturition to allow clearance of any infection, although there is always the possibility that a bull may become infected by serving an infected cow on the property.

Where these measures are not feasible, the disease may be controlled by the removal of old bulls and any proven carriers, and the use of young clean bulls less than 4 years old which are less susceptible to infection than older bulls.

Further reading

Bon Durant, R.H. (1985). Diagnosis, treatment and control of bovine trichomoniasis. *The Compendium on Continuing Education*, **7**, 179–188.
Skirrow, S.Z. (1988). Bovine trichomoniasis. *Veterinary Bulletin*, **58**, 591–603.

A.G.H.

TRYPANOSOMOSIS

The trypanosomoses are a group of diseases of man and animals caused by parasitic trypanosomes. The trypanosomes of veterinary and medical importance are subdivided into two sections, the Stercoraria and the Salivaria, on grounds of mode of development in their insect vectors and vertebrate hosts. These are summarized in Table 13.

Table 13 Trypanosomes of veterinary and medical importance

Trypanosome spp.	Animals affected	Mode of transmission	Distribution
1. Salivaria			
T. brucei, T. vivax, T. congolense, T. simiae, T. suis	All domestic animals (Nagana)	Cyclically by tsetse flies	Sub-Saharan Africa
T. b. rhodesiense, T. b. gambiense	Man (Sleeping sickness)	Cyclically by tsetse flies	Sub-Saharan Africa
T. vivax	Domestic ruminants	Mechanically by haematophagous flies	South America, Mauritius, Africa
T. evansi	All domestic animals (Surra)	Mechanically, principally haematophagous flies	Tropics except sub-Saharan Africa
T. equiperdum	Equidae (Dourine)	Venereally	Tropics and subtropics
2. Stercoraria			
T. cruzi	Man, dogs, cats, pigs (Chagas' disease)	From faeces of infected triatomid bugs	Central and South America

Tsetse-transmitted animal trypanosomoses

The trypanosomoses of domesticated livestock in Africa are diseases caused by infection with several different species of trypanosomes transmitted by tsetse flies of the genus *Glossina*. The diseases caused by these organisms vary considerably in severity and duration and depend on a number of factors associated with both the host species and the species of trypanosome involved. For instance, there are differences in susceptibility to infection among different species of host animals, e.g. *T. congolense* readily infects cattle causing disease but rarely causes problems in pigs. Certain West African breeds of small, humpless cattle are less susceptible (tolerant) to the effects of trypanosomosis than humped, Zebu breeds. There are many different serodemes (strains) of each species of trypanosome and they can show a widely differing range of virulence, even within the same trypanosome species. Thus certain isolates of *T. vivax* in East Africa cause a severe, rapidly fatal disease with a characteristic haemorrhagic syndrome; *T. brucei* usually produces only mild disease in cattle, while *T. congolense* varies in virulence. All species of domesticated livestock are affected by the trypanosomoses and the disease is characterized by a relapsing parasitaemia, anaemia, loss of condition, abortion, alterations in ovarian cyclicity leading to infertility and, if left untreated, a high mortality.

Aetiology

Trypanosomes are flagellated, blood-borne protozoa belonging to the section Salivaria (Table 13). Three species which affect cattle, namely *T. vivax*, *T. congolense* and *T. brucei*, are widely distributed throughout Africa and are frequently encountered in infected livestock. Mixed infections with these three species often occur in individual animals. *T. simiae*, a parasite of pigs, has a more limited distribution and *T. suis*, also found in pigs, has been seen only rarely. Trypanosomes are found in blood, but some species such as *T. brucei* are found in tissue spaces. Multiplication takes place by longitudinal fission and can occur extravascularly as well as in the blood. *T. brucei*, *T. vivax* and *T. congolense* can be readily distinguished both by their morphological appearance and their characteristic behaviour in wet blood films.

   T. brucei is a pleomorphic organism, the trypanosomes showing a variation in size so that individuals in the population can be classified as long and slender (24–38 μm), intermediate (20–24 μm) and short and stumpy (18 μm). The slender and intermediate forms have a long, free flagellum, pointed posterior end, subterminal kinetoplast and a conspicuous undulating membrane. The stumpy forms are short and broad, with a short or absent flagellum and a prominent undulating membrane. Long and slender *T. brucei* are highly active when viewed microscopically, but do not show any movement across the microscope field: short, stumpy forms are less active.

   T. vivax is a long, slender monomorphic parasite (18–28 μm) with a rounded posterior end and a terminal kinetoplast. The flagellum is long but the undulating membrane is inconspicuous. In fresh blood preparations, these parasites move rapidly back and forth across the microscope field.

   T. congolense is the smallest of the pathogenic trypanosomes (8–14 μm), with a marginal kinetoplast, no free flagellum and an inconspicuous undulating membrane. Its movement in fresh preparations is very slow and it is often found in close proximity or attached to erythrocytes. *T. simiae* is morphologically indistinguishable from *T. congolense*, varying from 12 to 14 μm in length.

   The rarely observed *T. suis* resembles the stumpy forms of *T. brucei*.

Occurrence

The diseases associated with the African trypanosomoses are usually related to the distribution of tsetse flies between latitudes 14°N and 29°S. Overall, some 40 African countries are affected and 10 million km² of land are infested with tsetse flies. The occurrence of trypanosomosis depends on the degree of contact between cattle and particular species of tsetse flies. Animal husbandry practices can affect contact by moving cattle into wet, tsetse-infested regions during the dry season for instance. Different species of tsetse fly differ in their ability to transmit pathogenic trypanosomes: *G. morsitans*, an efficient vector of pathogenic trypanosomes, can completely prevent use of land by livestock, so that trypanosomosis only occurs at the edges of the fly belt.

   T. vivax is the only one of the tsetse-transmitted species of trypanosomes which has established itself in areas where tsetse flies are absent, i.e. South America and Mauritius.

Species affected

Economically, the tsetse-transmitted trypanosomoses are of most importance in cattle, with some 50 million head at risk. However, in addition to infections in domesticated livestock, trypanosomes are found in many species of African wild mammals. Tsetse flies frequently feed on wild mammals which are infected with trypanosomes, and parasites may then be transmitted to domesticated animals which come into close association with them. Animals such as the warthog (*Phacochoerus*), bush pig (*Potamochoerus*), duiker (*Silvicapra* spp.), eland (*Taurotragus*), bushbuck (*Tragelaphus*) and buffalo (*Syncerus*), in which trypanosome infections are mild and symptomless, act as reservoir hosts from which domesticated livestock can be infected.

All species of domestic animals are susceptible to infection with one or more species of the salivarian trypanosomes (Table 14), but trypanosome infections are economically of greatest importance in cattle. The pathogenicity of each trypanosome species varies in different host species and within species other factors such as breed, age, level of challenge, parasite strain and stress can affect the clinical picture. Table 14 summarizes the commonly accepted patterns of infectivity and pathogenicity of tsetse-transmitted trypanosomes in different species of domestic animals.

Table 14 The infectivity and pathogenicity of tsetse-transmitted trypanosomes to domestic animals[a]

Animal	T. vivax	T. congolense	T. simiae	T. brucei	T. suis
Zebu cattle	***	***	R	**	R
West African dwarf cattle	**	**	R	**	?
Sheep	**	*	**	*	R
Goats	***	*	***	*	R
Pigs	R	*	****	*	***
Horses	* or ***	*	R	***	?
Donkeys	* or ***	*	R	**	?
Camels	* or ***	*	* or ***	***	?
Dogs	R	* or ***	R	***	?

[a]Adapted from Stephen (1986), Trypanosomiasis: A veterinary perspective. Pergamon Press, Oxford.
* ** *** ****, Pathogenicity; R, refractory to infection.

Transmission

Salivarian trypanosomes are normally maintained in wild animals by transmission cycles involving tsetse flies (*Glossina* spp.). Adult flies derive all their nutritional requirements from vertebrate blood and seek out suitable hosts in the daylight by sight and smell. Within their ecological habitats, different species of tsetse flies often have favoured hosts if these are available. Thus, warthog blood constitutes 60% of feeds by *G. morsitans* in some parts of Africa. Other studies have shown that *G. pallidipes* and *G. fuscipes* favour bovidae, particularly bushbuck (45%). This latter species has a wide range of acceptable hosts, including reptiles. *G. brevipalpis* feeds on bushpig (45%), bovids and hippopotamus.

Animals are infected with trypanosomes by the bite of an infected tsetse fly. Tsetse flies themselves become infected when they feed on an infected animal host: the ingested trypanosomes undergo a cycle of development in the fly lasting between 8 and

35 days before infective metacyclic trypanosomes are produced. Once infected, a fly is usually capable of transmitting trypanosomes for the rest of its life. Infection rates in wild populations of tsetse flies are characteristically low, varying from 1 to 20%. Mixed infections can occur.

Many factors influence the level of trypanosome infections in tsetse flies, including species of *Glossina*, sex, age of the fly at infective feed, trypanosome species and ecological factors including environmental temperature and source of the infected blood meal. Thus, work in Uganda has shown that infected *G. pallidipes*, *G. fuscipes* and *G. brevipalpis* derived *vivax*-type infections from bovidae and *congolense*-type infection from both bovidae and suidae. Trypanosome infection rates and transmission characteristics differ: *G fuscipes* is a poor transmitter of *T. congolense* compared with *G. morsitans* and *G. pallidipes*, but a good transmitter of *T. vivax*.

Tsetse flies can be divided into groups broadly associated with their preferred habitats, namely forest, riverine and savannah species. Trypanosomosis becomes important when man and domestic livestock compete with wild animals and tsetse for grazing land, or come into contact with tsetse as a result of other activities. The forest tsetse are of least economic importance as their habitat is frequently unsuitable for raising livestock. Riverine tsetse are more important because they infest vegetation near essential water supplies. Savannah tsetse have the greatest impact on livestock production and development because they occupy vast areas of land otherwise suitable for grazing animals.

Mechanical transmission by both tsetse and other biting flies can also take place, but good evidence for its occurrence in the field is sparse. Normally, when tsetse are eradicated, trypanosomosis also disappears. However, the disease is prevalent in certain areas in Africa where possible tsetse habitats are negligible and no tsetse can be demonstrated, but large populations of other biting flies exist. Transmission of *T. vivax* also occurs in the absence of tsetse flies in Central and South America. Prenatal infection is possible, but is not considered important. Lions, hyaenas, dogs and cats can be infected with *T. brucei* by feeding on the carcases of infected animals.

Clinical features

Animals exposed to infection by tsetse flies develop patent infections after incubation periods of variable length depending on the strain and species of the infecting trypanosomes and on the number of trypanosomes introduced by the tsetse flies. Trypanosomes appear in the blood of most animals exposed to infection with *T. vivax* after 8–10 days and with *T. congolense* after 12–16 days. In the case of *T. simiae* in pigs, the prepatent period is 4–5 days. The prepatent period with *T. brucei* is less well defined, but the parasites can sometimes be detected in the blood as early as 3–4 days after exposure to infection.

The invasion of the blood by actively dividing trypanosomes is associated with increased body temperature, and the initial parasitaemia and fever usually persist for several days before a trypanolytic crisis occurs, parasites become scanty in the blood and the temperature returns to normal. The first trypanolytic crisis is usually followed by further intermittent periods of parasitaemia, associated febrile attacks and remissions of infection.

The subsequent course and outcome of the disease varies considerably and is influenced by the breed, background and management of the stock concerned, the nature and severity of the trypanosome challenge, the pathogenicity of the infecting trypanosome and the period of exposure to infection.

Acute infections may be seen occasionally in all domestic animals, notably with *T. vivax* in cattle and with *T. brucei* in the horse and dog, leading to death after 1–3 weeks. Infections with *T. simiae* in pigs are also usually particularly severe and short-lasting and infected animals die 12–36 hours after the onset of signs, which include high fever, respiratory distress and prostration.

Trypanosomosis is more commonly seen as a chronic disease with intermittent fever, an increasing degree of anaemia and progressive loss of condition. Infected animals are dull, they have a staring lustreless coat, lose weight and are easily exhausted, lagging behind the herd. Superficial lymph nodes are enlarged and prominent. Cattle infected with *T. vivax* often show photophobia and excessive lachrymation, and in the horse and dog infected with *T. brucei* corneal opacity may occur. Oedema of the limbs, ventral surface of the abdomen, scrotum or vulva is a feature of infection in the horse. Severe trypanosomosis resulting from repeated exposure to infection leads to increasing weakness, debility and emaciation and results in recumbency and death in many cases after periods of 1–6 months.

Trypanosomosis is not an invariably fatal disease. Some animals, particularly those of trypanotolerant breeds, given good feeding and management may recover after transient infections lasting a few weeks, particularly after limited periods of exposure to infection with low numbers of trypanosomes and strains of low virulence. Occasionally, animals recover more slowly over periods of weeks or months from more severe trypanosome infections which progress through a state of premunity (co-infection immunity) to complete self-cure.

Pathology

The pathogenesis and pathology of tsetse-transmitted trypanosomoses are complex and not fully understood and differ according to the species causing the infection. *T. vivax*, *T. congolense*, *T. simiae* and *T. suis* are essentially parasites of the blood plasma, but *T. brucei* is more widely distributed in the host, infecting blood plasma, the intercellular fluids of connective tissue of various organs, and the extracellular fluids of the body cavities.

Tissue damage due to trypanosomosis is probably multifactorial in aetiology, but the underlying feature is the progressive anaemia throughout the course of the disease, even in the later stage when the parasites are present in either very low numbers or apparently absent altogether. In the live animal infected with trypanosomes, the level of anaemia estimated by measurement of erythrocyte numbers, packed cell volume percentage and blood haemoglobin content, can be related to the severity of the clinical disease.

In the early stage of the disease, which can last up to 12 weeks in cattle, a fluctuating parasitaemia together with anaemia are the main features. The cause of the anaemia is complex but is believed to be haemolytic, caused primarily by erythrophagocytosis due to stimulation and expansion of the mononuclear phagocytic system throughout the reticulo-endothelial system. As a result, splenomegaly occurs. The severity of the anaemia is directly related to the level of parasitaemia, and trypanotolerant breeds of cattle such as the West African N'dama are able to suppress the parasitaemia following infection, thereby reducing the resulting anaemia and attendant clinical signs.

If animals survive the early parasitaemic phase, the disease becomes chronic during which the parasitaemia is low and the parasites are difficult to detect or even apparently absent altogether. Despite this, the anaemia persists.

Death can occur at any time, but in chronic disease when animals are weak and cachexic, the final cause of death may be due to secondary complications.

Post-mortem examination of animals after acute trypanosomosis may show extensive small haemorrhages involving mucous and serous surfaces, areas of emphysema in the lungs and mild gastroenteritis. After more chronic infections, the carcase may be anaemic and emaciated, with an enlarged spleen and lymph nodes. Subcutaneous oedema and accumulations of pericardial and thoracic fluid containing trypanosomes are found particularly in horses and dogs infected with *T. brucei*.

Histologically, aggregates of *T. congolense* occur in the capillaries of the heart, skeletal muscle and brain causing impairment of the microcirculation and frequently the development of focal polioencephalomalacia in the brains of cattle. Death caused by *T. vivax* may be associated with extravascular coagulation of blood elements and aggregates of trypanosomes in the vascular system. *T. brucei* infections result in extravascular accumulations of trypanosomes associated with cellular infiltration and necrosis in many tissues and organs, notably heart, skeletal muscles, brain, pericardial and serosal surfaces. Examinations of lymph nodes and spleens from infected animals reveal a progression of changes after different periods of infection. Increased numbers of lymphoblasts and marked plasma cell hyperplasia occur in the early stages of infection, but these cells are depleted as infections progress and are replaced by macrophages and reticular cells. Such cellular changes have been linked in experimental studies with the production of abnormal amounts of immunoglobulin and the occurrence of immunosuppression in trypanosome-infected animals.

Diagnosis

The history of the affected animals, the geographical incidence of the disease and the clinical signs of infection may arouse suspicions of trypanosomosis, but definite diagnosis depends on the detection of the parasites.

A number of techniques are available for the parasitological diagnosis of trypanosomosis, some of which are more suited to the laboratory than the field. In the field, examination of blood smears is routinely used, although lymph node biopsies are considered to be useful in some instances. Blood smears can be examined as wet films, or as stained thin or thick films. With wet films examined under high-power magnification, the motility of the organisms can readily be seen but morphological characteristics are less easily distinguished. Thin and thick blood smears are stained with a suitable Romanowsky stain before examination. This smears can be used to identify a trypanosome species; thick films are more useful for detecting the presence of trypanosomes, but the staining procedures used tend to distort the parasites and they are difficult to identify. Modifications of the basic staining method, utilizing methylene blue, can however enhance preservation of morphology. In acute cases of trypanosomosis where parasites are present in large numbers, trypanosomes can be detected in peripheral blood samples. In chronic trypanosomosis, parasites may be difficult to demonstrate because the numbers of organisms present is low. The sensitivity of the various diagnostic techniques differs with each trypanosome species (see Table 15), hence the use of a particular diagnostic technique can lead to a bias in the species of trypanosome detected. Thus, where chronic infections are encountered, thick film examination is more suitable for *T. congolense*, but the technique often fails to detect *T. vivax* or *T. brucei*.

When diagnosis of infection in individual animals is required, thick films prepared on several consecutive days are used. Diagnosis of infection on a herd basis may be carried out by examining a proportion of the animals on a single occasion.

Examination of lymph node smears is often more useful for *T. vivax* than examination of blood smears, but such techniques are less easily applied to large numbers of animals.

A number of other tests are more usually carried out under laboratory conditions because they may require use of centrifuges. However, small hand-held, battery-powered, haematocrit centrifuges are available which allow field application of some of these techniques. For detection of low numbers of parasites in blood, concentration techniques involving centrifugation of blood in haematocrit tubes are highly sensitive (Table 15). After centrifugation, the haematocrit tubes can be examined directly using a low-power objective ($\times$ 10) to visualize trypanosomes at the buffy coat/plasma junction. Alternatively, the haematocrit tube can be cut a few millimetres below the junction of the buffy coat/plasma, and the erythrocytes, buffy coat and plasma expressed on to a slide and examined by dark ground phase-contrast microscopy. Separation of trypanosomes from blood by anion-exchange chromatography (e.g. diethylaminoethyl cellulose) can be accomplished using purpose-built columns or adapting 2-ml plastic syringes. Trypanosomes can often be detected in column eluate, but centrifugation of eluates is usually necessary. Inoculation of blood into laboratory rodents is a useful method and with *T. brucei* is particularly sensitive (Table 15). Some isolates of *T. congolense* can also infect rodents, but these animals are completely refractory to *T. vivax*. *T. congolense* and *T. brucei* can be isolated in culture medium, but in practice this technique is rarely used.

A large number of serological tests have been used to indicate infections with trypanosomes. However, few of them have found practical application.

Interpretation of the results of serological diagnostic tests are made difficult because antigens from different trypanosome species show considerable cross-reactivity and antibodies persist for several months after trypanocidal drug treatment. Hence, the specific diagnosis and determination of current infection status serologically is problematic. Fluorescent antibody tests have been used successfully for differentiation of antibody responses to different trypanosome species, but the most promising tests in use are those based on enzyme-linked immunosorbent assays (ELISA). Species-specific monoclonal antibodies are currently being developed which should allow preparation of defined antigens for use in assays for antibody detection. In addition, monoclonal antibodies could be used in sandwich ELISA to detect trypanosomal antigen and thus the presence of active infections. ELISA kits might also be produced with would enable assays to be conducted under field conditions.

Trypanosomosis can be confused superficially with any other chronic wasting disease, notably helminthosis and malnutrition, but a firm diagnosis can be made on the basis of the demonstration and identification of trypanosomes of pathogenic species. These parasites must be distinguished from *T. theileri* which occurs in a high proportion of cattle in some areas and which may be seen as an isolated organism in approximately

Table 15 Sensitivity of different parasitological diagnostic techniques for detection of *Trypanosoma* spp.[a]

Numbers of trypanosomes (ml^{-1})	DG			HCT			WF			TF			I
	Tb	Tv	Tc	Tb	Tv	Tc	Tb	Tv	Tc	Tb	Tv	Tc	Tb
5×10^4	+	+	+	+	+	+	+	+	+	+	+	+	+
1×10^4	+	+	+	+	+	+	+	−	+	+	+	+	+
5×10^3	+	+	+	−	+	−	−	−	−	+	−	−	+
1×10^3	−	+	+	+	+	−	−	−	−	−	−	−	+
5×10^2	−	+	+	+	−	−	−	−	−	−	−	−	+
1×10^2	−	−	−	−	−	−	−	−	−	−	−	−	−

[a]Based on Paris, Murray and McOdimba (1982), *Acta Tropica*, **39**, 307–316.
DG, dark ground phase contrast microscopy; HCT, haematocrit centrifuge technique; WF, wet film; TF, thick film; I, rodent sub-inoculation.

1% of blood films submitted to the laboratory for the diagnosis of protozoal disease. *T. theileri* is considered non-pathogenic and is recognized by its large size (60–70 μm), pointed posterior end, subterminal kinetoplast, much folded undulating membrane, and free flagellum.

Treatment

The names and proprietary synonyms of drugs in current use for the treatment of tsetse-transmitted trypanosomal infections, and indications for their use in animals infected with organisms of different species, are shown in Table 16. No curative is available for *T. simiae* infections, although pigs at risk can be protected prophylatically with a complex of suramin and quinapyramine which can be made up as required.

Table 16 Drugs used in the control of tsetse-transmitted trypanosomosis in domestic animals

Drug	Proprietary preparations	Host	Indications (trypanosomes)
Curative drugs			
Diminazene aceturate	Berenil (Hoechst), Trypazen (Virbac)	Cattle	*T. vivax, T. congolense, T. brucei*
Homidium chloride	Ethidium "C" (Boots), Novidium (May and Baker)	Cattle, horses	*T. vivax, T. congolense, T. brucei*
Homidium bromide	Ethidium bromide (Boots)		
Isometamidium chloride	Samorin (May and Baker), Trypamidium (SPECIA)	Cattle, horses, dogs	*T. vivax, T. congolense, T. brucei* / *T. congolense, T. brucei*
Suramin	Naganol (Bayer)	Horses, camels, dogs	*T. brucei*
Prophylactic drugs			
Isometamidium chloride	Samorin (May and Baker), Trypamidium (SPECIA)	Cattle	*T. vivax, T. congolense, T. brucei*
Quinapyramine-suramin complex		Pigs	*T. simiae*
Quinapyramine dimethyl sulphate 10 g		Inject subcutaneously behind the ear	
Suramine anhydrate 8.9 g		at 20–40 mg/kg body weight	
Distilled water q.s. 200 ml		for quinapyramine sulphate	

No new drugs for treatment or prophylaxis have been developed for nearly 30 years and, in recent years, some have either been withdrawn or are contraindicated because of resistance to them. Consequently, those remaining in use require careful management to minimize resistance problems.

Curative drugs can be used for the treatment of individual animals, but cattle are frequently treated on a herd or area basis to circumvent the problems of identifying individual infected animals, e.g. in endemic areas where infection is inevitable, or to "clean up" transhumant cattle moving from tsetse-infested to tsetse-free grazing areas.

Resistance by trypanosomes to all available drugs has been recorded, but, of the curative drugs, diminazene aceturate has had the least problems. Consequently, if curatives are being used regularly, e.g. to treat cattle in endemic areas, diminazene should be kept in reserve to act as a "sanative" in the event of resistance occurring to other drugs. A regimen for curatives in cattle to minimize the risk of resistance was developed in Kenya in the early 1960s and is still recommended for present-day use (Table 17).

Table 17 A regimen for curatives in cattle

Risk of trypanosomosis	Curative drug alternatives	
	Homidium	Diminazene
High	1 year	1 year
Medium	2 years	1 year
Low	As long as possible	1 year

Sheep and goats can be treated with the same curative drugs as cattle.

Cattle herds may be protected against trypanosomosis prophylactically providing they are under good management, as it is essential that the timing of administration and the dosage of the drugs are correct to prevent resistance. If used at irregular or infrequent intervals, there is a risk that blood levels of the prophylactic will fall below therapeutic levels, resulting in the appearance of drug-resistant trypanosomes. Recent analyses of the performance of cattle in the Mkwaja Ranch in Tanzania has shown the value of chemoprophylaxis when correctly administered.

Cattle temporarily exposed to tsetse challenge may also be protected prophylactically, e.g. *en route* to an abattoir or moving to fresh grazing.

Chemoprophylaxis is contraindicated in areas of high tsetse challenge or in migratory cattle whose movements cannot be followed.

Immunology

A major reason for the success of the pathogenic trypanosomes is the ease with which they can evade the host defence mechanisms. Bloodstream forms of trypanosome are able to switch their surface antigens, the phenomenon known as antigenic variation, and thereby establish persistent infections. Variation occurs spontaneously and does not require antibody as a stimulus. The number of antigens which a trypanosome may express is unknown but, theoretically, could run into many hundreds. In addition to the multiple variable antigen types expressed during a single infection, there is also evidence for existence of different strains or serodemes, each capable of expressing a different repertoire of variable antigens. Recent work has shown that there is also a number of metacyclic variable antigen types, but these are more limited in number than those found in bloodstream trypanosomes.

Acquisition of protective immunity can readily be achieved against individual trypanosome populations by a number of techniques, including infection followed by trypanocidal drug treatments. Cattle thus treated are immune to homologous challenge but remain susceptible to challenge with heterologous strains or serodemes. This type of immunity can be effected easily with *T. brucei* or *T. congolense*, but less so with *T. vivax*. Animals infected with several different serodemes of trypanosomes, when treated may not acquire resistance to all the serodemes with which they were infected. The antigenic composition of the metacyclic trypanosomes is constant for any one serodeme and immunity can thus be effected against cyclically transmitted trypanosomes. Protective immunity against metacyclic trypanosomes appears to occur at the skin, because in immune animals no detectable development of trypanosomes takes place in dermal chancres.

Despite the multiplicity of antigenic types and serodemes, cattle kept in tsetse-infested areas under chemotherapy can acquire resistance. Presumably, this is due to acquisition of immunity to those serodemes present in the local tsetse fly population. Evidence for the build up of immunity can be shown by the decreased need for trypanocidal drug treatment in the cattle at risk.

Among the wild bovidae in Africa, many are unsusceptible or resistant to trypanosomosis. There are also a number of trypano-tolerant breeds of West African cattle such as the N'Dama and West African Shorthorn. These animals are often able to survive in areas of tsetse infestation without the need for chemotherapy. The mechanisms of resistance are not known and are not absolute, and N'Dama can become ill and die of trypanosomosis. Nevertheless, they do appear to have the ability to control parasitaemia more effectively than Zebu cattle and to develop a less severe anaemia.

Chronic trypanosomosis causes a number of pathological disturbances including immunosuppression. This is very pronounced in laboratory animals, but there are indications that disruption of immune mechanisms can occur in ruminants as well. Evaluation of the responses of trypanosome-infected cattle to a variety of viral and bacterial antigens have sometimes shown lowered antibody responses. There is also experimental evidence that cattle infected with *T. vivax* or *T. congolense* and immunized against *Mycoplasma mycoides* remained susceptible to infection with the live organism. There is no evidence from the field that immunosuppression caused by trypanosomosis is a problem affecting immunization against other diseases.

Control

The prevention and control of tsetse-transmitted animal trypanosomosis depend on minimizing contact between livestock, wild animals and tsetse infestations, the destruction of tsetse vectors, diagnosis and chemotherapy, chemoprophylaxis, and the control of animal movements. The exploitation of trypano-tolerant breeds of livestock may have a greater role to play in the future. The antigenic diversity of trypanosomes has prevented the development of immunization techniques.

T. vivax in Central and South America, the West Indies and Mauritius

T. vivax infections occur in cattle in the absence of tsetse flies in Central and South America and the West Indies and was probably introduced in the last century with infected cattle imported from Africa. Trypanosomes in cattle in Mauritius were mistakenly identified as *T. evansi* until the mid-1930s, when it was realized that *T. vivax* was also present, but the source of infection is not known and no recent studies have been carried out.

Aetiology

Morphologically, New World and African *T. vivax* parasites are similar and limited studies have indicated similar isoenzyme and antigenic patterns. The New World parasites, however, have apparently lost the ability to infect tsetse flies and it has been suggested they should be regarded as a subspecies.

Occurrence

Infection has been recorded in Bolivia, Ecuador, Colombia, Venezuela, Panama, Brazil, Guyana (French, Dutch and British), and the Caribbean Islands of Martinique and Guadaloupe. In addition, serological surveys indicate its presence in El Salvador, Costa Rica, Peru and Paraguay.

Species affected

In the New World, infection is found in cattle, buffalo, sheep and goats. The situation in Mauritius is unclear, but infection was recorded in cattle and possibly equidae.

Transmission

Infection in the New World is probably transmitted mechanically by biting flies. Studies in Colombia show an association of infection with low-lying swampy areas where cattle and deer, thought to be reservoirs, congregate and where biting flies are common. The parasite has been found in deer in Venezuela.

Clinical features

The pathogenicity of New World *T. vivax* is very variable but tends to be lower than African strains. Reports of symptomless infections are not unusual and mixed infections are common (e.g. with babesiosis and anaplasmosis), thereby confusing the clinical picture. Clinical signs are similar to those of tsetse-transmitted trypanosomosis and include intermittent fever, anaemia and loss of condition. Mortality rates of 40% and more have been recorded in Venezuela. Advanced cases in cattle have a swaying gait which may be confused with rabies. Animals in good condition may recover spontaneously.

Diagnosis

Diagnosis is based on the demonstration of the organism in blood smears. The swaying gait of advanced cases may be confused with rabies, and diagnosis can be differentiated by response to treatment with trypanocidal drugs.

Treatment and control

The economic importance of the disease in the New World is unknown and little is recorded on treatment and control. Diminazene aceturate is the drug of choice for treatment.

Further reading

Paris, J., Murray, M. and McOdimba, F. (1982). *Acta Tropica*, **39**, 307–316.
Stephen, L.E. (1986). Animal trypanosomiasis beyond the distribution of *Glossina*. In *Trypanosomiasis – A veterinary perspective*, pp. 171–183. Pergamon Press, Oxford.
Wells, E.A. (1984) Animal trypanosomiasis in South America. *Preventive Veterinary Medicine*, **2**, 31–41.

Surra

Surra is a disease affecting horses, camels, buffalo, goats, sheep and pigs caused by *Trypanosoma evansi*, and the closely related organism *T. equinum*.

Aetiology

Trypanosoma evansi is morphologically indistinguishable from the long slender and long slender-intermediate forms of *T. brucei*. *T. evansi* is thought to have evolved from *T. brucei* following its introduction into camels when they entered the tsetse belt and its subsequent adaptation to direct transmission by tabanids. *T. evansi* is incapable of cyclical development in *Glossina* spp. because it lacks the genes needed for formation of the mitochondrion, which is a prerequisite for cyclically transmitted members of the *brucei* group. It is not markedly pleomorphic, although a small proportion of short stumpy trypanosomes may be present. Isolates of the trypanosomes can vary in length from 15 to 34 μm with an average of 24 μm.

The parasite multiplies by longitudinal binary fission in the trypanosome form in the blood and tissue fluids of the vertebrate host. Strains of *T. evansi* in which a percentage of organisms lack a kinetoplast occur spontaneously in nature or can be produced by treatment with certain drugs. Therefore, there is no need to regard the South American akinetoplastic variant *T. equinum*, which is otherwise identical to *T. evansi*, as a separate species. Strains of *T. evansi* from different geographical localities vary greatly in virulence for domestic animals.

Occurrence

The disease occurs within a wide range of climate and vegetation in the Middle East, Asia, the Far East, Central and South America, and in areas of Africa north of the distribution of tsetse. The distribution of surra overlaps that of tsetse-transmitted animal trypanosomosis, and delineation is difficult because of similarities of morphology and pathogenicity between *T. evansi* and *T. brucei*. *T. equinum* is reported only from South America. In certain countries, particularly in Africa and Asia, surra has a marked seasonal incidence in association with wet and humid climatic conditions which favour the development of large biting fly populations, the so-called "surra season".

Species affected

Surra is economically important in the camel and the horse, but the relative importance in both hosts varies in different countries. In the Sudan, for example, the disease occurs almost exclusively in camels, but in Asia and South America infections in the horse are often more important. The dog may also suffer acute disease. Possible explanations include the existence of trypanosome strains of different pathogenicity and differing susceptibilities of breeds of animals.

Cattle and buffalo in endemic areas are usually considered to harbour subclinical infections and, indeed, may act as reservoirs of infection. There are reports that buffalo recover spontaneously from surra and become serologically and parasitologically negative. However, apparently healthy animals may be a potential source of infection to other susceptible livestock. Epidemics of surra can occur in cattle and buffalo. In North Vietnam, in the Red River Delta area and in the southern states of China, many thousands of buffalo have died from acute trypanosomosis. In Indonesia, cattle and buffalo imported from Australia or New Zealand or animals moved into new endemic areas rapidly succumb to surra if not treated with trypanocidal drugs.

Wild animal infection, unlike the tsetse-transmitted trypanosomosis, seems to be rare, or at least, only rarely reported. Species infected include wild pigs (*Sus philippinensis*) in the Philippines, deer (*Cervus* spp. and *Axis* spp.) in Mauritius and Indonesia, and the capybara (*Hydrochoerus capybara*) in South America.

Transmission

T. evansi is transmitted mechanically by haematophagous flies and several different genera have been implicated, including *Tabanus*, *Stomoxys*, *Haematopota*, *Chrysops* and *Lyperosia*. The most important genus is *Tabanus*, and the presence of large numbers of biting flies in the wet season is widely associated with an increased prevalence of surra. Transmission can also be influenced by the degree of parasitaemia, high numbers of parasites in the blood of camels and horses increasing the likelihood of flies spreading infection. Close herding or stabling of animals can also increase transmission. Experimental studies have identified nearly 30 species of *Tabanus* capable of transmitting *T. evansi*.

The morphological adaptation of tabanid mouthparts ensures that small volumes of blood are trapped after the fasicle is withdrawn from the host. Tabanids are also persistent, aggressive feeders, annoying the host so that feeding is often interrupted, thus ensuring that several new hosts may be bitten, thereby increasing the possibility of multiple infections occurring. For effective transmission, flies should feed within a few hours of an infective feed.

Evidence suggests that *T. evansi* can be maintained by transmission cycles involving only domestic animals, and the epidemiological importance of infections in wild animals is thought to be low. The level of parasitaemia in recovered domestic animals is characteristically low and an explanation is still required of how infections in susceptible animals can be initiated by non-cyclical transmission.

Experimental work has shown that the vomit drop from lapping flies which have fed on parasitaemic blood and exudates from wounds caused by biting flies can also be infective to laboratory rodents. Cyclical transmission by a species of soft tick has been claimed but not subsequently confirmed by other investigators. Carnivores can be infected by eating meat from parasitaemic animals, and in South America the vampire bat *(Desmodus rotundus)* can be infected from blood feeds. The vampire bat can also act as a vector, transmitting the trypanosome in its saliva when it feeds on a new host.

Clinical features

Infections of camels in Africa, notably in the Sudan, result in many deaths within a few months in the absence of treatment. A few camels die in 2–3 weeks. Infected animals show signs of fever and progressive emaciation, and may develop anaemia, oedema of dependent parts and paralysis. Some African camels have mild and protracted infections and Asian camels exhibit chronic symptoms which persist for years.

Severe infections occur in horses in North Africa and in Asia, with fever, emaciation, oedema and high mortality as the main features. The oedema varies from plaques on the neck and flanks to oedema of the muzzle, chest wall, sheath, scrotum and legs up to the knees and hocks. Death may occur within a few days or a few months. A high mortality in horses occurs in Central and South America following a more chronic syndrome lasting a period of months and progressive paralysis of the hindquaters is reported as an important feature.

In dogs, oedema is well marked, particularly in the scrotum, ears and neck. Opacity of the cornea is frequently present. Emaciation is rapid and death can occur within 2 weeks.

Although cattle and buffalo in endemic situations usually carry a subclinical infection, it is possible for overt disease to develop in response to environmental stress or intercurrent infections. Acute disease is characterized by fever, emaciation and anaemia and death may occur within 24 hours of the onset of clinical disease. Chronic trypanosomosis can affect reproductive performance, including delay in oestrus, abortion and stillbirth.

Pathology

Post mortem lesions are not well defined. Necrosis of the skin may occur on the thorax and abdomen. The carcase is anaemic and ascites and hydrothorax may be present. Petechiae are seen on any serous surface, and within liver and kidney parenchyma. Lymph nodes are enlarged.

Histologically, the lesions seen may resemble those associated with infection with *T. brucei*.

Diagnosis

Trypanosomes are readily seen in blood films from animals suffering acute disease, but low parasitaemias occur in chronic infections. In such cases, thick and thin blood smears from individual animals taken on consecutive days or lymph node puncture smears should be attempted. Other good laboratory methods of diagnosis include concentration of trypanosomes in peripheral blood by centrifugation and the injection of blood samples from suspected cases into rodents.

A number of non-specific tests indicating increased serum protein levels in cases of trypanosomosis have been used widely, although they have now been supplanted by more specific serological assays for demonstrating the presence of trypanosomal antigen or antibody. Increased serum protein levels were demonstrated by using mercuric chloride, formol gel or stilbamidine. This test, using mercuric chloride, was used for many years for camels in the Sudan.

Complement fixation, passive haemagglutinaion, indirect fluorescent antibody tests and enzyme-linked immunosorbent assays (ELISA) have all been used to demonstrate serological evidence of infection with *T. evansi*. In some areas, serology could detect infection unequivocally, as *T. evansi* is the only pathogenic species present, but where other species of pathogenic trypanosome co-exist with *T. evansi*, problems of identification of infecting species of trypanosome could occur. ELISA could provide a possible means of overcoming such problems by the use of species-specific monoclonal antibodies. ELISA could also be used to monitor for the presence of trypanosomal antigen, hence identifying active infections. However, none of the newer serological tests are in general field use.

Treatment

The drugs commonly used are shown in Table 18. Repeated underdosing using suramin has induced populations of resistant trypanosomes. These, however, are still sensitive to quinapyramine sulphate. Quinapyramine sulphate may have pronounced toxic effects in the horse and dog and the therapeutic dose may be diluted or divided into two or more parts given at 6-hourly intervals.

Chemoprophylaxis is not in general use, but animals can be protected for short periods with suramin or quinapyramine (prophylactic). A quinapyramine – suramin complex drug has also been used for prophylaxis in horses in India.

Immunology

Antigenic variation occurs in *T. evansi*, leading to a relapsing parasitaemia in infected animals. *T. evansi* may be more limited antigenically than tsetse-transmitted trypanosomes, possibly by the absence of developmental stages in an insect vector which could preclude the opportunity for genetic exchange. Characterization of predominant antigen repertoires of isolates of *T. evansi* in the Sudan, collected from geographically widely dispersed locations, has shown the existence of only three serodemes. In Indonesia, too, it is likely that antigenic diversity is limited. It is possible that in areas where few serodemes occur and the incidence of clinical disease is low, the development of immunity may be important in regulating natural infections. Premune carrier states can be disturbed under conditions of environmental stress.

Control

The measures include detection and treatment of infected animals; removal of susceptible hosts from known infected areas, or areas known to be dangerous, at seasons of the year when biting fly populations are high; protection of animals from biting flies; the control of sale of meat from infected animals; and the control of stock movements. Direct measures against biting flies are not likely to be of practical use.

Further reading

Hoare, C.A. (1972). *The trypanosomes of mammals*, pp. 555–593. Blackwell, Oxford.

Table 18 Drugs available for treatment of *T. evansi* infections

Drug	Trade name	Species	Dosage	Remarks
Quinapyramine sulphate (curative)	Antrycide[a] (Alkaline Chemical Corporation of India)	Pigs, camels, buffalo	4 mg/kg	Prosalt should provide 3 months' prophylaxis
Quinapyramine prosalt (Prophylactic and curative)	Trypacide (M&B), Noroquin (Norbrook) Quintrycide (Gharda), Tribexin (Gharda)	Cattle, elephants	3–5 mg/kg s.c.	
		Horses	3 mg/kg s.c.	In horses, the dose should be divided
Suramin	Naganol (Bayer)	Horses, donkeys	6–10 mg/kg i.v.	Therapy
		Cattle, buffalo, camels	3.5–10 mg/kg s.c. or i.m.	1–4 months prophylaxis; temporary painful swellings may occur
		Dogs	30–50 mg/kg i.v.	Therapy
Diminazene aceturate	Berenil (Hoechst), Ganaseg (Squibb)	Cattle, buffalo	8–10 mg/kg i.m.	
		Camels	3.5 mg/kg i.m.	Potentially toxic to camels, do not exceed this dose
Isometamidium chloride	Samorin (M&B), Trypamidium (Specia)	Camels	2 mg/kg i.m.	High dosage necessary to be effective but causes painful local reactions; i.v. administration at this dosage causes shock
		Equidae	0.25 mg/kg i.m.	
		Dogs	0.5–1.0 mg/kg i.m.	

[a]Distributed by Bella Trading Company, Khartoum, Sudan.

Dourine

Dourine is a venereal infection of equids caused by *Trypanosoma equiperdum* and characterized by a slow progressive course, genital oedema, dermal plaques and terminal paralysis. It is the only trypanosome of veterinary importance that does not require an arthropod vector.

Aetiology

T. equiperdum is morphologically similar to *T. evansi* and strains vary in length from 25 to 28 μm. The organism is thought to have evolved from *T. brucei*, possibly through an intermediate stage as *T. evansi*, and become monomorphic in the course of repeated direct transmission. The trypanosome divides by longitudinal binary fission in various tissue fluids, particularly in the reproductive system and in subcutaneous urticarial plaques.

Occurrence

The disease occurs in North and South Africa, Central and South America, the Middle East, Asiatic Russia, Asia Minor and parts of South East Asia. It has been eradicated from Europe and North America.

Species affected

Natural infection is known to occur only in horses and donkeys.

Transmission

T. equiperdum is transmitted at coitus. If other transmission mechanisms occur naturally, they are of little significance.

Epidemics originate from the introduction of infected "carrier" breeding animals into a susceptible population. An infected stallion may infect many mares before the disease is recognized because of the slow onset of symptoms.

Clinical features

The onset of the disease is insidious and the incubation period may extend from 1 to 20 weeks. The first sign of infection is a mucoid vaginal or urethral discharge. A low recurrent fever may be detected and oedema of the genitalia follows. In the mare, the swelling of the vulva slowly extends to the udder and ventral surface of the abdomen, while in the stallion the oedema of the scrotum and prepuce may extend forward as far as the chest. Ulceration of the genital mucosae may leave depigmented scars. The trypanosomes are carried by the bloodstream to other parts of the body and invade the skin; urticarial plaques 2-10 cm in diameter appear on any part of the body, but particularly the flanks and any one plaque may last only a few hours, but alternatively can persist for days. Plaques are not an invariable feature, but if they appear they are considered pathognomonic. The animal loses condition, becomes weak and lame in one or both hind limbs, and muscular atrophy occurs, particularly in the gluteal region. The parasites may invade the central nervous system and nervous symptoms become manifest, first as inco-ordination progressing terminally to ataxia and paralysis. The course of fatal forms of the disease may last from 1 to 12 months, or longer.

The disease may take an acute course, and animals die within a few weeks to 2 months. In some instances, infection is entirely symptomless, but the animals remain lifelong carriers.

Pathology

There is pronounced anaemia and oedematous infiltration of the perineal tissues and ventral abdominal wall. The urogenital tract is inflamed and hydrothorax, hydropericardium and ascites are often pronounced. In longstanding cases, the external genitalia may be fibrosed.

Diagnosis

Diagnosis is usually based on the history of the animal and on lesions and clinical signs, as parasitological confirmation can be very difficult. The detection of trypanosomes by microscopical examination of blood, oedema fluid from the genitalia and urticarial plaques, and vaginal washings can be attempted, but is often unsuccessful despite attempted concentration of the organisms by centrifugation. The primary isolation of the trypanosome by inoculating similar material into laboratory rodents is also difficult, unless special routes of inoculation, e.g. into rabbit testes, or splenectomized or immunuosuppressed animals are used.

The complement fixation test provides a very efficient method of diagnosis, except in areas where other trypanosomes of the subgenus *Trypanozoon* (*T. evansi* and *T. brucei*) occur, because such organisms have antigens in common with *T. equiperdum*.

Treatment

Quinapyramine sulphate is the drug of choice but the response to therapy may be poor. Successful treatment with diminazene aceturate has recently been reported from the USSR.

In general, measures to control breeding should take precedence over attempts to treat clinical cases.

Immunology

The trypanosome undergoes antigenic variation and infected animals produce humoral antibodies. The antibodies can be transferred passively in the colostrum and they persist in the foal for about 4 months. Although dourine is characteristically a chronic and progressive disease, some animals appear to have symptomless infections leading to a lifelong "carrier" state in which they are infective to further hosts.

Control

Strict control of breeding, of movements of horses, and quarantine and slaughter in clinical outbreaks has a marked effect on the incidence of the disease. Detection of carrier animals by the complement fixation test and slaughter or castration leads to eventual eradiction. In-contact animals are declared free after three consecutive monthly negative complement fixation tests.

The complement fixation test can also be used for the examination of horses to prevent the importation of dourine into a clean area.

Further reading

Barrowman, P.R. (1976). Observations on the transmission, immunology, clinical signs and chemotherapy of dourine in horses with special reference to cerebrospinal fluid. *Onderstepoort Journal of Veterinary Research*, **43**, 55–66.
Stephen, L.E. (1986). *Trypanosoma (Trypanozoon) equiperdum* Doflein, 1901. In *Trypanosomiasis – A veterinary perspective*. Pergamon Press, Oxford.

Chagas' disease (*T. cruzi* infection)

This important disease of man in Central and South America is essentially a zoonosis, and a wide range of wild and domestic animals are naturally infected providing a reservoir of infection to man. Infection is transmitted by bloodsucking reduviid bugs.

Aetiology

The causative agent, *T. cruzi*, has different morphological forms in the mammalian and vector hosts. In blood films of infected mammalian hosts, *T. cruzi* is morphologically a typical trypanosome with a free flagellum, a poorly developed undulating membrane and an average length of 20 μm. In stained preparations, the kinetoplast is large and prominent, the posterior extremity is pointed and many of the organisms are characteristically curved in a crescent shape. The parasites are essentially histotropic and penetrate cells of various tissues, particularly myocardium and striated muscle. Within the cells, the parasite shortens, loses the free flagellum and becomes a rounded amastigote form. These multiply to produce a "pseudocyst" or intracellular nest of amastigotes which periodically elongate, reacquire flagellae and are released into the blood from which they are either taken up by a vector or invade further muscle cells.

Occurrence

Chagas' disease is widespread throughout South and Central America, extending into the southern states of the USA.

Species affected

Although its main importance is in man, *T. cruzi* also infects many wild animals, notably armadillos (*Dasypus* spp.) in South America, opossums (*Didelphis* spp.)

throughout its area of distribution and wood rats (*Neotoma* spp.) in the southern USA. Domesticated animals, notably dogs, cats and pigs, may also be infected, thus providing a reservoir of infection for man.

Transmission

The vectors of *T. cruzi* are bloodsucking bugs of the family Reduviidae. Many different bugs are involved in the transmission of the trypanosome, notably *Rhodnius* spp., *Triatoma* spp. and *Pan strongylus* spp.

Trypanosomes ingested by a bug multiply as epimastigotes in the alimentary canal. Infective trypanosomes develop in the hind gut and are passed in the faeces. The infection is transmitted to the definitive host by contamination of mucous membranes and skin with reduviid faeces.

A reservoir of the disease is maintained by a primary sylvatic cycle involving bugs and wild animals, and man and domestic animals become infected when they interrupt the natural transmission cycle.

Clinical features

Acute cases of Chagas' disease occur in young dogs and children. The onset of symptoms is marked by fever followed by a progressive anaemia, emaciation and oedema. The trypanosome has a predilection for heart muscle, resulting in heavy infection of tissues with amastigotes causing a necrotizing granulomatous myocarditis accompanied by pulmonary oedema, and passive congestion and enlargement of the liver. Other less frequent lesions include visceral lymphadenopathy, splenomegaly and renal congestion. Death due to heart failure may occur. Survivors of acute disease may become chronically infected for several years. Chronic infections in man may be symptomless or associated with cardiac and other disorders of variable severity, sometimes resulting in heart failure and death without the obvious presence of trypanosomes. Chronic disease in the dog has only been described in experimental infections in which the picture of chronic myocarditis is similar to that of man, but it probably also occurs naturally.

Pathology

A reaction often occurs at the site of infection, characteristically subcutaneously or in the region of the eye, marked by local swelling, inflammation, oedema and degenerative changes in the tissue. Death from acute disease is associated with extensive inflammatory oedema and degeneration in parasitized tissue, particularly in the heart. Intracellular nests of parasites can be found histologically in many other tissues and organ sites. In chronic and longstanding cases in man, degenerative changes occur in the heart and other organs, sometimes in the apparent absence of parasites, but in association with extensive lymphocytic infiltration. More rarely, chronic infection is associated with degenerative changes in the nerve supply of the alimentary tract resulting, for example, in the development of megaoesophagus and megacolon.

Diagnosis

In acute cases, the trypanosome can be demonstrated microscopically in blood films and lesion smears. The organism can also be isolated by inoculating blood and tissue fluids into young laboratory rodents and in various culture media.

In chronic infections, these methods are less efficient and more reliance is placed on xenodiagnosis and serological tests. Xenodiagnosis is performed by feeding clean, laboratory-bred bugs on the suspected animal, and examining the bugs by trituration or dissection 40–60 days later when any ingested trypanosomes have had time to develop. The serodiagnostic tests in field use include complement fixation, immunofluorescence and haemagglutination procedures.

Treatment

No satisfactory treatment of the intracellular stages of *T. cruzi* has been developed.

Immunology

A premunition often develops following a clinical or symptomless primary infection. Both cell-mediated and humoral immune mechanisms are involved.

Circulating antibody formation is important in the context of serodiagnostic tests.

Although many infections appear clinically insignificant for periods of several years and satisfy the criteria of premunity, there is evidence in some cases that underlying progressive pathological changes occur which eventually become overt and result in fatal disease.

Control

In the absence of satisfactory drugs for the treatment of infections, a degree of control over Chagas' disease is effected by insecticidal elimination of bugs from dwellings and by discouraging and destroying wild mammalian hosts in peridomestic habitats.

Full control requires economic measures to improve living standards, in particular the replacement of primitive dwellings with better housing.

Further reading

Losos, G.J. (1986). Trypanosomiases. In *Infectious tropical diseases of domestic animals*, pp. 182–318. Longman, London.

Stephen, L.E. (1986). The Stercoraria. In *Trypanosomiasis – A veterinary perspective*, pp. 330–336. Pergamon Press, Oxford.

Williams, G.D. *et al.* (1977). Naturally occurring trypanosomiasis (Chagas' disease) in dogs. *Journal of American Veterinary Medical Association*, **171**, 171–177.

Zeledon, R. (1974). Epidemiology, mode of transmission and reservoir hosts of Chagas' disease. In *Trypanosomiasis and leishmaniasis with special reference to Chagas' disease*. Ciba Foundation Symposium 20, pp. 51–85. Associated Scientific Publishers, Amsterdam.

A.G.H.
A.G.L.

Diseases caused by rickettsia

G.R. Scott

ANAPLASMOSES

The anaplasmoses are arthropod-transmitted rickettsial infections of ruminants and, perhaps, the horse, by species of the *Anaplasma* genus in the Anaplasmataceae family of the Rickettsiales order. They are obligate intracellular parasites which multiply by binary fission in erythrocytes inside membrane-lined vacuoles. The infective elementary (initial) bodies are 0.3–0.4 μm in diameter, whereas the round intraerythrocytic inclusions may reach a diameter of 1.0 μm. When stained with Giemsa the inclusions are dense bluish-purple.

Five named species are recognized: three, *A. marginale*, *A. centrale* and *A. caudatum*, parasitize cattle; one, *A. ovis*, parasitizes sheep and goats; and one, *A. mesaeterum*, is apparently restricted to sheep. In addition, two other ill-characterized anaplasms have been reported, *A. buffeli* in domesticated buffaloes and *A. equi* in horses. The host responses to most of the species are subclinical, but major clinical episodes may occur when cattle are moved from infection-free areas to areas where *A. marginale* is endemic. Mild reactions occur under similar circumstances when naive cattle are infected with *A. centrale*, and naive sheep and goats are infected with *A. ovis*. Clinical signs may also be induced in persistently infected ruminants that are stressed by malnutrition, concurrent infection or splenectomy.

Bovine anaplasmosis

Also known as gall sickness, bovine anaplasmosis infects domesticated and wild ruminants reared in the tropics and subtropics. Infections in the sucking young are usually clinically inapparent and, once infected, animals remain carriers for life. Clinical reactions characterized by fever and progressive anaemia occur in naive cattle infected for the first time. Similar but less acute reactions may occur in stressed persistently infected animals.

Aetiology

The pathogenic anaplasm is *A. marginale*. *A. centrale* and *A. caudatum* induce subacute infections and frequently occur together. Although all three species possess common generic antigens, they are distinct. In addition, *A. marginale* is closely related to *A. ovis*.

Occurrence

Bovine anaplasmosis is prevalent in the tropics and subtropics of all continents.

Species affected

The economically important hosts of bovine anaplasmosis caused by *A. marginale* are cattle; in other domesticated and wild ruminants, *A. marginale* usually produces an inapparent infection. Infections have been reported in camels and African giant rats and disease has been observed in giraffes.

Transmission

Bovine anaplasmosis is not contagious. The major vectors are numerous species of ticks which are themselves infected and there is trans-stadial and transovarian transmission in ticks. A tick cycle, however, is not essential, and many species of biting diptera will transmit anaplasms mechanically. Similarly, iatrogenic spread readily occurs with blood-contaminated needles and instruments. Ox-pecker birds are also capable of transmitting anaplasmosis. Transplacental transmission of extraerythrocytic elementary bodies occurs in naive pregnant cows infected in the second or third trimesters of gestation.

Clinical features

Natural selection for high innate resistance to anaplasmosis has occurred in cattle reared for many generations in association with anaplasms. When their progeny are infected they undergo clinically inapparent reactions. They remain persistently infected and stress may exacerbate the latent infection producing a transient low-grade fever, a transient anaemia and loss of condition. In contrast, cattle reared in areas free of the rickettsia may react severely when infected, the case mortality rate being highest in the oldest animals. Calves infected *in utero* may be actively and acutely ill when born, whereas other calves infected *in utero* throw off the infection and are born with antibodies.

Illness is first evident 2–12 weeks after infection, the duration of the clinical incubation period being inversely related to the dose. Erythrocytes are first patently parasitized 5–10 days before the onset of fever, but the number of parasitized cells is low. The fever steadily increases over the next 2–3 days as the parasitaemias become more intense. The onset of illness is manifested by a slight fever and a drop in the milk yield of lactating cows. The fever peak and the peak parasitaemia tend to occur on the same day. Other clinical signs are now evident – affected animals are depressed, stop eating, develop a rapid pulse, lose their co-ordination and, if exerted, become breathless. The visible mucous membranes are first pale and then yellow. The lymph nodes are enlarged. Although the urine may be brown, there is no haemoglobinuria. A few animals become aggressive. Pregnant animals abort and death supervenes within a few days. Convalescence in survivors is spread over several weeks, but recovered animals remain carriers. Some survivors never regain full health, become emaciated and stay unproductive. The clinical picture is often complicated by concurrent infections, in particular, by babesiosis.

Clinical pathology

At the peak of parasitaemia in acute cases, 15–30% of erythrocytes are parasitized but, on occasion, up to 65% of parasitized erythrocytes have been observed. Over the next few days, the fevers and the parasitaemias fall dramatically and the anaemic crisis becomes evident, the macrocytic anaemia being induced by opsonic stimulation of auto-immune phenomena which leads to the intracellular destruction of erythrocytes in tissue macrophages. The erythrocyte count, the haematocrit readings and the haemoglobin concentrations fall. The reticulocytes enter the circulation producing a macrocytic anaemia with moderate anisocytosis and a slight polychromasia. A transient leucopenia coincides with the onset of fever but thereafter leucocyte values are either normal or marginally increased. Apparently recovered animals have a persisting non-responsive, normocytic, normochromic anaemia in which parasitized erythrocytes are rarely observed.

High levels of unconjugated bilirubin are present in the serum by the time of the peak of parasitaemia. In contrast, the serum transaminase, SGOT, is decreased significantly at this time, but then rises sharply thereafter. Changes in the serum transaminase, SGPT, are not significant.

Pathology

Carcases of animals dying at the time of the anaemic crisis are in good condition, whereas animals that die after persistent chronic infection are emaciated. There are no pathognomonic gross lesions. The carcase is pallid or jaundiced and the blood is thin and watery. The spleen is enlarged and mushy with prominent splenic follicles, the liver is mottled and yellow, the gall bladder is distended and the bile is thick and brownish-green. The hepatic and mediastinal lymph nodes are brown in colour. Epicardial and pericardial petechiae and ecchymoses are usually present. The significant microscopic finding is widespread erythrocyte phagocytosis in reticulo-endothelial organs. *A. marginale* organisms are scant in number.

Lesions in aborted foetuses include hepatomegaly with capsular petechiae, splenomegaly, epicardial and endocardial petechiae and haemorrhagic lung lobules. An examination of films of heart blood will reveal parasitized erythrocytes.

Diagnosis

A presumptive diagnosis based on an assessment of the history, clinical signs and *post mortem* lesions is relatively easy in acute cases, the significant markers being a history of recent animal or tick movement into the area and an anaemia without haemoglobinuria. Confirmation requires detection of the rickettsias in Giemsa-stained blood films; *A. marginale* inclusions are usually towards the periphery of the parasitized erythrocytes. In contrast, confirmation of a presumptive diagnosis of chronic anaplasmosis is difficult and must be based on the detection of antibody; similar techniques are used to identify carriers.

Treatment

Treatment is effective if drugs are administered during the early febrile phase of the disease. The drugs of choice are tetracyclines and imidocarb diproprionate. Techniques designed to eliminate the carrier states from cattle grazing marginally endemic areas include daily doses of a short–acting tetracycline for 10 days at the rate of 11 mg/kg body weight, four doses of long-acting tetracycline at the rate of 22 mg/kg administered 3 days apart, two doses of imidocarb proprionate at the rate of 4 mg/kg 2 weeks part or daily for 3 days at 5 mg/kg.

Immunology

Protection from reinfection is associated with persistence of the organism. It does not, however, prevent exacerbated relapses following stress. Both humoral and cell-mediated mechanisms are involved, but transfer of antibodies in the colostrum does not passively protect sucking calves. Several serological tests are available for detecting antibodies.

Control

Control measures in areas where anaplasmosis is endemic are aimed at limiting stress of indigenously reared animals. Newly purchased animals from disease-free areas should either be immunized immediately on arrival or be closely monitored clinically and haematologically for at least 3 months after arrival and treated when necessary. The most effective vaccines are either living attenuated strains of *A. marginale* coupled with treatment if required. Injection of the less pathogenic *A. centrale* rickettsia protects against *A. marginale* and is used extensively in Africa and Australia, but it sometimes produces severe reactions. Inactivated vaccines also protect, but a serious snag is the production of iso-antibodies against the recipient's erythrocytes.

Further reading

Kuttler, K.L. (1984). *Anaplasma* infections in wild and domestic ruminants; A review. *Journal of Wildlife Diseases*, **20**, 12–20.

Ovine anaplasmosis

Ovine anaplasmosis is a persistent but benign rickettsiosis of sheep and goats in Africa, Asia, Europe and the western USA. Infected animals are carriers and splenectomy and other stresses may provoke clinical episodes, some of which may prove fatal. Recently imported naive animals are at risk and, when infected, may develop severe anaemia and jaundice.

Aetiology

Of the two species of anaplasm that parasitize sheep and goats, *A. ovis* is more pathogenic than *A. mesaeterum*. They have antigens in common but are not identical. *A. ovis* is also related to the bovine anaplasm *A. marginale*, but it is not immunologically identical.

Occurrence

Ovine anaplasmosis caused by *A. ovis* is prevalent in sheep and goats in Africa, Asia, Europe and the western USA. In contrast, *A. mesaeterum* appears to be restricted to north-western Europe.

Species affected

Sheep, goats and deer are natural hosts of *A. ovis* and *A. mesaeterum*. In addition, *A. ovis* sometimes infects cattle.

Transmission

The primary mode of transmission is not known. *A. ovis*, however, has been shown to cross the placenta and iatrogenic needle transmission readily occurs. Experimental trials have shown that argasid and ixodid ticks may act as vectors, although keds do not.

Clinical features

Lambs infected *in utero* exhibit no clinical signs. Post-natal infections in sheep are likewise clinically muted despite the emergence of low patent parasitaemias 12 days after infection. The anaemia that develops is progressive. In contrast, clinical reactions in splenectomized sheep are acute, being manifested by early high fevers, anorexia and cachexia. Patent parasitaemias in splenectomized sheep are many times higher than in entire animals producing severe anaemia, jaundice, and, not infrequently, death.

Pathology

The gross pathology of splenectomized sheep that die mimics the pathology seen in fatal bovine anaplasmosis, jaundice being the dominant lesion.

Diagnosis

The detection of erythrocytes in blood films parasitized with *A. ovis* or *A. mesaeterum* is usually fortuitous but diagnostic in entire sheep. The former anaplasm is sited marginally in the infected erythrocyte and *A. mesaeterum* lies more centrally.

Treatment

The drug of choice is tetracycline if treatment is necessary.

Immunology

Recovered animals become carriers and may be identified serologically. The antibodies, however, are not in themselves protective.

Control

Control measures are seldom applied to indigenous sheep and goats with a long ancestral association with these anaplasms. Recently purchased naive animals should be monitored daily for 3 months.

Further reading

Zaugg, J.L. (1987). Ovine anaplasmosis: *in utero* transmission as it relates to stage of gestation. *American Journal of Veterinary Research*, **48**, 100–103

CHLAMYDIOSIS

Currently, chlamydias are classified in a monogeneric rickettsial order, the Chlamydiales. There are two species, *Chlamydia trachomatis* and *C. psittaci*. Three biotypes of the former cause diseases in man and one biotype infects mice. All chlamydias affecting animals are considered to be strains of *C. psittaci*, and two biotypes are recognized, one of which causes disease in birds and man and the other which infects a wide range of domesticated animals. The mammalian and avian biotypes do not cross-react serologically. Within the mammalian biotype there are two serovars – one attacks the alimentary, respiratory and reproductive tracts, and the other causes polyarthritis, conjunctivitis and encephalitis. The economically significant chlamydial infection in farm livestock is enzootic abortion of ewes.

Enzootic abortion of ewes

Synonyms for enzootic abortion of ewes (EAE) include ovine enzootic abortion, ovine chlamydial abortion and kebbing. EAE is a placentitis that causes late abortions, stillbirths and premature delivery of weak lambs. Infected ewes remain carriers but rarely abort twice.

Aetiology

The infective elementary bodies of *C. psittaci* are tiny cocci 300 nm in diameter which multiply only inside membrane-bound vacuoles in the cytoplasm of mammalian cells. They turn light blue with Giemsa and bright red with modified Ziehl-Neelsen stains. They are heat labile but will survive on pasture for several days.

Occurrence

In Europe, EAE has been known for more than 100 years. Epidemics have also been recognized in Africa, Asia and North America.

Species affected

Clinical signs are only seen in pregnant ewes.

Transmission

A few lambs are infected *in utero*, but most are infected orally at birth or shortly thereafter through contact with infected placentas and foetal fluids. An inapparent enteric infection follows and persists for years up until the fourth month of pregnancy, when it moves from the alimentary tract to the reproductive tract and invades the cotyledons.

Clinical features

Usually, the first sign of trouble is the discovery of dead lambs 2–3 weeks before lambing is due. Some lambs are aborted, some are premature stillbirths, some are full-term stillbirths, some are born alive but moribund, and others are weak. Most weak lambs fail to survive. Some infected ewes give birth to normal live lambs which they rear successfully.

There are no premonitory signs of impending abortions. Afterwards, ewes expel a discoloured uterine discharge but are otherwise clinically normal. If the placenta is retained, a metritis is liable to develop and may cause death of the ewe from secondary infection.

Aborted lambs are well grown and fresh but some are oedematous, some have their fleece stained by pink-brown debris from the infected placenta, and a few have found to be mummified by not putrefied.

Pathology

Gross changes in aborted or stillborn foetuses are limited to blood-tinged subcutaneous and intramuscular oedema. Foetal membranes, however, show characteristic changes. Necrosis of the cotyledons and chorion is manifested by accumulations of red-creamy discharges. The cotyledons themselves lose their normal purple colour and are dark red, pink or clay-coloured. The chorion is either oedematous or thick and leathery being covered with a dirty pink exudate containing flakes.

The microscopic lesion is a placentitis with loss of epithelial cells and progressive necrosis of the underlying villi and tips of the caruncular septa. The chlamydias multiply within the cytoplasms of the trophoblastic epithelial cells and the resulting inclusions are readily visible.

The uterus is unaffected.

Diagnosis

In virgin epidemics, the morbidity is up to 30% and persists for 1–2 years. Moreover, all ages are affected. A presumptive field diagnosis is therefore easy. In contrast, the morbidity in endemically infected flocks is about 5% and suspicions may not be aroused. The diagnosis is confirmed by demonstrating the chlamydias in smears of the cotyledons stained with Giemsa or modified Zeihl-Neelsen stain. They usually occur in clusters but many single organisms will also be seen. In a flock diagnosis, the demonstration of a rising antibody titre is diagnostic.

Treatment

Prompt treatment of the ewes at risk with the long-acting oxytetracycline may limit the severity and the extent of the outbreak.

Immunology

Aborting ewes remain carriers and are infectious but they rarely abort a second time. They also resist reinfection. The carrier state is associated with the production of humoral antibodies which may be detected by complement fixation, immunodiffusion or ELISA.

Control

Aborting ewes should be segregated and their placentas destroyed. If the infection in the flock is limited, the affected animals should be culled, but if the infection has been widespread, affected ewes should be retained.

An inactivated adjuvanted vaccine is available and should be used to protect new lambs before mating, with revaccination every 3 years thereafter. The vaccine, however, only mitigates the worst effects of EAE and it does not eliminate infections. Clean flocks should be kept closed if possible. Replacement stock should only be obtained from flocks known to be free of EAE.

Further reading

Shewen, P.E. (1980). Chlamydial infections in animals: A review. *Canadian Veterinary Journal*, **21**, 2–11.

COWDRIOSIS

Cowdriosis or heartwater, is the most feared rickettsial infection of ruminants in Africa. Every year it decimates the calf and lamb crops of nomadic stockmen after the flocks and herds are moved from the arid tick-free areas where parturition occurs on to tick-infested dry-season grazing. Official prevalence data are conspicuous by their absence because the stockowners recognise the early clinical signs of heartwater and slaughter the affected animals for food. Heartwater has also nullified many attempts to raise the productivity of indigenous African livestock through the importation of hypersusceptible exotic breeds.

The causative rickettsia, *Cowdria ruminantium*, is the sole species of the *Cowdria* genus in the Ehrlichieae tribe of the Rickettsiaceae family. Isolates possess common antigens but cross-protection between them is not complete. Serological cross-reactions have been noted between *C. ruminantium* and *Ehrlichia (Cytoecetes) equi*, *E. canis* and, perhaps, *E. bovis*, but the epidemiological significance of the reactions is not known.

Heartwater is a relatively benign rickettsiosis of domestic and wild ruminants reared in Africa in the presence of infected *Amblyomma* ticks. In naive weaned animals, it manifests itself as a severe febrile illness that usually terminates fatally after the onset of dramatic nervous signs.

Aetiology

Cowdria ruminantium is a pleomorphic rickettsia which multiplies in mammalian hosts in vascular endothelial cells, forming clusters of small cocci inside intracytoplasmic vacuoles. It circulates in the cytoplasms of neutrophils. In vector ticks, the organism first develops in gut cells and later in haemocytes, salivary glands and malpighian tubules.

Occurrence

Heartwater is endemic in Africa south of the Sahara, Malagasy, Mauritius and the West Indies, areas infested with the vector *Amblyomma* ticks. There is a seasonal prevalence, clinical cases tending to occur during the "rains".

Species affected

Heartwater parasitizes many species of wild and domesticated ruminants in Africa. There is also an unconfirmed report of infection in camels. Immature stages of *Amblyomma* ticks are usually found on small mammals, ground birds and occasionally reptiles and some of them are suspected of playing a role in the maintenance of the infection; for example, ground guinea-fowls and leopard tortoises are both proven hosts of *C. ruminantium*. Some isolates have been propagated experimentally in mice.

Indigenous animals, both domesticated and wild, usually undergo inapparent infections, particularly if they are infected while young. Animals introduced from heartwater-free areas react severely when infected.

Transmission

Heartwater is not contagious and it is transmitted by three-host bont ticks of the genus *Amblyomma*. Of the 12 species of *Amblyomma* known to be capable of transmitting *C. ruminantium*, the tropical bont tick *A. variegatum* is the most important. In southern Africa the vector is *A. hebraeum*, and in the West Indies the vectors are *A. variegatum* and *A. cajennense*. Trans-stadial transmission occurs readily in ticks and transovarian transmission rarely. *C. ruminantium* may survive for 3 years in one generation of ticks infected as larvae.

Clinical features

The incubation period following exposure to infected ticks ranges from 7 to 28 days. Clinical reactions in the very young are mild and are often not observed. Reactions in older animals are acute, being manifested first by a sudden onset of fever that remains high until shortly before death. Other signs are minimal until nervous symptoms become obvious. Affected animals chew constantly, lick their lips, and flick their eye-lids while circling with a high-stepping gait or standing with legs straddled and head lowered. The nervous signs worsen. The stricken animals subside into sternal recumbency and then into lateral recumbency and die during a galloping convulsion. The course of the disease in peracute cases is measured in hours after the onset of nervous signs; in acute cases, the course lasts 3–6 days.

Clinical pathology

Haematological changes are not marked, but there is a neutropenia, an eosinopenia and a lymphocytosis. There is a proportional drop in both haemoglobin and haematocrit, possibly linked to a normocytic, normochromic anaemia.

Bilirubin levels are increased shortly after the onset of fever, darkening the plasma. Widespread effusion leads to a fall in plasma protein levels.

Pathology

The dominant gross feature is effusion into the body cavities together with oedema of the lungs and lymph nodes and splenomegaly. The nervous signs are attributable to brain oedema. There are few microscopical changes other than the presence of colonies of *C. ruminantium* in the cells lining the capillaries.

Diagnosis

A history of the recent movement of naive animals into a known *Amblyomma* infested area together with the clinical signs and *post mortem* lesions are very suggestive. Confirmation, however, is not easy, and it depends upon the detection of the rickettsias in vascular endothelial cells using squashed smears of the cerebral grey matter stained with Giemsa. The rickettsias occur as clusters of cocci in the cytoplasm of the vascular endothelial cells and stain bluish-purple to reddish-purple. It is not essential to open the brain case and a suitable grey-matter specimen may be obtained by entering the brain through the *Foramen magnum* using a long handled spoon.

Differential diagnosis

Peracute deaths should be differentiated from anthrax and acute theileriosis. Nervous cases should be differentiated from tetanus, strychnine poisoning, cerebral theileriosis, cerebral babesiosis and hypomagnesaemia. Attention should also be paid to the possibility of the presence of *E. bovis* and/or *E. ovina*.

Treatment

Tetracyclines are useful if administered in the early days of the fever. In animals exhibiting nervous signs, supportive therapy should include the use of diuretics, dimethyl sulphoxide and a non-steroidal anti-flammatory agent.

Immunology

A carrier state of several weeks duration develops in recovered animals. Resistance to the reinfection persists for longer, from 6 months to 4 years. Humoral immunity does not appear to play a specific role in resistance to reinfection and it is believed cell-mediated immune mechanisms are the important factor. Antibodies are transferred in the colostrum to the sucking young but they are not protective.

Control

Systematic dipping with reliable acaricides at weekly intervals may reduce the incidence of the disease. The introduction of *Amblyomma*-infested stock or fodder into clean areas should be avoided. In areas where the disease is endemic, adult animals are normally immune and hence it is only necessary to immunize the annual calf or lamb crop. Animals purchased from heartwater-free areas should also be immunized. Infected sheep blood or a suspension of infected nymphal ticks is used as the immunizing agent and is administered intravenously. Severe post-immunization reactions are abated with tetracyclines.

Further reading

Bigalke, R.D. *et al.* (1987). Heartwater: Past, present and future. *Onderstepoort Journal of Veterinary Research*, **54**, 163–546.

CYTOECETOSES

Most of the common tick-borne rickettsias parasitizing livestock are classified in the *Ehrlichieae* tribe of the Rickettsiaceae family. They differ fundamentally from the common human rickettsias by their low or non-pathogenicity for man, by multiplying inside cytoplasmic vacuoles of host cells, by not retaining the red colour of modified Ziehl-Neelsen stain, by not inducing Weil-Felix antibodies and by their inability to grow in yolk sacs of embryonated hen eggs. They resemble the human rickettsias by their susceptibility to tetracyclines.

Two genera in the Ehrlichieae tribe parasitize circulating leucocytes, viz. *Cytoecetes* and *Ehrlichia*. The former parasitize mainly granulocytes and, occasionally, monocytes. The latter affect monocytes and tissue macrophages. There are five, perhaps seven, species in the *Cytoecetes* genus but only two are economically significant, viz. *C. ondiri*, the causative agent of bovine petechial fever, and *C. phagocytophila*, the causative agent of tick-borne fever in sheep and pasture fever in cattle.

Bovine petechial fever

Synonyms for bovine petechial fever include ondiri disease and ondiriitis. Bovine petechial fever is an aberrant rickettsiosis of cattle, characterized by a high fluctuating fever, depressed milk yield and widespread petechiation of visible mucous membranes. Pregnant animals abort.

Aetiology

Cytoecetes ondiri parasitizes granulocytes and, more rarely, monocytes multiplying within membrane-lined cytoplasmic vacuoles. In addition, it multiplies in similar intracytoplasmic vacuoles in capillary endothelial cells and Von Kupffer cells. *C. ondiri* is serologically related to *C. phagocytophila*, which resembles it morphologically and tinctorially.

Occurrence

Restricted endemic foci of *C. ondiri* occur in the highland areas of East Africa characterized by being forest edges or thick bush. Experienced farmers have learned to know the danger spots on their farms and avoid grazing cattle in those areas.

Species affected

C. ondiri is an endemic rickettsiosis of wild animals, particularly the bushbuck, *Tragelaphus scriptus*. Cattle are accidentally infected when they graze or browse the same thick bush as bushbuck. Sheep and goats may be infected experimentally and probably natural infections occur in both these species.

Transmission

Bovine petechial fever is not contagious and a tick vector of restricted distribution is believed to be responsible, but it has not yet been identified.

Clinical features

Illness has not been observed in the true natural host, the bushbuck. The incubation in cattle following natural exposure is believed to range from 5 to 14 days. Reactions in recently imported animals are peracute, being characterized by sudden high fever, abrupt agalactia, petechiation of visible mucous membranes, and pulmonary oedema. Affected cows collapse and die within 3 days.

Most cattle develop longer acute reactions. There is a high fluctuating fever and the milk yield drops but other clinical signs are muted. Petechiation of the mucous membranes becomes evident 24 hours after the onset of fever; they are transient, fading within hours only to be replaced by fresh petechiae, the cycles continuing for 7–10 days. A few animals develop a unilateral conjunctivitis known as "poached-egg eye", in which the cunjunctival sacs are swollen and everted around a tense and protuberant eyeball containing a pool of blood in the lower part of the aqueous humor. Affected animals continue to eat but pregnant cows may abort. The case mortality rate may reach 50%.

Subacute reactions are characterized by their transient non-fatal course. Some cattle present no clinical signs other than a loss of condition and perhaps anaemia.

Clinical pathology

The significant haematological changes are leucopenia and thrombocytopenia. Patent parasitaemias are evident at the onset of fever and for the first few days of fever.

Pathology

Opening the carcase, which is normally in good condition, reveals widespread submucosal and subserosal haemorrhages. The heart, in particular, is intensely involved with sheet haemorrhages underlying the epicardium and endocardium, together with ecchymoses below the serous covering of the fat around the coronary vessels. Haemorrhages are present along the mucosal surfaces of the respiratory, alimentary and urogenital tracts. Lymph nodes are enlarged and oedematous and often contain cortical and subcapsular petechiae. The spleen may or may not be enlarged.

The characteristic microscopic change is hyperplasia of the cells of the lymphoid series.

Diagnosis

A presumptive diagnosis is relatively easy in areas where the infection is known to exist but diagnosis of cases occurring in new areas is difficult. Confirmation of the diagnosis depends on the detection of *C. ondiri* organisms in granulocytes of blood films stained with Giemsa, but it is essential that the blood films be made shortly after the onset of fever because the visible parasitaemias wane within a few days. It may be necessary to subinoculate blood collected in EDTA into a sheep or a susceptible calf using the intravenous route. The inoculated animals should be clinically and haematologically monitored daily for 10 days.

The diagnosis may be confirmed in fresh carcases by making impression smears of the cut surface of the spleen, lung and liver. The smears are fixed and stained with Giemsa and examined for the presence of *C. ondiri*.

Differential diagnosis

Cases of bovine petechial fever tend to be sporadic and its importance lies in the difficulty in differentiating it from other haemorrhagic diseases of cattle. In African highland areas, blood films of bovine haemorrhagic fevers should be scrutinized for granulocytophilic rickettsias. The causes of diagnostic confusion include bracken and arsenic poisoning, haemorrhagic septicaemia, heartwater, acute trypanosomosis and acute theileriosis.

Treatment

Tetracycline formulations are the drugs of choice and if administered during the incubation period will prevent the development of the disease. Normal therapeutic doses of tetracyclines, however, have little effect in overt cases; long-acting formulations are more effective.

Immunology

Most recovered animals become carriers and relapses may occur. Resistance to reinfection persists for a variable period up to 2 years after recovery.

Control

In recent years, the incidence of bovine petechial fever has declined because extensive development of farmland has eliminated the bushbuck habitats. Fresh foci, however, are likely to emerge wherever land covered in shrub or forest is being cleared for grazing.

Further reading

Snodgrass, D.R., Karstadt, L. and Cooper, J.E. (1975). The role of wild ruminants in the epidemiology of bovine petechial fever. *Journal of Hygiene, Cambridge*, **74**, 245-250.

Tick-borne fever/pasture fever

Tick-borne fever (TBF), a benign rickettsiosis of domestic and wild ruminants, is characterized by a minimal constitutional disturbance despite a prolonged parasitaemia and high fever. Lactating animals stop milking and pregnant animals abort. Defence mechanisms in affected animals are depressed allowing potentiation of other pathogens.

Aetiology

Cytoecetes phagocytophila parasitizes granulocytes and, on occasion, monocytes where it multiplies in intracytoplasmic vacuoles recognizable in Giemsa-stained blood films as either slate-blue coloured single coccobacilli about 0.5 μm in diameter, open morulae 2 μm in diameter or clusters of minute cocci. European isolates are antigenically related but they are not identical. *C. phagocytophila* also shares antigens with *C. ondiri* and *C. (Ehrlichia) equi*, present in horses in North America and Europe. *C. ovis*, a rickettsia observed in the blood of sheep on the Deccan Plateau of India, is probably related to *C. phagocytophila*.

Occurrence

Infection with *C. phagocytophila* is limited to the temperate areas of Europe, Africa and Asia where suitable exotic vector ticks are available. The prevalence of the organism in ticks appears to be very high and there is a clear-cut seasonal prevalence associated with questing-tick activity.

Species affected

The domesticated animal hosts are cattle, sheep and goats. Domesticated and wild deer are also susceptible. Most clinical cases are seen in young lactating cows turned out on to tick-infested pastures and in sucking lambs born on tick-infested grazing. The abortion rate is high when naive pregnant animals are moved on to tick-infested areas.

Transmission

The natural tick vectors are *Ixodes ricinus* in Europe and *Rhipicephalus haemophysaloides* in Asia. The vector in southern Africa is not known. Although *C. phagocytophila* allegedly multiplies in the ooplasm and mitochondria of developing oocytes, only trans-stadial and not transovarian transmission in ticks has been demonstrated. Multiplication of the rickettsia in the tick, however, is not essential, and accidental iatrogenic transmission readily follows the transfer of a minute drop of blood from a parasitaemic ruminant to a susceptible ruminant; re-used hypodermic needles, tattooing instruments and ear-punches are particularly incriminated.

Clinical features

The natural incubation period following infestation with infected ticks ranges from 3 to 13 days. All sucking ruminants possess a high innate resistance and most primary infections in such animals are not observed. In older animals, the onset of illness is sudden, being manifested by a high fever which fluctuates between 40.5 and 42°C for 4–22 days. The systemic disturbance, nevertheless, in non-pregnant and non-lactating animals is minimal. The prolonged fevers are claimed to impair spermatogenesis, but this has been disputed. Naive pregnant animals usually abort while still parasitaemic 2–8 days after the onset of fever, but occasionally the foetus mummifies and is expelled weeks later.

The pasture fever syndrome occurs in young lactating cows turned out to grass. Milk yields fall dramatically, fevers are high, appetites are depressed, coughing is frequent and the ears droop. Death is rare except in aborting animals which die later from post-parturient sepsis.

Many, if not all, affected animals become carriers and relapses of up to 2 days duration commonly occur. Relapses are characterized by overt parasitaemia with or without transient fever.

The importance of tick-borne fever in non-pregnant animals lies in its ability to exacerbate latent infections and to influence adversely the course of concurrent and super-infections. The most common and economically troublesome sequel is tick pyaemia, a crippling staphylococcal infection of young lambs. The list of potentiated pathogens, however, is long and includes viruses, other rickettsias, bacteria and protozoa.

Clinical pathology

The haematological picture is characteristic and diagnostic. Leucopenia and thrombocytopenia are both pronounced. The leucopenia is derived first from a lymphocytopenia and then, 2–3 days later, from a profound neutropenia. The overt parasitaemia which is restricted to granulocytes and monocytes is patent at the onset of fever and persists throughout the fever.

Pathology

Animals that die as a result of infection with *C. phagocytophila* exhibit the lesions of the exacerbated latent infection or super-infection, e.g. ewes dying after abortion have a purulent metritis. The dominant lesion in an animal killed during an acute primary reaction is splenomegaly. Often there are no visible macroscopic lesions. Occasionally, there is hydropericardium, hydrothorax and ascites. Microscopic examination of impression smears of cut surfaces of the spleen, liver and lung reveals the presence of *C. phagocytophila* rickettsias in the cytoplasm of neutrophils, von Kupffner cells and perhaps alveolar macrophages.

Diagnosis

The crucial factor in arriving at a presumptive diagnosis, based on the sudden appearance of fever, drop in milk yield or abortion, is the recent arrival of naive animals on to pastures infested with infected ticks. The diagnosis is confirmed by demonstrating the presence of the rickettsias in Giemsa-stained blood films or impression smears of the cut surface of the spleen. Recent infections may also be identified by the detection of antibodies in the serum by counter-immunoelectrophoresis or indirect immunofluorescence tests.

Treatment

Affected lactating cows should be treated immediately with oxytetracycline, which abates the fever and clears the parasitaemia but does not prevent a mild relapse occurring later ensuring resistance to reinfection. The treatment of an uncomplicated tick-borne disease in sucking lambs is not warranted.

Immunology

Recovered animals are carriers and most resist homologous reinfections but the duration of the acquired resistance varies and appears to be related to the level of humoral antibodies. Passive protection of the sucking young, however, does not occur. Reinfections are rarely observed, but if detected, affected animals have fever, lymphocytopenia, neutropenia and a patent parasitaemia. The severity of the reinfection reaction, however, and its course are never as severe as the primary reaction. Reinfected pregnant ewes allegedly do not abort.

Control

In areas harbouring the vector ticks, the essential control measure is exposure of the sucking young to the ticks as soon as possible. On farms where the prevalence of tick pyaemia is high, losses may be mitigated by dipping lambs in an acaricide and by injecting them with a long-acting antibiotic. Pregnant animals should not be moved from tick-free to tick-infested areas.

Further reading

Scott, G.R. (1984). Tick-borne fever in sheep. *Veterinary Annual*, **24**, 100–106.

EHRLICHIOSES

Most, if not all, livestock in the tropics exposed to ixodid vector ticks harbour ehrlichias. Although they were once thought to be protozoa, ehrlichias are leucocytophilic bacteria and they only multiply inside cytoplasmic vacuoles of circulating monocytes and tissue macrophages. They may be propagated, therefore, *in vitro*, unlike the other closely related leucocytophilic cytoecetes. They are classified as a genus of the Ehrlichieae tribe of rickettsias. The best characterized species is *Ehrlichia canis*, the aetiological agent of canine ehrlichiosis and its immunologically mediated sequel known as tropical canine pancytopenia. Two other tropical species, *E. bovis* and *E. ovina*, are less well studied and their economic significance is greatly underrated.

Bovine ehrlichiosis/nofel

Also known as nofel (Jembrana disease?), bovine ehrlichiosis is a rarely reported but nevertheless widespread tick-borne rickettsiosis of cattle characterized by irregular fever, lymphadenosis, depression and loss of condition. Recovered animals are persistently infected and, if stressed severely through malnutrition and/or intercurrent disease, relapse and develop severe illnesses that may end fatally after exhibiting neuronal signs that mimic heartwater.

Aetiology

Ehrlichia bovis is a rickettsia that primarily parasitizes tissue macrophages and, to a lesser extent, circulating monocytes forming dense cytoplasmic clusters of small cocci. Morphologically, *E. bovis* resembles *E. canis* and *E. ovina*. Serologically, cross-reactions have been reported between *Cowdria ruminantium* and *E. bovis*, but cross-challenge experiments in calves failed to show any relationship between the two rickettsias.

Occurrence

Bovine ehrlichiosis has been identified in Africa from north to south, in Asia, South America and some of the Caribbean islands.

Species affected

Natural infections have been observed in cattle and pigs. Both failures and successes have been reported in attempts to infect sheep experimentally. On the other hand, *E. bovis* produces fever and depression in injected monkeys. A Brazilian isolate of

E. bovis has been propagated *in vitro* in normal bovine leucocyte cultures and proved infective for cattle after 48 hours.

Transmission

Bovine ehrlichiosis is not a contagious disease and transmission is primarily affected through the bites of ixodid ticks. Proven vectors include *Amblyomma variegatum* in West Africa, *Rhipicephalus appendiculatus* in southern Africa and *Hyalomma excavatum* in Iran. The vector in Brazil is believed to be *A. cajennense*. Trans-stadial transmission in ticks is known to occur but there is no information regarding transovarial transmission.

Clinical features

E. bovis is a persistent parasite of low pathogenicity in healthy cattle reared in tick-infested areas where the parasite is endemic and primary infections in indigenous animals are usually not observed. Potentiation of chronic persistent infections follow stress, producing clinical signs of nofel in 10–50% of animals in a herd with case mortality rates ranging from 5 to 25%. Morbidity and mortality also occur in primary infections in imported cattle or in virgin soil epidemics where imported cattle introduce infected ticks to previously disease-free areas.

Incubation periods appear to range from 1 to 6 weeks. In acute primary cases in naive animals, fevers fluctuate between 39 and 41°C for 7–10 days. Affected animals neither eat nor ruminate and develop diarrhoea. They stand depressed and immobile with lowered heads. Many develop transient nervous signs which disappear on recovery. The most severely affected animals usually die during a convulsion about 8 days after the onset of illness.

Nofel is an exacerbation of a persistent *E. bovis* infection and is characterized by enlarged superficial lymph nodes, swollen drooping ears and a bilateral suppurative otitis. Affected animals have fevers, congested mucous membranes, ocular and nasal discharges, inappetence and constipation. Most die if not treated promptly.

Clinical pathology

Although clusters of *E. bovis* are rarely seen in the cytoplasms of circulating monocytes, the haematological changes are nevertheless diagnostically significant. The monocytes usually increase in number and are bizzare; their cytoplasms are filled with vacuoles of varying size, most of which appear empty but some contain rickettsias. The nuclear membranes of the monocytes are ragged and torn and the nuclei themselves often contain vacuoles. Lymphocyte numbers are not affected, but neutrophils and eosinophils both decline. In addition, there are many immature cells in the circulation and cells in mitosis are usually present. There is also a thrombocytopenia.

Pathology

The dramatic lesions in naive cattle that die from primary infections are hydropericardium, lung oedema, hydrothorax and hydroperitoneum. The perilobular oedema is sometimes so severe that it mimics the lesions seen in cases of contagious bovine pleuropneumonia. Lymph nodes are hypertrophied, oedematous and congested. Likewise, the spleen is reactive and the kidneys are congested. Changes in the central nervous system, however, are not marked.

E. bovis is most readily detected in organ smears, particularly lung and liver smears, taken fresh at death. It is never found in vascular endothelial cells. The dramatic microscopic changes occur in the convoluted tubules of the kidneys.

Diagnosis

The history, clinical signs and *post mortem* lesions of primary infections in naive animals are readily confused with heartwater. They may be differentiated by haematological examinations despite the difficulty of detecting *E. bovis* in blood films, because bizarre monocytes do not occur in heartwater.

The history and clinical signs of nofel warrant the immediate administration of tetracyclines.

Immunology

Recovered animals become carriers and relapses may occur. Previously infected cattle will resist challenge doses of *E. bovis* isolated in the same area.

Treatment and control

Tetracycline formulations have been used with spectacular success in the treatment of clinical cases of nofel. Presumably they would also be as efficacious in primary infections in naive animals. The essential prophylactic measure, however, is tick control and any introduced animals moved into an endemic area should be monitored and treated if fevers ensue.

Further reading

Rioche, M. (1966). La rickettsiose générale bovine au Sénégal. *Revue de l'Elevage et de Medécine Vétérinaire des Pays Tropicaux*, **19**, 485–494

Canine ehrlichiosis/tropical canine pancytopenia

Synonyms include canine rickettsiosis, Lahore canine fever and Nairobi bleeding disease. Canine ehrlichiosis is a tick-borne rickettsiosis of dogs characterized by fever, purulent nasal and ocular discharges, anaemia and emaciation. Tropical canine pancytopenia (TCP) is an immunologically mediated sequel to canine ehrlichiosis in naive adult dogs characterized by fatal acute epistaxis and pancytopenia.

Aetiology

Ehrlichia canis is an obligate intracellular parasite multiplying inside membrane-lined cytoplasmic vacuoles in circulating mononuclear cells where it is found in clusters or morulae. Individual organisms are about 0.5 μm in diameter, whereas clusters and morulae range in size up to 4 μm in diameter. They stain bluish-purple with Giemsa stain.

TCP is an immunoproliferative syndrome which develops several weeks after the primary clinical episode; a persistent latent infection by *E. canis* stimulates the reticuloendothelial system, producing pathological numbers of plasma cells which accumulate in the meninges, kidneys and lymphopoietic tissues.

E. canis is not related to two other rare rickettsial parasites of dogs, namely *Ehrlichia platys* which parasitizes platelets and *Cytoecetes (Ehrlichia) canis* which parasitizes granulocytes. *E. canis*, however, is closely related, if not identical, to a human ehrlichia, *E. sennetsu*. It is also related to *Cytoecetes (Ehrlichia) equi*, which parasitizes granulocytes in North American and European horses. In addition, there is weak evidence that *E. canis* and *Cowdria ruminantium* may cross-react.

Occurrence

The global distribution of the vector tick delineates the distribution of canine ehrlichiosis which involves most of the tropics and subtropics of the world with the exception of Australasia. Some areas have a seasonal prevalence linked to tick activity.

Species affected

All species of wild and domesticated canids are probably susceptible. Primary infections in endemic areas occur in young puppies and are usually clinically inapparent. Severe clinical reactions occur in exotic dogs imported as adults from tick-free areas. Cases of human infection with *E. canis* have recently been detected in the USA and they may be identical with *E. sennetsu* infections in man reported from Japan.

Transmission

The natural vector is the common brown dog tick, *Rhipicephalus sanguineus*. Transstadial transmission occurs but not transovarian transmission. Infected dogs are infected for life; consequently, iatrogenic transmission may occur with any drop of infected blood.

Clinical features

Canine ehrlichiosis: In areas where the disease is endemic, infections in puppies are clinically inapparent. The puppies, however, become carriers, and stress such as malnutrition, pregnancy, major surgery or concomitant infection will precipitate overt relapses manifested by vague clinical signs which include weight loss, poor appetite and intermittent lethargy.

An acute syndrome occurs in naive dogs within 3 weeks of exposure to infected ticks. The onset of illness is sudden and is manifested by depression, anorexia, fluctuating fever and vomiting. Splenomegaly and lymphadenitis are present. Mucous membranes may be pale or congested. Some affected dogs recover without incident within 1–2 weeks of the onset of illness, but most develop haemorrhages, manifested by petechiae and ecchymoses on visible mucous membranes and over the relatively hairless areas of the skin. Clotting abnormalities lead to epistaxis, haematuria and blood in vomit and faeces. Bleeding into joints may cause lameness. Death may occur within a week of the onset of illness. Other dogs develop ureamia manifested by polyurea, polydipsia, oedema of the limbs and oral ulceration. The breath is fetid because the gums and teeth are coated with a foul brown deposit. Some ureamic cases make a complete recovery, but others have to be maintained on a low protein diet for life.

Some dogs apparently recover but then develop repeated heamorrhagic episodes and anaemia and are refractory to treatment. Others waste away and die over a period of weeks.

Tropical canine pancytopenia: TCP occurs suddenly as an unexpected nose bleed several weeks after recovery from a primary clinical episode. The epistaxis may be unilateral or bilateral and it may be the only clinical sign. Usually, however, it is accompanied by fever, inappetence, dyspnoea, ventral oedema, petechiation of visible mucosae, corneal opacity, lethargy and wasting. If the initial haemorrhage is severe, death may occur within a few hours.

Clinical pathology

Leucopenia, thrombocytopenia and, in time, anaemia develop in acute cases of canine ehrlichiosis. A low-grade parasitaemia precedes the onset of fever and persists throughout the fever.

Dogs that develop TCP have leucopenia, erythrocytopenia and thrombocytopenia. There is bone-marrow depression and plasmacytosis with hypergammaglobulinaemia.

Pathology

The gross lesions of uncomplicated acute canine ehrlichiosis are typical of acute rickettsioses; the changes include oedema, ascites, hydrothorax, splenomegaly, lymphadenopathy and haemorrhagic mottling of the liver and kidney. Microscopic examination of lung impression smears reveals numerous parasitized macrophages.

The gross pathology of TCP is dominated by lymphadenopathy and the presence of petechiae, ecchymoses on serosal and mucosal surfaces. The lungs often exhibit a brownish mottling with some areas of consolidation. Microscopically, bone-marrow depression and plasmacytosis predominate.

Diagnosis

Ante mortem diagnosis of canine ehrlichiosis is difficult and depends upon the detection of *E. canis* in the cytoplasm of circulating mononuclear cells. Overnight incubation of buffy coats and plasma in culture vessels containing flying coverslips greatly enhances the detection rate of infected mononuclear cells. The preferred stain is Giemsa, but direct immunofluorescence is particularly useful when the parasitaemia is scanty. *Post mortem* confirmation is most easily accomplished by examining Giemsa-stained impression smears of cut organ surfaces, particularly the lungs.

The diagnosis of TCP is based on an assessment of the history, clinical signs and haematological findings. *Post mortem* confirmation rests on the histopathological evidence of widespread plasmacytosis; *E. canis* organisms are only rarely observed in tissue sections.

Differential diagnosis

The most common diagnostic problem is concomitant babesiosis. The clinical signs are equivocal and in areas where both conditions are endemic it is wise to assume that the two infections are present simultaneously. Other differential problems are auto-immune haemolytic anaemia, Warfarin poisoning, canine distemper and trypanosomosis.

Treatment

Tetracycline is the drug of choice. Uraemic cases, however, may not tolerate oral tetracyclines and they should be switched to doxycycline. Imidocarb dipropionate has also been advocated, but its efficacy has been questioned. Treatment is of little or no avail in chronic cases and in cases of TCP.

Immunology

Most surviving dogs become carriers and relapses follow stress despite the presence of humoral antibodies detectable by immunofluorescent techniques.

Control

Naive dogs moved from tick-free areas to tick-infested areas should be carefully monitored over the first few weeks, particularly in the rainy season. When illness and parasitaemias occur, they should be treated. Attempts should also be made to control the tick population.

Further reading

Price, J.E., Sayer P.E. and Dolan, T.T. (1987). Improved clinical approach to the diagnosis of canine ehrlichiosis. *Tropical Animal Health and Production*, **19**, 1–8.

Ovine ehrlichiosis

Ovine ehrlichiosis is a persistent rickettsial infection to sheep in Africa and Asia, usually detected accidentally in the course of other disease investigations. Once infected, sheep are carriers for life. When carrier animals are severely stressed, either by malnutrition or concurrent disease, a fatal clinical syndrome that mimics heartwater may ensue.

Aetiology

Ehrlichia ovina was the first haemorickettsia to be recognized, parasitizing circulating monocytes and tissue macrophages forming clusters of cocci in intracytoplasmic vacuoles. It possesses the characteristics of the better known *E. canis* and its modes and sites of replication are the same. Neither the complete natural host range nor the antigenic relationship to other ehrlichial species is known.

Occurrence

Sightings of *E. ovina* are few in number. The organism has been detected in sheep in North, West and southern Africa, the Middle East and Sri Lanka. Fatal exacerbations in carrier sheep have been reported from south-west Africa and North Africa.

Species affected

E. ovina has only been isolated from sheep and its antigenic relationship to other *Ehrlichia* spp. is not known.

Transmission

Tick transmission is suspected but it has yet to be confirmed. Experimentally, *E. ovina* has been transmitted with adult *Rhipicephalus evertsi* ticks fed previously as nymphs on infected sheep. The disease is not contagious.

Clinical features

Incubation periods in susceptible sheep following infestation with infected adult ticks range from 15 to 18 days. The onset of illness is manifested by a sharp rise in the rectal temperature (up to 41 °C) and the fever persists for 3–10 days and sometimes as long as 17 days. Affected animals, however, are depressed and anorexic for only 3–4 days after the onset of fever. Anaemia has been observed towards the end of the febrile phase. Recovery is rapid but the haematological pictures takes 4–6 weeks to return to normal.

The clinical signs in fatal exacerbations mimic those seen in cases of heartwater. The onset is sudden and the course short; affected animals rapidly develop signs of ataxia and then paraplegia before sinking into sternal recumbency and unconsciousness. Death rapidly supervenes.

Clinical pathology

Clusters of cocci occur in the cytoplasms of circulating monocytes and tissue macrophages 2–3 days after the onset of fever. Relapse parasitaemias of short duration are not uncommon. An eosinopenia and a monocytosis have both been reported.

Pathology

Primary infections of sheep with *E. ovina* are not fatal. Activated carrier infections, however, are fatal in animals that are severely stressed from intercurrent disease, malnutrition or shortage of water. The gross changes *post mortem* simulate those of heartwater, the conspicuous lesions being hydropericardium, hydrothorax, hydroperitoneum, lung oedema, splenomegaly and cardiac haemorrhages.

Diagnosis

Primary infections are fortuitously detected while examining blood films being screened for other conditions. It is impossible to differentiate fatal ovine ehrlichiosis from heartwater in areas where *Amblyomma* ticks are present without a microscopic search. *E. ovina* occurs exclusively in monocytes and macrophages and does not parasitize vascular endothelial cells.

Immunology

The immune response of sheep parasitized by *E. ovina* is unknown.

Control

Primary infections are benign and do not warn the institution of control measures. Exacerbation in carrier animals are associated with severe stress and treatment is to no avail.

Further reading

Neitz, W.O. (1968). *Ehrlichia ovina* infection. *Bulletin de l'Office International des Epizooties*, **70**, 337–340.

EPERYTHROZOONOSES

Eperythrocytic rickettsias in the *Eperythrozoon* genus of the Anaplasmataceae family commonly parasitize pigs, rodents and ruminants. They are minute organisms, less than 1.5 μm in diameter. When stained with Giemsa they appear light blue or pinkish-violet. They are very pleomorphic, the common shapes being spheres, commas, rings, rods and chains. They lie on the surfaces of erythrocytes, often in depressions, and also occur free in the plasma. The major modes of transmission have not been clearly elucidated; experimental transmission by inoculation of susceptible hosts with blood from an infected host readily occurs and natural transmission has been attributed to the activities of bloodsucking diptera. Some may be transmitted by the oral route and others across the transplacental barrier.

Most eperythrozoon species are well adapted and equilibrated with their hosts, but two that affect domesticated animals are economically important, viz. *Eperythrozoon ovis* and *E. suis*.

Ovine eperythrozoonosis

Ovine eperythrozoonosis is a worldwide infection of sheep and goats, caused by *E. ovis*. Infections are normally clinically inapparent but, on occasion, induce anaemia. In Australia, for example, ovine eperythrozoonosis is considered to be the major cause of ill-thrift in lambs and weaners.

Occurrence

E. ovis has been reported from all continents wherever sheep are husbanded.

Species affected

Natural infections have been observed only in sheep and goats, but several species of African wildlife have been infected experimentally. Cattle are refractory.

Transmission

Iatrogenic transmission occurs through the misuse of re-used hypodermic needles, tattooing and castration instruments. In temperate areas, transmission is blamed on the tabanids and keds and in the tropics on mosquitoes. Ixodid ticks are also capable of transmitting the infection. Recently, transplacental transmission has been demonstrated and may be the major mode of transmission.

Clinical features

Lambs infected *in utero* show no clinical signs unless stressed. The exacerbated latent infections are manifested by fever, anaemia, sometimes jaundice, and perhaps death. Parenterally inoculated animals may or may not develop fever but many become anorexic and depressed. Visible mucous membranes are pale and occasionally jaundiced as the result of a progressive haemolytic anaemia. Haemoglobinuria occurs but it is usually missed. Affected weaners lose weight and fail to thrive.

Clinical pathology

The erythrocyte count, the haematocrit readings and haemoglobin values are all severely depressed. Most of the erythrocytes are parasitized and others show anisocytosis, poikilocytosis and basophil stippling. Haemoglobin is present in the urine.

Pathology

The dramatic feature of the gross pathology is the splenomegaly, spleens being twice their normal size. The haemolymph nodes are also enlarged. On occasion, a hydropericardium has been observed. A significant microscopic finding is the heavy deposits of haemosiderin in many of the organs, particularly in the convoluted tubules of the kidneys.

Diagnosis

Case of ill-thrift should always be examined haematologically for the presence of parasitized erythrocytes and, if this is negative, checked for the presence of antibodies.

Treatment

The recommended treatment if required is chloramphenicol administered subcutaneously. Tetracycline formulations are not as effective, but imidocarb dipropionate will abate parasitaemias transiently.

Immunology

Infected sheep remain carriers for life but patent parasitaemias are often but not always transient. Infected animals, however, are protected against reinfections and the protection is associated with the production of antibodies, detectable by indirect immunofluorescence or ELISA.

Control

Practical measures that limit the risk of spread of infection include controlling insects, avoiding stress and taking care while using instruments.

Further reading

Gretillat, S. and Gevrey, J. (1983). Note preliminare sur l'anemie infectieuse des agneux a *Eperythrozoon ovis* (Neitz, Alexander et du Toit, 1934) en France. *Revue de Medecine Veterinaire*, **134**, 399–405.

Swine eperythrozoonosis

Swine eperythrozoonosis is a common disease of fattening pigs exacerbated by stress and manifested as a febrile ictero-anaemia. In addition, subclinical eperythrozoonosis in gilts and sows increases the number of stillborn piglets.

Occurrence

Swine eperythrozoonosis has been observed in every major pig-raising area of the world.

Species affected

E. suis appears to be restricted to domesticated pigs.

Transmission

The major routes of transmission are believed to be across the placenta and by the oral route. Biting lice and biting diptera have also been incriminated. Iatrogenic transmission is common through the medium of blood-contaminated needles and instruments.

Clinical features

Some newborn piglets infected *in utero* show signs of skin pallor and even jaundice, but they recover within a few days. Most *in utero* infections are subclinical.

Exacerbations of latent infections are common in fattening pigs, stressed through malnutrition and concurrent diseases such as mange, louse infestation and helminthiasis. Exacerbations also occur in sows near to farrowing. Affected pigs suddenly stop eating, become depressed and develop high fever for a few days. In parturient sows, the fever tends to persist until farrowing is complete. Some, moreover, are unable to nurse their piglets because of agalactia. Many animals recover within a few days after regression of the fever. Others develop a progressive haemolytic anaemia which may lead to jaundice and bile-stained faeces. Affected pigs are weak and inco-ordinated, and they may die. Some become chronically affected, have recurrent relapses, and eventually became debilitated, pale and jaundiced. Chronically affected animals do not gain weight despite *ad lib* feeding and many die as a result of concurrent infections.

Clinical pathology

Blood films taken from pigs in the early febrile stage of the disease contain massive numbers of *E. ovis* rickettsias on and near the surfaces of the erythrocytes. There is a severe hypoglycaemia, a moderate bilirubinaemia and a mild anaemia. The patent parasitaemia declines rapidly with the regression of the fever. The anaemia worsens and a transient thrombocytopenia occurs. Thereafter, there is a transient hyperglobulinaemia.

Pathology

The carcase in acute deaths is jaundiced, the liver is yellow, and the spleen is soft and enlarged. Lymph nodes are swollen and oedematous. Sometimes hydropericardium, hydrothorax and ascites are present. The carcases of chronically affected pigs are also pale or jaundiced, but the dominant *post mortem* findings relate to the super-infection that killed.

Microscopic examination reveals a hyperplastic bone marrow, extensive haemosiderosis of the liver with necrosis of the lobules and lymphocyte infiltration.

Diagnosis

A presumptive diagnosis is not easy in the early stages of the disease. Haematological examinations, however, will readily identify the cause; there is a massive parasitaemia, together with the dramatic fall in erythrocyte numbers, haematocrit readings and haemoglobin values.

A presumptive diagnosis is easier when pigs develop jaundice but confirmation is difficult. The most reliable technique is reverse passive haemagglutination and titres of 140 are considered diagnostic.

Treatment

Effective treatment regimens have yet to be developed despite the abatement of the parasitaemia by single doses of tetracyclines. In the USA, arsenilic acid is frequently added to the rations for sows and fattening pigs on an intermittent basis, although there is risk of accumulative arsenic toxicosis.

Immunology

Infected pigs are infected for life, although patent parasitaemias only develop after stress. The persistent infection is associated with the continuous production of IgM antibodies, detectable by a reverse-phase passive haemagglutination.

Control

Because the prevalence of *E. suis* infection is so widespread, control efforts are directed towards elimination of mange, lice and helminth infections, i.e. the avoidance of stress. The risk of iatrogenic spread should be minimized by the careful use of needles and surgical instruments within the herd.

Further reading

Zachary, J.F. and Smith, A.R. (1985). Experimental porcine eperythrozoonosis: T-lymphocyte suppression and misdirected immune responses. *American Journal of Veterinary Research*, **46**, 821–830.

Q FEVER

The causative agent of Q fever is *Coxiella burnetii*, an obligate intracellular bacterium currently classified as a rickettsia in the Rickettsieae tribe of the Rickettsiaceae family within the Rickettsiales order. It is wrongly classified because unlike other members of the tribe it multiplies in intracytoplasmic vacuoles and, moreover, it undergoes sporogenesis. It is therefore very tough, resisting chemical and physical insults and surviving for years in dust.

Q fever is a zoonotic infection of little economic significance to the agricultural industry despite widespread persistent and silent infection of domesticated ruminants. Man, however, is an aberrant host who acquires infection through contact with animals, both live and dead.

Aetiology

C. burnetii is a tiny Gram-negative bacterium that is usually described as being a bipolar rod. There are, however, two distinct morphological forms; namely, a compact small rod about 0.2 μm in diameter and a larger pleomorphic vegetative bacterium about 1.0 μm long. In addition, some of the large vegetative forms contain an endospore. Like chlamydial elementary bodies, *C. burnetii* stains bright red by the modified Ziehl-Neelsen methods.

Occurrence

C. burnetti has a worldwide distribution; everywhere it has been sought it has been found. In its basic ecological niche, *C. burnetii* cycles silently between ticks and small free-living ground mammals. It has, however, overspilled into domesticated animals, both directly from tick bites and indirectly from contact with dried infected faeces. Tick-free cycles have evolved in herds and flocks in which *C. burnetii* localize, and multiplies in the genital tract and udder to be shed intermittently or, sometimes, continuously in milk, faeces and urine.

Species affected

C. burnetii has been isolated from an enormous range of animals, but disease is largely limited to man. The presence of the organism in the placenta does not lead to abortion. In its sylvatic niche it is tick-borne. In contrast, transmission in infected herds and flocks occurs at parturition when enormous numbers of the organisms are voided on to pastures and bedding. In-contact susceptible animals become infected by inhaling aerosols of the infected fluid discharges or dust loaded with dried discharges. *C. burnetii* is also shed in milk. Animal handlers, however, are exposed to a greater risk of inhaling the organism while handling infective animals.

Clinical features

Overt disease in animals is conspicuous by its absence. Despite periodic claims to the contrary, abortion is not considered to be a feature of infection in animals. It may, however, affect fertility.

Infections in man acquired by drinking infected milk or eating infected milk products are clinically inapparent. In contrast, infections acquired by inhalation of infective droplets often develops into disease meriting medical attention. The disease in man is influenza-like, starts abruptly after an incubation period of 2–3 weeks and lasts for 1–2 weeks. Some patients develop pneumonia and a few hepatitis. Death is rare, but convalescence is prolonged over several months. The most serious sequel is an endocarditis.

Pathology

Reports of pathological changes in infected domesticated animals are rare. Mild to severe placentitis has been observed in sporadic cases, the placental lesions being most conspicuous in the intracotyledonary zone where they are covered by abundant inspissated white to red exudates. The placenta under the exudate is thickened and leathery with multifocal areas of white mineralization. Necrosis of the cotyledonary vili and intracotyledonary epithelium is extensive. Microscopically, there is a heavy neutrophilic infiltration and clusters of *C. burnetii* are present in the trophoblasts of the chorion.

Diagnosis

There are no clinical signs in domesticated animals warranting a presumptive diagnosis of Q fever. Diagnostic confusion arises when ewes abort, necessitating laboratory investigations to differentiate between the presence of *C. burnetii* and *Chlamydia psittaci*.

Treatment

Treatment of infective animals is seldom attempted.

Immunology

Recovered animals remain infected and infective for many years and sometimes for life. The persistent infection is associated with the presence of humoral antibodies, detectable by complement fixation, microagglutination, indirect immunofluorescence and ELISA.

Control

The spread of infection in domesticated animals may be limited by adopting hygienic precautions at the time of parturition. In particular, placental membranes should be destroyed. Recently, routine vaccination of cattle, sheep and goats has been advocated to prevent epidemics of Q fever in man. Vaccination of naive animals limits the shedding of *C. burnetii* at parturition but does not prevent it.

Further reading

Little, T.W.A. (1983). Q fever – an enigma. *British Veterinary Journal*, **139**, 277–283.

Diseases caused by viruses

G.R. Scott

AFRICAN HORSE SICKNESS

African horse sickness (AHS) is a seasonal, midge-borne viral infection of horses, mules and donkeys characterized by fever and oedema of the subcutaneous tissues and lungs.

Aetiology

The causal virus of AHS is a member of the *Orbivirus* genus of the Reoviridae family of double-stranded RNA viruses. Nine serotypes of the virus are known. They are remarkably stable in the presence of protein.

Occurrence

AHS virus cycles silently in what is believed to be the major host, the zebra, in Africa south of the Sahara. Clinical episodes in horses occur after the onset of the rains. Periodically, the virus is introduced with wind-borne midges into neighbouring continents causing sharp short-lived epidemics.

Species affected

All African equids and camels are susceptible. In addition, AHS virus has been isolated from dogs in Egypt and in Kenya. Antibodies have been detected in the sera of East African elephants, but the epidemiological significance of this finding is as yet unknown.

Equine races vary in their innate resistance to AHS virus. Thus zebras, African donkeys and African horses undergo clinically inapparent or subacute infections, whereas non-indigenous horses and mules develop overt signs of disease, Newly imported exotic horses, in particular, are at risk and, if not vaccinated, are likely to die.

Transmission

AHS virus is transmitted by night-flying midges (*Culicoides* sp.). The disease, therefore, has a seasonal prevalence. The epidemiological role of other biting diptera is negligible. Dogs acquire infection through eating infected horse flesh.

Clinical features

Although incubation periods may range from 2 to 21 days, most last 5–7 days. Four clinical forms of the disease are described; namely, an acute pulmonary syndrome, a subacute systemic circulatory form, a mixed form, and an uncomplicated fever.

The acute disease has a short course of a few hours duration and is characterized by high fever (41°C), cough, conjunctivitis and pulmonary oedema that leads to respiratory distress and induces a copious frothy nasal discharge. The appetite is not lost until the affected horse collapses and dies. In diseased dogs, the pulmonary form predominates.

The course of the subacute systemic circulatory syndrome lasts several days longer. The onset is manifested by a fever (40°C) and its attendant signs. Later, petechiae appear in the injected conjunctivae and cyanosis commonly affects the tongue and gums. The critical sign is a bilateral bulging of oedematous tissues overlying the supra-orbital fossae. As the disease progresses, the temperature falls and the subcutaneous oedema extends from the sites of the supra-orbital fossae to involve the whole head inverting the eye-lids. In severe cases, the oedema also involves the neck and brisket. Affected horses are restless. Many die, death being preceded by respiratory distress.

The mixed form in which lung oedema and subcutaneous oedema occur is probably the most common syndrome.

Horse sickness fevers occur in indigenous equids. They are low grade and transient with full recovery being the norm.

Pathology

Gastritis is commonly seen in all forms of the disease. The dominant features in animals affected with the acute pulmonary syndrome, however, are the voluminous hydrothorax and the massive pulmonary oedema that involves both the inter lobular and pleural tissues distending them with a yellow gelatinous fluid. The bronchi and trachea are filled with froth. in contrast, the dominant feature in the circulatory syndrome is subcutaneous, subserous and intermuscular oedema. The heart has subepicardial and subendocardial haemorrhages. The significant microscopical finding is lymphoid depletion and necrosis in germinal centres.

Diagnosis

A presumptive diagnosis based on a history of the recent arrival of exotic horses, mules or donkeys into a humid environment favouring midge activity in Africa south of the Sahara, together with an assessment of the clinical signs and *post mortem* lesions is relatively easy. A history of previous vaccination, moreover, should be discounted. In contrast, the cause of an explosive outbreak in a previously disease-free country recently invaded by wind-borne infected midges is usually not suspected until after many deaths have occurred.

Confirmation is readily achieved in an agar-gel immunodiffusion test in which a concentrated spleen suspension is diffused against a known positive antiserum. If the affected animal has a history of earlier vaccination, an attempt should be made to isolate the virus to identify the serotype. Blood from febrile cases should be collected in an anticoagulant which should be EDTA rather than heparin. The specimen container should be forwarded to the laboratory in water-ice.

Differential diagnosis

All cases of sudden death give rise to differential diagnostic problems. These include babesiosis, equine arteritis and anthrax.

Immunology

Viraemias of several months duration may occur in zebras and African horses. Thereafter, recovered animals have a durable immunity to the serotype that infected them but they remain susceptible to the other serotypes. Foals of immune mares are protected passively for several months after birth. Antibodies are readily detected by ELISA.

Control

Horses, mules and donkeys imported into Africa should be vaccinated against African horse sickness before shipment. If prior vaccination is not possible, arrangements should be made for the horses to arrive in Africa during daylight and to be transferred immediately to midge-proof stabling where they should be vaccinated and held for 2 weeks. Thereafter, the imported horses and other high-risk horses are protected by annual vaccination and during the rains are housed at night. Supplementary precautions are designed to limit the numbers of midges by adequate drainage near buildings, by lighting smoke fires at night, by use of repellent chemicals and insecticides and by installing ultra-violet "insectecutors".

The nine serotypes of AHS virus necessitate the use of polyvalent vaccine to protect animals at risk. The vaccine comprises a mixture of live attenuated serotypes of the virus and, consequently, competitive interference between the attenuated viruses may, on occasion, leave vaccinated horses susceptible to one or more serotypes. Vaccination of foals should be delayed until they are 8 months old.

Outbreaks outside Africa are caused by a single serotype and horses at risk in such outbreaks are better vaccinated with the appropriate monovalent vaccine. The virus does not persist in exotic countries, presumably because of the absence of a maintenance host.

Further reading

Newsholme, S.J. (1983). A morphological study of the lesions of African horse sickness. *Onderstepoort Journal of Veterinary Research*, **50**, 7–24.

AFRICAN SWINE FEVER

African swine fever (ASF) is a symptomless tick-borne viral infection of warthogs that has spilled over into domesticated pigs either through the bites of infected soft ticks or through the feeding of infected pig-meat scraps. The acute disease in domesticated pigs is characterized by fever, widespread visceral haemorrhages and death. Surviving pigs become chronically ill, exhibiting an undulant fever, progressive wasting and oedema before dying within 2–15 months.

Aetiology

Though clinically and pathologically similar to hog cholera (HC), ASF is caused by a completely different virus with no taxonomic or immunological relationship to HC virus. ASF virus is a DNA virus belonging to the *Iridovirus* group. It has a very distinctive ultrastructure more reminiscent of an insect virus than an animal virus. It is one of the toughest viruses known, and survives for years in frozen infected carcases, for 18 months in infected refrigerated blood, for 6 months in hams and for more than 18 weeks in decomposed blood held at room temperature.

Occurrence

ASF is endemic in Africa between the equator and the Tropic of Capricorn, its distribution being governed by the distribution of the vector tick *Ornithodoros moubata porcinus*. In 1957, the virus spread from Angola to Portugal and then to Spain and a new endemic focus was created, being maintained by feral pigs and by infection of a European soft tick. Spread from this European focus has occurred at regular intervals into various countries in Europe, the Caribbean and South America.

Species affected

The true natural host of ASF is the soft tick *O. moubata porcinus*. Events in Europe have created another true natural host in a soft tick, *O. erraticus*. The natural mammalian hosts are the wild pigs of Africa, in particular the warthog, of which approximately 60% are infected at any given time. The wild boar of Europe is also susceptible to ASF, but unlike the wild pigs of Africa it develops clinical disease when infected. The North American wild pig, the peccary, however, is resistant to ASF. All species of domesticated pig appear to be susceptible, except for a resistant line of large white pigs recently developed in Portugal.

Transmission

ASF virus is spread or maintained in night-feeding *Ornithodoros* tick populations by transovarian transmission and venereal transmission. Warthogs are infected shortly after birth through the bites of infected ticks. In pig herds kept behind pig-proof fences, infection gains entry in infected pig-meat scraps being fed to the pigs. Once established in a domestic pig herd, the virus spreads rapidly, being shed in large quantities in the nasal pharyngeal secretions, faeces and urine. Susceptible pigs become infected through the ingestion of fomites.

Clinical features

The incubation period in domesticated pigs ranges from 3 to 15 days. The clinical syndromes range from the peracute to the acute, subacute, chronic and inapparent. In the peracute syndrome, death may occur before any clinical signs appear. In the acute syndrome, affected pigs develop a high fever up to 42°C, which persists for 3–4 days. Clinical signs appear 1–2 days after the onset of fever. Affected animals stop eating and lie huddled together. If forced to move they appear weak and wobbly. Red skin blotches often occur on the extremities and on the flanks. Other signs that may be present are mucopurulent nasal and ocular discharges, respiratory distress, vomiting and blood-stained diarrhoea. Pregnant sows abort. Death usually occurs within 7 days of the onset of fever. A subacute syndrome is characterized by a course ending in death or recovery after a period of 3–4 weeks. It begins with a high fever which persists for several days and thereafter fluctuates irregularly throughout the course of the disease. Abortions are common and may be the only sign of the disease. Surviving pigs remain carriers of the virus for life.

Chronic ASF is extremely variable and rare, but may last for up to 15 months. Often the only signs are stunting and emaciation. Death can occur at any stage, usually following a secondary bacterial infection, commonly a pneumonia.

Pathology

The gross pathology of ASF is indistinguishable from that of hog cholera. The most typical lesions in peracute and acute ASF are an enlarged dark coloured spleen and haemorrhages in all organs. Petechiae are found in the mucosae of the intestines and urinary bladder, in the myocardium, on the subendocardial surfaces of the heart, and in the renal cortex. Lymph nodes are swollen, red and haemorrhagic and many look like blood clots. The tonsils are also swollen and haemorrhagic.

Subacute ASF is also characterized by widespread haemorrhages in the lymph nodes and kidneys. In addition, the lungs often show areas of consolidation and sometimes interstitial pneumonia.

In chronic ASF, gross lesions are very variable but usually include enlarged lymph nodes, fibrinous pericarditis and pleurisy, and small hard white nodular masses in the lungs. Arthritis in one or more joints is usual.

Diagnosis

ASF cannot be differentiated from hog cholera on clinical or pathological findings. Laboratory confirmation is therefore essential. The samples that are required are blood in EDTA or heparin, blood for serum from live animals and, from carcases, spleen, lymph node, tonsils, livers, kidneys and lung. All samples should be sent to the laboratory without preservatives.

Differential diagnosis

Differentiation of ASF from hog cholera is the major problem. Other conditions that cause diagnostic confusion are acute bacteraemias and septicaemias, pseudorabies, thrombocytopenic purpura and warfarin poisoning.

Immunology

ASF virus does not stimulate production of neutralizing antibodies in infected pigs and, consequently, passive immunity does not protect the young against infection. Nevertheless, antibodies are detectable by a variety of serological tests and thus have a diagnostic role. Surviving pigs remain infected and probably infectious for life.

Control

Low-risk countries maintain their freedom from the disease by a total prohibition of imports of live or dead pigs. Similarly, high-risk countries that are geographically or commercially adjacent to endemically infected countries, protect themselves by prohibiting imports of live or dead pigs. If an outbreak occurs in a high-risk country, it is controlled by a stamping-out policy with slaughter and destruction of carcases. In warthog-associated endemic areas, domestic pigs are protected by housing them behind pig-proof fences and forbidding the feeding of swill. In the endemic focus in Europe, control is virtually impossible where pigs are allowed free range. Individual farmers, however, may protect their herd by strict segregation and a ban on the feeding of swill.

Attempts to control the soft tick vector have failed.

Further reading

Genovesi, E.G., Knudsen, R.C., Whyard, T.C. and Mebus, C.A. (1988). Moderately virulent African swine fever virus infection: Blood cell changes and infective virus distribution among blood components. *American Journal of Veterinary Research*, **49**, 338–344.

AKABANE DISEASE

Synonyms for Akabane disease include epizootic abortion, epizootic congenital arthrogryposis and hydranencephaly syndrome. Akabane disease is a seasonal arthropod-borne teratogenic viral infection of ruminants manifested only by abortion, premature births and congenital abnormalities.

Aetiology

The causative agent of Akabane disease is a member of the Simbu sero-group of the *Bunyavirus* genus of the Bunyaviridae family of RNA viruses. It is a labile virus, being rapidly inactivated by ambient temperatures above 37°C, by acidic pH and by lipid solvents.

Occurrence

Seasonal outbreaks of congenital abnormalities in cattle were first recognized in Australia in the 1950s. Their viral aetiology was ascertained in similar episodes in Japan in the 1970s and, since then, the infection has been detected in Africa, Eastern Europe and the Middle East.

Species affected

Teratologic incidents have been observed in cattle, sheep and goats. In addition, antibodies have been identified in the sera of buffaloes, camels, horses, zebras and many African wild ruminants.

Transmission

The common vectors of Akabane disease virus are mosquitoes in Japan and midges in Australia. Infected midges have initiated epidemics in previously disease-free districts of Australia after being wind-blown for more than 1500 km. When pregnant animals are infected, the virus passes through the placenta to infect the foetus. The virus may be shed with semen.

Clinical features

Systemic signs of infection in adult animals other than abortion are conspicuous by their absence. In contrast, the responses of infected foetuses are dramatic. In animals born alive, clinical signs include inco-ordination, inco-ordination with mild arthrogryposis manifested by retention of one or more joints in a flexed position, severe arthrogryposis, and hydranencephaly with or without arthrogryposis.

Pathology

The lesions range from a generalized mild encephalomyelitis and polymyositis to severe congenital abnormalities that include arthrogryposis, cervical scoliosis, hydranencephaly and microencephaly.

Diagnosis

A provisional diagnosis based on a history of an epidemic of abortions, stillbirths and congenital abnormalities with a seasonal prevalence should be confirmed by demonstrating the presence of specific antibodies in pre-colostral sera.

Differential diagnosis

Several other arthropod-borne viruses infecting ruminants are teratogenic and their differentiation from Akabane disease requires laboratory facilties. They include bluetongue, Rift Valley fever and Wesselsbron viruses. The non-arthropod-borne flaviviruses in the *Pestivirus* genus, viz., bovine virus, diarrhoea virus and Border disease virus, are likewise teratogenic.

Immunology

Akabane disease virus induces the production of specific neutralizing antibodies in the sera of immunologically competent animals including foetuses older than 3 months. The antibodies apparently persist for life.

Control

Inactivated and attenuated vaccines are available commercially in Japan to protect animals at risk in the known areas where the infection is endemic. Both vaccines are alleged to be safe for use in pregnant animals, but neither stimulates a high level of antibodies and booster doses are recommended before the onset of the warm, wet season. In addition, active steps should be taken to limit the numbers of midges and mosquitoes.

Further reading

Haughey, K.G., Hartley, W.J., Della-Porta, A.J. and Murray, M.D. (1988). Akabane disease in sheep. *Australian Veterinary Journal*, **65**, 136–140.

BLUETONGUE

Bluetongue is a *Culicoides*-borne virus disease of sheep and goats characterized by fever, ulcerative stomatitis, muscle oedema and lameness. Subclinical infections are widespread in other domesticated and wild ruminants and camels.

Aetiology

Bluetongue virus belongs to the *Orbivirus* genus of the Reoviridae family of double-stranded RNA viruses. Serum neutralization tests have differentiated 24 serotypes with some cross-reactions between them. They share a group antigen demonstrable by complement fixation, agar gel diffusion and fluorescent antibody tests. In addition, the same tests reveal that the viruses of epizootic haemorrhagic disease of deer and Ibaraki disease of cattle are related to the bluetongue. All orbiviruses are very stable and survive for years at most shade temperatures.

Occurrence

Bluetongue virus probably has the widest global distribution of any arthropod-borne virus infection of domesticated animals. It cycles in Africa, Asia, America and the southern fringes of Europe between 40°N and 35°S. Being a *Culicoides*-borne virus, there is a seasonal prevalence associated with the periods of maximal activity by the vectors.

Species affected

Most mammalian infections with bluetongue virus are silent, being identified serologically. Clinical disease is restricted to sheep and goats that live in countries at the limits of the geographical distribution range. When naive animals are imported into endemic areas, epidemics result. Infections of naive pregnant cattle may result in congenital abnormality or early foetal death.

Transmission

Bluetongue virus latently maintained in cattle is activated into a viraemic state by the bites of *Culicoides*. There are numerous species of *Culicoides*, but only a few are implicated in the transmission of bluetongue virus. In Africa the vector is *C. imicola*, in the USA *C. variipennis* and in Australia *C. brevitarsis*. These species of *Culicoides* are preferential cattle feeders. Infected *Culicoides* prefer warm, moist conditions and are highly nomadic, moving over vast distances, thereby allowing the virus access to a constant supply of susceptible hosts.

Transovarian transmission in *Culicoides* is not known, but there is vertical transmission in infected mammalian hosts, which can produce congenital abnormalities and foetal death. In addition, venereal transmission from affected bulls to naive heifers and their offspring has been observed. Otherwise, bluetongue is not a contagious disease.

Clinical features

The incubation period in sheep and goats is about 1 week and the onset of illness is manifested by a high fever, which fluctuates for about 1 week. The attendant signs of fever are congestion of the buccal and nasal mucosae, excessive salivation with licking of the lips and a clear nasal discharge. Within a few days the discharge becomes mucopurulent and dries, encrusting the nostrils.In the meantime, the lips swell and are very tender and bleed when handled. The encrustation that may follow mimics orf. Sometimes a swollen blue tongue is evident. Deep ulcers filled with white necrotic debris appear at any site where there is irritation. Towards the end of the fever, lameness and stiffness develop. The lameness stems from a coronitis manifested by the development of a red or purplish band which travels down the hoof with the growth of the horn. The stiffness is due to degeneration of skeletal muscle fibres. Severely affected animals become recumbent and will only move on their knees if forced. Some exhibit torticollis. Thereafter, emaciation and weakness are rapid.

Secondary infections of the respiratory system commonly occur. Diarrhoea, which is often bloodstained, is sometimes seen.

The mortality rate varies from 0 to 20%, though in isolated epidemics it can be up to 90%. The severely affected animals die within 1 week of the onset of fever but others will linger on and die after 1 month. Convalescence in surviving sheep is prolonged and such animals frequently exhibit a moth-eaten appearance caused by breaks in the wool.

Pathology

Gross changes in the alimentary tract are most prominent in the mouth where the mucous membranes are oedematous, hyperaemic and sometimes cyanotic. Ecchymoses and excoriations which are often covered with grey necrotic tissue are present on the lips, hard palate, cheeks and tongue. The fore-stomachs are hyperaemic. Congestion, catarrhal inflammation and petechial haemorrhages occur throughout the small and large intestines.

The nostrils are partly occluded by encrusted nasal discharge. The upper respiratory tract exhibits a catarrhal inflammation and occasionally the lungs show oedema.

Widespread hyperaemia, oedema and haemorrhage characterize the changes in the vascular system. Subepicardial and subendocardial haemorrhages are common.

Skin and muscles show the most constant and most suggestive lesions. Exposed areas of the skin have irregular encrusted exanthematous eruptions. The subcutaneous and intramuscular connective tissues are infiltrated with a red gelatinous fluid. Tiny haemorrhages are found scattered throughout the muscles, together with grey areas of necrosis producing a mottled appearance.

Damage to the endothelium of the small blood vessels is the essential microscopic finding.

Diagnosis

The history, clinical signs and *post mortem* findings in acute cases are highly suggestive, but in areas where fatalities are low a presumptive diagnosis is often difficult and requires laboratory confirmation. The samples required from live animals are coagulated and non-coagulated blood. The tissues to be harvested from dead animals include the spleen and mesenteric lymph nodes. Spleen specimens should also be collected from aborted or deformed foetuses. All specimens should be forwarded to the laboratory on wet-ice, and blood samples in particular should not be frozen.

Differential diagnosis

Early cases of bluetongue are often misdiagnosed as orf. Other common early differential problems are goat plague and foot-and-mouth disease. In addition, abortions and congenitally deformed lambs may be confused with those caused by the Akabane, border disease and Rift Valley fever viruses.

Immunology

Sheep that survive develop humoral antibodies and a cellular immune response to the serotype that infects them, but they remain susceptible to a second serotype. However, there is some heterotypic cross-protection between some of the serotypes. Cattle, when infected, undergo persistent and later latent infections. The duration of the persistent infection appears to be about 50 days, but there are no data on the duration of latency.

Control

Control measures are rarely implemented in endemic areas to protect indigenous stock. However, imported animals are at risk and should be vaccinated. Similarly, sheep and goats in high-risk areas adjacent to the endemic areas should be vaccinated regularly. The vaccines in common use are live attenuated virus vaccines, which are usually polyvalent. In South Africa, three pentavalent vaccines covering 15 serotypes are used at intervals of 3 weeks. In East Africa, two pentavalent vaccines are recommended. Naive pregnant animals should not be vaccinated.

Vector control is difficult. Nevertheless, infection can be avoided by moving stock during the rains to high, well-drained ground where there are no *Culicoides* or by housing at night. Smoke-fires at night and the use of insecticides have a role to play. In addition in southern Africa, it is the practice to kraal sheep along with cattle on the grounds that the *Culicoides* prefer cattle blood to sheep blood.

Further reading

Jeggo, M.H., Wardley, R.C., Brownlie, J. and Corteyn, A.H. (1986). Serial inoculation of sheep with two bluetongue virus types. *Research in Veterinary Science*, **40**, 386–392.

BORDER DISEASE

Synonyms for Border disease (BD) include pestivirus teratomata of sheep, hairy-shaker disease, congenital trembles and fuzzy lambs. BD is a congenitally acquired viral disease of lambs characterized by an abnormally hairy birth coat, abnormal pigmentation, cerebellar tremors and a low survival rate. Superinfection of recovered hairy-shakers with Border disease virus precipitates a fatal acute lymphoproliferative reaction.

Aetiology

The causative teratogenic virus is a member of the *Pestivirus* genus of the Flaviviridae family of RNA viruses. It is closely related to the other members of the genus, in particular, to the virus of bovine virus diarrhoea. Cytopathic and non-cytopathic strains of BD virus exist. It is a fragile virus.

Occurrence

BD has been widely recognized in all the major sheep-rearing countries of the world.

Species affected

The natural hosts of BD virus are sheep and goats. BD virus, however, will also infect cattle and, conversely, bovine virus diarrhoea virus may infect sheep.

Transmission

BD virus is shed in the secretions and excretions of persistently infected animals. Susceptible pregnant ewes in contact with shedders become infected presumably by the aerosol route and, in turn, the virus passes through the placenta to the foetus. The infected ewes throw off the primary infection and develop neutralizing antibodies, but in lambs infected *in utero* the virus persists. Some persistently infected progeny survive to conceive and they either abort or produce affected lambs over a period of many years. Affected male lambs that reach maturity are subfertile but many transmit the virus in their semen.

Clinical features

Primary post-natal infections in non-pregnant animals are subclinical. A placentitis develops when the susceptible pregnant ewe is infected and it may be preceded by a low-grade fever and leucopenia. When the placentitis is diffuse abortion follows, but if it remains focal the foetus survives to be born prematurely. The abnormal hairy birth coat is readily recognized as soon as the lamb has been licked dry. Similarly, the abnormal brown-black pigmentation is obvious. The rhythmic tremors start as soon as the lamb is able to stand. Most affected lambs are small and some exhibit skeletal abnormalities. The survival rate is low, but with careful nursing a low proportion of hairy-shaker lambs may be reared, although it takes 4–5 months before the tremors disappear. About 10–20% of congenitally affected lambs do not show clinical signs.

Pathology

The acute necrotizing placentitis may be diffuse or remain as multiple small foci of necrosis. In hairy-shaker lambs, the significant pathological changes are in the central nervous system and skin. The histopathological lesion in the brain and spinal cord is hypomyelination and gliosis. An examination of affected skin reveals an increased size of primary wool follicles together with a decreased number of secondary wool follicles.

Diagnosis

The clinical signs are suggestive and can be confirmed histopathologically. A more rapid confirmation is the demonstration of specific antigen in cryostat sections of affected tissues.

Differential diagnosis

It may be necessary to differentiate BD abortions from those caused by bacteria, chlamydia and toxoplasma. Difficulties may also arise in differentiating BD central nervous system disturbances from bacterial meningo-encephalitis and swayback.

Immunology

Recovered adult animals develop neutralizing antibodies to BD virus, but lambs infected before the 50th day of gestation do not produce neutralizing antibodies. Although lambs infected late in gestation produce antibodies, persistence of the virus is not prevented.

Control

Disease-free flocks have to be closed to maintain a disease-free status. If new genetic material is desired, it should be restricted to embryo transplants. If a previously susceptible flock becomes infected, it is probable that the damage will be done before the disease is diagnosed. Nevertheless, in-lamb ewes should be segregated from ewes with affected lambs. Susceptible flock replacements should be exposed before breeding to surviving hairy-shaker lambs to immunize them. All surviving lambs from a flock in which BD has occurred should be slaughtered before the next breeding season. Commercial vaccines are not available.

Further reading

Horner, G.W., Hunter, R. and Smart, S.H. (1986). Epidemiological studies on a hairy shaker virus infected flock. *New Zealand Veterinary Journal*, **34**, 194–196.

BOVINE EPHEMERAL FEVER

Synonyms for bovine ephemeral fever (BEF) include three-day sickness, stiff sickness and bovine epizootic fever. BEF is an athropod-borne virus infection of cattle and domestic buffaloes characterized by transient fluctuating fever, shifting muscular pain, lameness and rapid recovery.

Aetiology

BEF virus is a member of a serogroup of an unnamed genus within the Rhabdoviridae family of RNA viruses. It is related to the other members of the serogroup, namely Kimberley, Berrimah and Adelaide River viruses cycling in Australia and FUK-II virus in Japan. A recent report classifies these viruses as serotypes of rabies virus. BEF virus is pH-labile and the pH changes in muscles following death inactivate the virus.

Occurrence

BEF virus infections are widespread in ruminants in the tropics of Africa, Asia and Australia. Clinical disease, however, tends to be limited to cattle and water buffaloes in the subtropics and the temperate areas of South Africa and Japan.

Species affected

Although clinical disease has only been observed in cattle and domesticated buffaloes, serological surveys have revealed a high prevalence of infection in a wide range of wild African ruminants and domestic and feral red deer in Australia. Natural infections of sheep have not been detected, but the experimental infection has been induced.

Transmission

BEF virus is transmitted by several species of *Culicoides* and mosquitoes. In Australia, wind-borne dissemination of infected *Culicoides* over a distance of 2000 km has been suspected.

Clinical features

Most infections are subclinical, many are subacute and a few are acute. Dangerous paralytic episodes do occur, but they are rare. The incubation period following the intravenous injection of infected blood is 4–7 days; the natural incubation period, however, is unknown.

Subacute reactions last for 1–2 days and are characterized by a slight fever, stiffness and/or lameness. Recovery is sudden and complete. The acute reaction includes a high fluctuating fever, loss of appetite, lacrimation, rhinorrhoea and a sharp fall in the milk yield which is never regained in that lactation. Peri-anal oedema may be evident, and there are often cutaneous muscle tremors together with stiffness and lameness. Most animals lie down but are able to rise if stimulated. Recovery is sudden, rapid and complete within 2 days.

Severe cases suffer temporary or permanent paralysis of all the limbs. Sternal recumbency becomes lateral recumbency and bloat is a common sequel. Affected animals salivate but are unable to swallow. Coma and death follow within 1–4 days.

Complications include abortion in pregnant cows and temporary infertility in bulls lasting up to 5 months. The infertility is associated with a high incidence of abnormal mid-pieces in spermatozoa.

Pathology

The pathological changes in BEF are often mild and often inapparent. The common finding is fibrinous exudate in the pleural, pericardial and peritoneal cavities. Lymph nodes are oedematous and the lungs may show patches of oedema. Localized necrosis may occur in skeletal muscles.

Microscopically, there is evidence of hyperplasia of vascular endothelium with perivascular neutral infiltration and perivascular oedema leading to focal necrosis of vessel walls, thrombosis and perivascular fibrosis causing focal infarcts in muscles.

Diagnosis

The diagnosis is usually made on the history and clinical signs. When necessary, confirmation is sought by isolating the virus by inoculating BHK-21 cells with leucocytes from sick cattle. The isolated virus is identified by immunofluorescence. A retrospective serological diagnosis may well be impossible because of cross-infection with other serotypes.

Differential diagnosis

Differential diagnostic problems arise when sporadic cases of BEF occur. A rapid supportive test is examination of Giemsa-stained blood smears which, if BEF is present, will reveal a neutrophilia with band forms.

Treatment

Symptomatic treatment helps to avoid complications. Good nursing is essential and anti-inflammatory drugs are beneficial. Australian workers recommend treatment with calcium borogluconate.

Immunology

Recovery is linked with the production of neutralizing antibodies and one attack of the disease is believed to induce a durable immunity. Infections with the other four serotypes of the virus are subclinical, but they sensitize the host to BEF virus.

Control

Quarantine and movement restrictions have no role in the control of BEF. The range of insect vectors capable of transmitting BEF virus renders insect control on a large scale difficult. Vaccination is considered by many to be the method of choice, but an ideal vaccine has yet to be developed. Inactivated vaccines combined with adjuvants give little or no protection. Some success has been achieved using virus grown in cell cultures and mixed with adjuvants shortly before injection. High titres of neutralizing antibodies have been induced by injecting live virus into animals followed by booster doses of killed vaccines.

Further reading

St. George, T.D. (1988). Bovine ephemeral fever: A review. *Tropical Animal Health and Production*, **20**, 194–202.

BOVINE LYMPHOSARCOMA

Synonyms for bovine lymphosarcoma include bovine leukaemia, bovine leucosis, malignant lymphoma and enzootic bovine leucosis. Enzootic bovine leucosis (EBL) is a multicentric malignant tumour of the lymphoid tissues of adult cattle that often involves other organs.

Aetiology

EBL virus is an oncovirus of the Retroviridae family of single-stranded RNA viruses. It is heat-labile, being destroyed within 16 sec at 74°C and in 30 min at 56°C. Freezing and thawing also destroy the virus.

Three other forms of lymphosarcoma are recognized in cattle; they occur sporadically in young animals and there is no evidence that they are caused by infectious agents.

Occurrence

EBL is prevalent in continental Europe and North and South America. It also occurs in New Zealand, Australia and the UK, but is rare.

Species affected

The natural hosts are cattle and domesticated buffaloes. There is some evidence that sheep are also naturally infected.

Transmission

Both vertical and horizontal transmission occurs. The major mode is excretion of the virus in the colostrum and milk and its ingestion by the sucking calf. Occasionally, foetuses are infected *in utero* and the virus has been transmitted venereally. Horizontal transmission requires the transfer of infected lymphocytes from a donor animal to a susceptible animal by bloodsucking insects or by contaminated instruments or syringes.

Clinical features

Two clinical syndromes are described, namely, a persistent lymphocytosis and a lymphosarcoma. Cattle with persistent lymphocytosis often do not show clinical signs other than poor fertility.

Lymphosarcoma cases have an incubation period of 4–5 years. The onset of disease is insidious and starts as a lymphocytosis. Productivity declines and many animals are culled at this stage. A slow progressive loss of weight ensues. The lymph nodes enlarge and the mucous membranes become pallid. Metastases produce a variety of clinical signs. Death usually occurs within weeks of the clinical signs being evident, but some animals may linger on for several months.

Pathology

Tumours involving lymphoid tissues and other organs are widespread. Microscopic examination reveals an excess of closely packed lymphoid cells in all the lymphoid tissues and in other affected organs.

Diagnosis

The age prevalence, the frank clinical signs and the *post mortem* lesions are suggestive. Confirmation is achieved by histopathological examination of the tumour masses which contain densely packed lymphoid cells.

The detection of apparently healthy carriers is best achieved by serological methods, such as the agar gel immunodiffusion test to demonstrate antibodies. A micro-ELISA test is also available.

Differential diagnosis

The histopathology of the tumour masses seen in sporadic leucosis is identical to that seen in EBL. The history – particularly the age prevalence and the distribution of the tumour masses – aid differentiation.

Immunology

Infected animals remain infected for life, carrying the virus in their B-lymphocytes. Nevertheless, antibodies develop 2–3 weeks after the initiation of infection. These include neutralizing antibodies which, when transferred in the colostrum, protect susceptible calves for several months.

Control

The absence of clinical disease does not rule out the presence of infection. Serological tests must be carried out before it is possible to acknowledge a disease-free status. If the prevalence of infection is low, reactors should be slaughtered and the herd re-tested every 3–4 months. Calves born to serologically positive cows should not be retained. If the prevalence is high, the herd should be split into positive and negative herds. Calves should not receive colostrum or milk from infected cows. Only seronegative bulls should be used and calves should be tested serologically at 6 months of age. The recent discovery that embryo transplants derived from sero-positive bulls and cows can be rendered free of the virus by thorough washing of the pre-implantation embryo, has enabled the salvage of valuable genetic material and the technique may be the method of choice for converting a positive herd into a negative herd.

Further reading

Burny, A., Cleuter, Y., Kettmann, R., Mammerickx, M., Marbaix, G., Portetelle, D., van den Broeke, A., Willems, L. and Thomas, R. (1987). Bovine leukaemia: Facts and hypotheses derived from the study of an infectious cancer. _Cancer Surveys_, **6**, 139–159.

BOVINE ORTHOPOX

Synonyms for bovine orthopox include cow pox/cat pox and vaccinia. Cow pox is a relatively rare, benign vesicular pox affecting the teats of lactating cows. Infection of domestic cats, however, is an increasingly recognized condition, and it is manifested by a primary lesion around the head, followed by secondary lesions elsewhere on the body. Vaccinia infections in cattle mimic cow pox and, in the past, explosive epidemics in cows infected by recently vaccinated stockmen were not uncommon. The use of vaccinia-vector virus vaccines therefore may not be without risk.

Aetiology

Cow pox/cat pox and vaccinia viruses are species of the _Orthopoxvirus_ genus of the Poxviridae family of DNA viruses. They are closely related. Both viruses resist environmental insults and are unaffected by lipid solvents.

Occurrence

Cases of cow pox/cat pox have only been authenticated in Western Europe. In contrast, vaccinia infections of cattle were widespread in the tropics and subtropics in the days when human smallpox vaccination was widely practised.

Species affected

Gerbils and other, as yet unknown, small wild mammals are believed to be the true natural hosts of cow pox/cat pox virus. Man is also susceptible and there have been more recorded cases of cow pox/cat pox in man than in cows. Vaccinia virus is the hybrid that evolved fortuitously in the nineteenth and twentieth centuries in laboratories producing smallpox vaccines.

Transmission

Index cases of cow pox/cat pox arise through direct or indirect contact with the wild mammal reservoir host. Transfer within a dairy herd is associated with milking procedures. Cat-to-cat transfer is relatively rare. Cat pox in Europe appears to have a seasonal distribution, most cases occurring in the autumn.

Transmission of vaccinia virus from intradermal sites of vaccinia-vector virus vaccinations seems possible. Experiments in the 1920s and 1930s detected systemic multiplication of vaccinia virus in cattle after inoculation of the skin.

Clinical features

Cow pox. Cow pock lesions are benign. They occur on the teats of the udder 5 days after exposure. The initial signs are an irregular prodromal fever and tenderness of the affected teats. Over a period of 4 days, macules become papules that develop into central vesicles which rapidly pustulate. The lesion ruptures and the exudate forms a thick red tenacious scab 1–2 cm in diameter. Healing takes place over 3 weeks, starting from the edges of the lesions. The site is scarred.

Cat pox. In cats a prodromal inappetance precedes the development of a single primary pock on the head, neck or a forelimb. Multiple widespread secondary skin lesions appear 4–16 days later. The character of the single primary lesions ranges from small ulcerated plaques or granuloma to extensive cellulitis. Secondary lesions start as small firm nodules 2–3 mm in diameter, which increase in size over 2–3 days to form discrete scabby pocks 0.5–2.0 cm in diameter. Fresh pocks continue to appear for up to 10 days. There are few systemic signs, and the scabs drop off 2–4 weeks later leaving healed scarred and hairless skin. Complete resolution with new hair growth soon follows.

Vaccinia. The evolution and character of vaccinia infections on the teats and udders of lactating cows is identical to that of cow pox.

Pathology

The gross pathological features of cow pox and vaccinia are restricted to the clinical sites. In cat pox, however, there is in addition marked oedema of the neck, thorax and abdomen.

The histopathology of the skin lesions is typical of pox infections and early lesions contain eosinophilic intracytoplasmic inclusions.

Diagnosis

In cow pox and vaccinia infections, the history and clinical signs are suggestive. Cat pox has only recently been identified, but it is being increasingly recognized from the clinical signs and evolution of the disease. A presumptive diagnosis is readily confirmed by electron microscopy of scabs and biopsies supplemented by histopathology.

Differential diagnosis

Differentiation of cow pox and vaccinia infections in cattle from pseudocowpox is difficult and may necessitate isolation of the causative virus and its identification in the laboratory. Similarly, laboratory techniques may be required to differentiate cat pox from other forms of feline cellulitis.

Treatment

The application of antiviral ointments is alleged to be efficacious, but the use of corticosteroids is contraindicated.

Immunology

Recovery is said to produce an immunity to reinfection and this resistance is associated with low titres of neutralizing antibodies.

Control

Specific control measures have yet to be formulated.

Further reading

Baxby, D. (1977). Is cow pox misnamed? A review of ten human cases. *British Medical Journal*, 1, 1379–1381.

Bennett, M., Gaskell, C.J., Gaskell, R.M., Baxby, D. and Gruffydd-Jones, T.J. (1986). Pox virus infection in the domestic cat: Subclinical and epidemiological observations. *Veterinary Record*, 118, 387–390.

Lum, G.S., Soriano, F., Trejos, A. and Llerena, J. (1967). Vaccinia epidemic and epizootic in El Salvador. *American Journal of Tropical Medicine and Hygiene*, 16, 332–338.

BOVINE PARAPOX

Synonyms for bovine parapox include pseudocowpox, bovine papular stomatitis (BPS), paravaccinia, milkers' nodules, proliferative stomatitis, erosive stomatitis, pseudoaphthous stomatitis, rat-tail syndrome.

Pseudocowpox and BPS are two benign clinical syndromes of a widely distributed parapox infection of cattle. Pseudocowpox is manifested by the development of eroded plaques on the teats and udders of lactating cows, whereas BPS is acquired by calves sucking cows with active pseudocowpox and it is manifested by the appearance of circular plaques in the peri-nasal and peri-oral regions and by a papular stomatitis. Man is susceptible and the disease in man is known as milkers' nodules.

Aetiology

The parapox virus of pseudocowpox and BPS is a member of the *Parapoxvirus* genus of the Poxviridae family of double-stranded DNA viruses. It resembles and is related to orf virus. It is heat-stable but it is inactivated by lipid solvents.

Occurrence

Pseudocowpox is the most common skin lesion of the teats and udders of cattle worldwide. BPS is equally common, but it is not so frequently recognized.

Species affected

Cattle are the natural hosts; however, on occasion, man is infected accidentally when handling affected calves or milking affected cows. The infection in man is usually dead-end.

Transmission

Calves are infected when they suck the teats of affected cows. They in turn infect in-contact susceptible calves by licking. Thereafter, the virus undergoes latency and recrudescence occurs whenever there is stress. It is suspected but not proven that the index case in a dairy herd is a recrudescence of a latent infection in a cow originally infected as a calf. Thereafter, the virus is spread to the teats of other lactating cows on the hands of the milkers or in the cups of the milking machine.

Clinical features

Pseudocowpox. Primary cases of pseudocowpox have an incubation period of about 6 days and a course of 6–8 weeks. In contrast, recrudescent pseudocowpox has a short course of 7–10 days. The disease is only seen in lactating cows and an essential precursor to both primary pseudocowpox and recrudescent pseudocowpox is trauma with breaks in the skin of the teats. Pocks first emerge as small macular erythemas which become oedematous, exude and form a glistening film over the lesion. The teats at this stage are painful. Within 48 hours the lesion has become papular in character, often light orange in colour at first but darkening as the papule becomes dry and scabby. The lesion enlarges centrifugally to reach a diameter of 1–2 cm and appears umbilicated. The central scab peels off leaving a characteristic horseshoe-shaped ring of minute scabs. The lesion heals from the centre slowly over several weeks. The evolution of the pocks of recrudescent pseudocowpox is similar, but the time span is much shorter.

A chronic form of pseudocowpox has been recognized in which a mild erythema of the teat is followed by profuse scabbing. The scabs are scurfy, yellowish grey in colour and are often rubbed off at milking. The teat surface becomes corrugated and tends to develop chaps and sores.

Bovine papular stomatitis. The incubation period is 3–7 days. Primary lesions develop on the margins of the nostrils, inner surfaces of the lips and on the edges of the tooth sockets. At first they are hyperaemic spots, a few millimetres in diameter. Within hours the primaries on the nostrils and lips become low round papules, the centres of which are white or grey. The papules increase in size daily until they are 1-2 cm in diameter with centres that are grey, roughened and necrotic. The rims are hyperaemic. The primaries on the edges of the tooth sockets stimulate the aformation of intensely hyperaemic granulation tissue, flecked with yellow necrotic debris that heaps up around the teeth.

The primary lesions persist for 3-4 weeks and then regress quickly. There is no scar formation, but often pallid, sometimes hyperaemic, spots persist for several weeks to mark the lesion sites. Secondary lesions develop 1-3 weeks after the onset of the primaries. They occur within the nostril, on the muzzle and in the mouth. On the ridges of the hard palate they tend to be elongated along the ridge rather than circular. The lesions expand centrifugally, forming concentric rings of different colours, yellow, grey and red. The ring lesions are particularly prominent on the muzzle and their presence aids differential diagnosis.

As old lesions regress further, new lesions may evolve. Consequently, the courses of the disease may be protracted for months. There is no systemic disturbance and the disease is not fatal.

Lesions in recrudescent papular stomatitis have a similar but accelerated evolution. In addition, stressed adult animals may develop a large ring lesion on the tongue known colloquially as a "fairy ring".

"Rat-tail syndrome". A necrotic dermatitis of the tail of feedlot cattle has been found to be associated with parapox virus. The switch of the tail is lost leaving a raw denuded area. Infected animals are chronically unthrifty and are usually culled.

Pathology

In pseudocowpox, lesions are seen rarely at sites other than the skin of the udder and teats. Lesions of BPS are in the peri-nasal and peri-labial regions and the oral cavity, and have been observed on the mucosae of the oesophagus and the fore stomachs. The histopathology of the lesions of pseudocowpox and BPS are the same, being characterized by hyperplasia of the dermopapillae, ballooning degeneration of epithelial cells and eosinophilic inclusions in the cytoplasm of degenerating epithelial cells.

Diagnosis

The appearance of the characteristic lesions is suggestive but differentiation from other conditions requires confirmatory tests. The specimens required are scabs and scrapings of the lesions and they should be submitted in dry containers. In addition, biopsies should be sent for histopathological examination in formol-saline. The easiest and quickest confirmatory test is the electron microscopical examination of negatively stained specimens of scab and scrapings.

Differential diagnosis

In the past, cow pox and vaccinia infections were often confused with pseudocowpox. The former still occurs in temperate areas but not in the tropics. Currently, vaccinia virus infections are not a problem. The lesions of herpes mammillitis tend to be more severe than those of pseudocowpox.

BPS and rinderpest have been confused and, on occasion, rinderpest has exacerbated latent BPS so that the lesions of both occur simultaneously. BPS has also been misdiagnosed as foot-and-mouth disease.

Treatment

The causative agent is a DNA virus and claims have been made regarding the effectiveness of frequent applications of ointments containing idoxuridine or acyclovir. These claims have yet to be substantiated.

Immunology

Recovered animals become latently infected and the latent infections may be activated by stress despite the presence of humoral antibodies.

Control

BPS is usually detected fortuitously too late for the application of effective control measures. In contrast, the public health implications of pseudocowpox infections warrant segregation of infected animals, the use of individual paper towels for washing udders and back-flushing of milking clusters to reduce cross-infection. Newly purchased cattle should be quarantined for at least 14 days and their teats inspected carefully for evidence of infection.

Further reading

Snider, T.G., McConnell, S. and Pierce, K.R. (1982). Increased incidence of bovine papular stomatitis in neonatal calves. *Archives of Virology*, **71**, 251–258.

BOVINE VIRUS DIARRHOEA/MUCOSAL DISEASE

Bovine virus diarrhoea (BVD) is an ubiquitous viral pathogen of cattle with a worldwide distribution. Post-natal infections are usually inapparent but, on occasion, are subacute, being manifested by transient febrile diarrhoea. In contrast, if an embryo survives early pre-natal infection, a live antibody-negative calf is born with a lifelong persistent viral infection. A late pre-natal infection produces either congenital abnormalities or a live calf that is virus-free but has antibodies.

Mucosal disease (MD) is a sporadic fulminating and fatal syndrome in cattle persistently infected with BVD virus that mimics cattle plague.

Aetiology

BVD virus is a member of the *Pestivirus* genus of the Flaviviridae family of RNA viruses. It is a non-arthropod-borne flavivirus and shares antigens with the other members of the genus, namely, Border disease and hog cholera viruses. BVD virus isolates vary in their ability to induce cytopathic effects in cell cultures. Most isolates from persistent viral infections are non-cytopathic, whereas those from fulminating fatal mucosal disease cases tend to be cytopathogenic. The virus is readily killed by environmental factors.

Occurrence

BVD infections in cattle have been recorded from all continents except Antarctica. The virus is an alarmingly frequent contaminant of cell cultures grown in maintenance medium supplemented with bovine foetal serum or calf serum.

Species affected

BVD virus and antibodies have been isolated from various species of the even-toed ungulates. The dominant natural hosts, nevertheless, are cattle.

Transmission

Pre-natal infections follow transplacental transmission of the virus from the cow to the foetus. Post-natal infections are acquired through aerosol contact with infected secretions and excretions shed by persistently viraemic animals. The virus is present in seminal fluids and venereal transmission may occur. There is a clear risk of iatrogenic transmission through multiple use of hypodermic needles and the inoculation of live virus vaccines inadvertently contaminated with the virus.

Clinical features

Non-pregnant cattle. Most post-natal infections of non-pregnant cattle are acute but silent. Often, the only signs after an incubation period of 3–5 days is a low-grade fever and loss of appetite. A few animals, in addition, may show oral erosions and transient diarrhoea. Recovery is associated with the development of neutralizing antibodies. Because BVD virus is immunosuppressive, a few animals develop complications induced by opportunist pathogens.

Pregnant cattle. The clinical response of pregnant cattle to infection with BVD virus is similar to that in non-pregnant cattle but, in addition, there is transplacental transfer of the virus to the foetus. The sequel depends upon the gestational age of the foetus when infected. If the gestational age is less than 100 days, the foetus is unable to mount an immune response and no antibody is produced and the calf is born with a persistent BVD viral infection.

If the gestational age of the foetus lies between 100 and 150 days, then an immune response is mounted producing immunologically mediated lesions associated with congenital abnormalities. Transplacental infection of the foetus at late pregnancy results in a typical acute viral infection which clears with the emergence of antibodies. Such calves are born free of virus and are antibody-positive before they have taken colostrum.

Foetal deaths may occur at any stage of pregnancy. Foetuses aborted in early pregnancy are either mummified or autolysed and the virus cannot be recovered from them. In contrast, abortions in late pregnancy yield fresh foetuses from which the virus can be isolated.

Persistently infected cattle. Fifty per cent of calves born persistently infected die within the first 2 years of life. Most die from mucosal disease, which develops either through super-infection with a cytopathic strain of BVD virus or by a mutation of the virus population within the animal itself. Mucosal disease mimics cattle plague, being characterized by fever, erosive stomatitis and watery diarrhoea. Some are lame and are reluctant to move. Death usually supervenes in 1–3 weeks, but sometimes chronic cases linger for several weeks.

Some persistently infected animals appear normal and breed successfully. A persistently infected cow, however, usually gives birth to a persistently infected calf.

Clinical pathology

Post-natally acquired clinically inapparent or subacute cases develop a profound leucopenia in the early stages. The leucocyte counts return to normal within 14 days. A severe leucopenia and a thrombocytopenia are also present in mucosal disease syndromes.

Pathology

Post-natal infections in virus-free animals rarely kill. Persistently infected animals developing the mucosal disease syndrome, however, die and the *post mortem* findings mimic those in cattle plague. The carcase is dehydrated, soiled and fetid. Erosions and ulcers occur throughout the alimentary tract which is congested and haemorrhagic. Zebra stripes in the colon are common. Erosions and ulcers also occur in the interdigital clefts of some animals. Chronic cases usually exhibit encrusted skin lesions.

The dramatic microscopic lesion is necrosis of the germinal centres of the lymph nodes and spleen.

Diagnosis

The retrospective presence of BVD virus infection acquired post-natally is usually suspected when animals give birth to congenitally abnormal calves or have unexplained abortions. Confirmation is most readily sought by examining paired serum samples. Antibody-negative animals should be retested for the presence of virus in heparinized blood samples. Slices of thyroid, spleen and salivary gland from fresh aborted foetuses are examined for antigen by immunofluorescence. Similar samples are used to confirm a diagnosis of mucosal disease.

Differential diagnosis

Differentiation between cattle plague and mucosal disease is essential, particularly in countries at risk from cattle plague or where cattle plague is prevalent. Therefore, investigators must be equipped to confirm the presence of either disease. The simplest technique which may be carried out in the field is to diffuse the suspect tissue samples against both hyperimmune anti-cattle plague serum and anti-hog cholera serum either through agar gel or in counterimmune electrophoresis preparations.

Immunology

Early pre-natal infections persist without inducing the production of antibodies. However, virus is cleared from animals that are infected late in the gestational period or after birth and recovery from infection is associated with the production of protective antibodies.

Control

Post-natally acquired BVD virus infections are trivial. Control measures, therefore, are directed to limiting the risk of transplacental infection. Persistently infected animals should be identified and removed and isolated from the breeding herd. Only virus-negative antibody-positive animals should be retained in the herd. Live and killed vaccines have been developed. The former have several disadvantages, such as the risk of transplacental infection. They are also immunosuppressive and epidemics of the mucosal disease syndrome have been recorded after the use of live virus vaccine. Killed vaccines, on the other hand, are safe but booster doses are necessary to achieve a good level of protected immunity.

Further reading

Duffell, S.J. and Harkness, A.W. (1985). Bovine virus diarrhoea-mucosal disease infection in cattle. *Veterinary Record*, 117, 240–245.

BUFFALO POX

Buffalo pox is a benign infection of domestic buffaloes characterized by the development of pocks on the teats, udder and perineum of lactating cows and on and around the lips and muzzles of sucking calves. Man is susceptible.

Aetiology

Buffalo pox virus is a member of the *Orthopoxvirus* genus of the Poxviridae family of DNA viruses and is related to the viruses of cow pox and vaccinia.

Occurrence

Buffalo pox has been reported in populations of domesticated buffaloes in Asia, Italy and Egypt.

Species affected

Natural infections appear to be restricted to domesticated buffaloes and their human attendants.

Transmission

Spread between lactating buffalo cows is attributed to milkers, and calves become infected through sucking affected buffalo cows. Other modes of direct and indirect contact probably occur.

Clinical features

There is no systematic disturbance. The pocks evolve through the classical stages of macule, papule, vesicle, pustule and scab formation, the course of the disease lasting 3-6 weeks. The common sites of the lesions in lactating buffalo cows are the teats, udder, perineum and inner thighs. In some epidemics, generalized skin infections have been reported with typical pock lesions at various stages of development present all over the body. The common sequelae in lactating cows are thickening of teats, stenosis of the milk ducts and mastitis.

Sucking calves acquire lesions in the oral mucosa and in the peri-labial, peri-nasal and peri-orbital areas of the head.

Latency occurs and may be exacerbated by stress and/or other infections such as cattle plague.

Pathology

Eosinophilic intracytoplasmic inclusions occur in epidermal cells early in the course of the disease.

Diagnosis and differential diagnosis

A presumptive diagnosis of a pock infection is based upon the clinical signs and can be most readily confirmed by electron microscopy of scab or biopsy samples. Vaccinia virus infections of buffaloes, however, are clinically and pathologically identical to buffalo pox and laboratory isolation of the virus is essential to differentiate them. The preferred samples are scabs and/or biopsies.

Immunology

Recovery from buffalo pox is associated with cellular and humoral immune responses being activated. Recovered animals resist reinfection with buffalo pox virus or cow pox virus.

Control

Although buffalo pox is an economically important disease, programmes to control it have yet to be formulated. Infected lactating animals should be segregated from other animals and should have separate attendants. The milk is not fit for human consumption. Symptomatic treatment measures should be applied with a view to preventing mastitis.

Further reading

Pandey, R., Kaushik, A.K. and Grover, Y.P. (1985). Biology of orthopox virus infections of domestic ruminants. *Progress in Veterinary Microbiology and Immunology*, **1**, 199–228.

CAMEL POX

Camel pox is a malignant pox of camels characterized by fever, generalized skin lesions and a low but significant mortality rate.

Aetiology

Camel pox virus is a member of the *Orthopoxvirus* genus of the Poxviridae family of DNA viruses. It is related antigenically to the viruses of variola and vaccinia. Like other orthopoxviruses, it is heat-stable at ambient temperatures.

Occurrence

Camel pox infections are widespread throughout Africa and Asia.

Species affected

Natural infections occur in both dromedary and bactrian camels and in humans.

Transmission

Camel pox virus spreads through camel herds by direct and indirect contact. Humans acquire infection by handling affected camels and perhaps by drinking milk from affected camels.

Clinical features

The natural incubation period is alleged to range from 10 to 15 days. Experimental inoculation, however, induces disease after an incubation of about 5 days. Malignant infections are most common in camel foals up to 3 years of age, whereas benign infections are more commonly seen in adults.

Illness is initiated by fever, which is followed by a rash 1–3 days later. The lesions thereafter progress through vesicular, pustular and scabbing stages. In fatal cases, the head is most affected with lesions concentrated around the mouth and eyes, often blinding the animals. In addition, there is widespread facial oedema. The case mortality rate is usually about 5% but may approach 30%. Deaths occur 3–15 days after the first emergence of the lesions. The sites of the lesions in survivors are scarred.

Pathology

Deaths appear to be associated with super-infections of generalized pocks by pyogenic bacteria. The carcase is emaciated, soiled and fetid and abscesses are found in many locations. Reports of detailed post-mortem examinations, however, are conspicuous by their absence.

Diagnosis and differential diagnosis

Diagnosis is usually based on the clinical signs. Clinical differentiation of benign camel pox from pustular dermatitis, a disease caused by a virus similar to that of orf, is impossible. The viruses, however, are readily distinguishable by electron microscopy. Camel pox virus will also grow on chorio-allontoic membranes of embryonated hen eggs, whereas the virus of pustular dermatitis does not. Histopathology of biopsies of lesions is a useful supplementary diagnostic aid. Camel pox is also readily confused with mange.

Immunology

Recovered animals develop antibodies and resist reinfection. Foals sucking immune dams are protected passively through ingestion of colostrum.

Control

Camel owners protect their foals by rubbing a suspension of crusts in milk into the pricked skin of the lips. Other control measures are palliative.

Further reading

Kriz, B. (1982). A study of camel pox in Somalia. *Journal of Comparative Pathology*, **92**, 1–8.

CAPRINE ARTHRITIS-ENCEPHALOMYELITIS

Synonyms for caprine arthritis-encephalomyelitis (CAE) include caprine arthritis-encephalitis, caprine encephalomyelomalacia and viral leucoencephalomyelitis of goats. CAE is a complex disease of goats characterized by progressive accumulations of mononuclear cells in many organs. The arthritic syndrome occurs in adult goats and the encephalomyelitic syndrome usually occurs in kids under 4 months of age.

Aetiology

The causal virus is a lentivirus of the Retroviridae family of RNA viruses. It is closely related to the lentivirus causing maedi-visna in sheep and goats. It resists irradiation but it is heat-labile and inactivated by lipid solvents.

Occurrence

CAE virus is distributed worldwide, but the prevalence of clinical disease is greatest in developed countries.

Species affected

Naturally acquired infections are restricted to goats. All breeds and ages are susceptible and infected goats are infected for life. Sheep infected experimentally develop lesions and young lambs fed on infected goats' milk will sero-convert. Natural cross-species transmission has not been observed.

Transmission

Newborn kids acquire the infection by drinking infective colostrum and milk. There is no transplacental transfer of the virus. Susceptible milking goats milked alongside an infected milking goat may become infected from aerosols generated by splashing milk.

Clinical features

Although the prevalence of infection is high, morbidity is low. The signs of disease depend on the site and the extent of the lesions. Arthritis occurs in sexually mature goats and commonly affects the carpal joints and less often the hocks and stifles. Affected animals are not necessarily lame despite having grossly enlarged joints. There is no fever and the appetite is maintained. Nevertheless, there is a gradual loss of condition identified by a poor hair coat.

The encephalomyelitic syndrome affects 2-to 4-month-old kids and the resulting neuronal derangement depends upon the site of the lesions which may be focal or diffuse. Common signs include blindness, head tremors, torticollis, opisthotonos, ataxia and paresis leading to recumbency and death.

Other significant syndromes include an indurated mastitis and a progressive pneumonia. The indurated mastitis affects the milk yield and may be diffuse or nodular. The progressive pneumonia is an interstitial pneumonitis similar to maedi in sheep and leads to a progressive weight loss over many months.

Pathology

The prominent pathological change in cases of arthritis is the development of hygromas. Microscopic examination of fluid withdrawn from affected joints reveals numerous mononuclear cells.

Gross lesions in the central nervous system, if they occur, are light brown or pink spots in the white matter. The microscopic changes are characterized by a disseminated perivenous accumulation of mononuclear cells together with a variable destruction of myelin. Mononuclear cells are also found free in the cerebrospinal fluid.

Diagnosis

The progressive nature of the clinical signs is diagnostically suggestive. The microscopic examination of synovial fluid aspirated from hygromas will reveal the presence of mononuclear cells. Similarly, examination of cerebrospinal fluid will reveal the presence of mononuclear cells. Histopathological studies will confirm the clinical pathological results.

Subclinically infected goats are identified by examining their sera for the presence of agar gel immunodiffusion antibodies or ELISA antibodies.

Differential diagnosis

Hygromas in mature goats are unlikely to be misdiagnosed. Neuropathies in kids, however, are difficult to differentiate and their aetiologies can only be identified in the laboratory. Problems also arise in cases with mastitis and progressive pneumonia, the latter being understandably confused with maedi which, on occasion, infects goats.

Immunology

CAE virus-infected goats are persistently infected despite the presence of antibodies. Sero-conversion, however, is slow to develop. Nevertheless, most kids infected in the neonatal period will be sero-positive by the time they are 1 year old. The antibodies are not protective.

Control

Vaccines are not available and are unlikely to be available in the foreseeable future. CAE virus infections, therefore, are controlled by limiting its transmission. Kids should be removed and separated from their does at birth and fed colostrum heated to 56°C for 1 hour. Thereafter, the kids should be fed pasteurized cows' milk.

If the number of antibody-positive goats is low the herd should be split into clean and sero-positive groups which should be managed separately. Thereafter, the clean herd should be tested serologically and any positives moved to the infected herd.

Stock purchases should only be made from herds which are tested regularly and have remained free of sero-positives. The high prevalence of sero-positives in developed countries has severely affected the export of goats to developing countries.

Further reading

Dawson, M. (1988). Lentivirus diseases of domesticated animals. *Journal of Comparative Pathology*, **99**, 401–419.

CATTLE PLAGUE

Synonyms for cattle plague include steppe murrain and rinderpest. Cattle plague is a contagion of wild and domesticated ruminants and pigs characterized by a short sharp fever, erosive stomatitis, gastroenteritis, fetid odour, dehydration and death. It is an ancient plague and regularly devastated the cattle and buffalo populations of Asia and Europe and occasionally wrought havoc in North Africa.

Aetiology

The causative virus is a member of the *Morbillivirus* genus of the Paramyxoviridae family of RNA viruses. The other members of the genus are the viruses of canine distemper, human measles and goat plague. Heterologous immunization between them is possible but not absolute. Serological tests will differentiate between the morbilliviruses because homologous neutralizing antibody titres are significantly higher than heterologous titres.

Cattle plague virus is heat-, light-and ultrasonic-sensitive. Infectivity is also readily destroyed by many chemicals including lipid solvents. Virus-infected carcases are rendered non-infectious by the pH changes that follow autolysis and inactivation is hastened by putrefaction. Air-borne cattle plague virus survives best at low and high relative humidities.

Occurrence

Cattle plague is endemic in most countries in northern equatorial Africa, in many countries of the Middle East and in parts of Pakistan and India.

Species affected

Although all cloven-hoofed animals are probably susceptible to cattle plague, overt disease most commonly occurs in cattle, domesticated buffaloes and Asiatic pigs. Clinical disease in goats and sheep is common in India but is seldom observed elsewhere. The list of proven cattle plague virus infections of wildlife grows annually. It includes the hippopotamus at one end of the spectrum and the giraffe at the other.

There are wide variations in innate resistance between and within species. A high innate resistance is often attributable to long, ancestral association with the disease; an anomaly, however, is the innate resistance of European breeds of pigs which when infected never react clinically. In contrast, the Asiatic pig frequently shows clinical disease and may die.

Transmission

Transmission requires close contact between sick and healthy animals. The virus is shed in the expired air, nasal and oral secretions and in the faeces. Infected droplets are inhaled and the virus penetrates through the mucosa of the upper respiratory tract. Pigs can also acquire the infection by eating infected offal, but the significance of this mode of spread is unknown.

Clinical features

The incubation period ranges from 1 to 15 days, being shortest in hypersusceptible animals and longest in animals with a high innate resistance. Clinical reactions may be peracute, acute, subacute or inapparent.

The onset of peracute reactions is sudden and the affected animals have a high fever, congested mucous membranes and respiratory distress. Death occurs 1–3 days later from cardiogenic shock.

Classical acute reactions occur in virgin epidemics involving animals with a low innate resistance. The clinical syndrome is divisible into four distinct phases. First, a prodromal fever which has a sudden onset which is often missed because other clinical signs are minimal except in lactating cows whose milk yield falls. Within 24–48 hours, overt illness is clearly evident; the animal is restless, stands depressed, apart and alone. Respirations are shallow and rapid and serous secretions are increased. The appetite is impaired, rumination is retarded and constipation is evident. Visible mucous membranes are congested but are still intact.

An erosive mucosa phase begins 2–5 days after the onset of the prodromal fever and is the first suggestive sign of cattle plague. Raised pin-heads of necrotic epithelium emerge from the surfaces of the mucous membranes lining the mouth, the nasal passages and the urogenital tract. The lesions abrade easily, exposing a shallow erosion with a red layer of basal cells. Salivation is stimulated and becomes profuse. The erosions enlarge and coalesce and the breath becomes fetid. Thick yellow patches of necrotic cells begin to coat the nasal passages and mix with nasal secretions producing a fetid mucopurulent discharge. A similar mucopurulent ocular discharge is now evident. Thirst is intense, but the appetite is lost. Soft faeces are voided frequently.

A spurting diarrhoeic phase starts as the fever regresses. The soft faeces become fluid, dark brown in colour and contain mucous and epithelial shreds. The smell is offensive. Affected animals arch their backs and strain, frequently exposing congested and eroded rectal mucosae. Respirations are now laboured and painful, being characterized by an audible grunt when exhaling.

In fatal cases, the diarrhoea worsens progressively, causing rapid dehydration. Affected animals waste visibly and stand with lowered heads, sunken eyes and arched backs. Sternal recumbency follows, and death supervenes 6–12 days after the onset of the prodromal fever.

In surviving animals, the onset of convalescence is insidious. The erosions heal and the diarrhoea stops, but recovery to full health takes many weeks. Pregnant animals usually abort in the convalescent period.

Subacute rinderpest occurs in young animals with a high innate resistance in areas where the disease is endemic. The evolution and course are similar to that of the classic syndrome but muted. One or more of the cardinal features of the classic syndrome are often absent. Most affected animals recover and convalescence is short.

A frequent sequel of subacute cattle plague infections is activation of latent pathogens, particularly protozoa. The onset of the activated infection is sudden, occurring 4–6 days after the onset of the prodromal fever. The signs of the activated infection often predominate.

Clinical pathology

A transient leucocytosis in the late incubation period is followed by a profound leucopenia that starts before the onset of fever, persists until death or for at least 5 weeks if the animal survives. The leucopenia is predominantly caused by a precipitous fall in both B-and T-lymphocyte populations. Erythrocytes fluctuate within normal ranges in surviving animals, but in fatal cases after the onset of diarrhoea, there is a 40–60% increase in the packed cell volume due to loss of body fluid which approaches 40%. The blood at death therefore is dark, thick and slow to clot. Serum separation is poor.

Total serum proteins decline, serum glutamic oxalacetic transaminase (SGOT) and serum urea nitrogen rise, but serum creatinine remains unchanged. Serum chloride levels fall terminally, but other electrolytes remain constant reflecting a net loss because of the haemoconcentration.

Pathology

While the gross pathology of cattle plague is suggestive, it is not pathognomic, being indistinguishable from that of the fatal mucosal disease syndrome of bovine viral diarrhoea and from goat plague infections. The virus has a primary predilection for lymphoid tissues and a secondary preference for the epithelium of the alimentary, upper respiratory and urogenital tracts.

The carcase is dehydrated, emaciated, soiled and fetid. The extensive desquamation of all oral surfaces extends into the pharynx and upper oesophagus but lesions in the fore-stomachs are rare. The folds of the abomasum are congested and oedematous with lines of erosions on their margins. The pyloric portion of the abomasum shows haemorrhagic ulceration. Although the congestion and oedema in the small intestine are less intense, the Peyer's patches are swollen and prominent, black in colour due to haemorrhage and friable from necrosis. The mucosal surface of the caecum is ulcerated with haemorrhages and spectacular striping, red in fresh carcases and greenish-black in old carcases, caused by distended capillaries, the so-called "zebra stripes". The caecal tonsil at the caecal-colonic junction invariably exhibits changes manifested as oedema, congestion, necrotic ulceration and haemorrhage. Zebra stripes extend throughout the colon as far as the rectum. In addition, the colonic mucosal surface is ulcerated and epithelial shreds and haemorrhages are evident.

The turbinates and nasal septa are coated with thick tenacious mucopurulent discharge. The mucosal surface itself is eroded and hemorrhagic. The upper trachea is congested with longitudinal haemorrhagic streaks. The lungs in early deaths are normal. In late deaths, there is conspicuous interlobular and alveolar emphysema.

In the kidneys, congestion is conspicuous at the corticomedullary junction. The urinary bladder is usually congested and its mucosal surface is often eroded.

The heart is usually normal, but in animals that die early in the course of the disease subendocardial ecchymoses in the left ventricle are common. Subepicardial petechiae may also occur on the base and along the coronary grooves.

In early deaths, the lymph nodes are swollen and oedematous, but in late deaths they are shrunken and grey with radial streaks in the cortex. The spleen is usually normal but occasionally there are subserosal haemorrhages along the margins. The gut-associated lymphoid tissues all show necrosis, ulceration and haemorrhage.

The dramatic histopathological changes are those found in the lymphoid organs and mucosal epithelium. They include the early formation of multinucleated giant cells containing intracytoplasmic and intranuclear inclusions and, later, necrosis of lymphocytes and epithelial cells.

Diagnosis

A presumptive diagnosis of cattle plague is based upon an assessment of the history, particularly a history of recent animal movement, the clinical signs and *post mortem* lesions. Confirmation is *not* essential in countries where the disease is prevalent or where the livestock are at risk. Outbreaks of disease in cattle and/or buffaloes characterized by FSE (fever-stomatitis-enteritis) must be regarded as cattle plague and immediate action taken to contain the outbreaks. In contrast, FSEs in previously disease-free countries should be confirmed or refuted as quickly as possible.

Confirmation of a provisional diagnosis is based (1) on the demonstration of the presence of specific antigens in the tissues, excretions and secretions of suspect cases, (2) on the isolation and identification of infectious virus from the tissues, excretions and secretions, and (3) on the detection of a rise in specific antibodies in the sera of suspect cases. The key to diagnostic success is the collection of suitable samples from several sick animals rather than many samples from one animal. Most cattle plague deaths are precipitated by fluid loss and electrolyte imbalance and, therefore, occur late in the syndrome after the diarrhoea has occurred. At this stage, viral antigens and infectious virus have fallen to low or undetectable levels. Thus dead animals should *not* be sampled. The clinical markers for selecting suitable donors for laboratory samples are:

1. High fever and/or early small erosions.
2. No mucopurulent ocular and nasal discharges.
3. No diarrhoea.
4. No soiled hindquarters.

The preferred samples from live animals are blood in EDTA anticoagulant, blood for serum, tears, gum scrapings, and lymph node biopsies. Useful additional samples from slaughtered animals are lymph nodes, spleen and tonsils. Aliquots of the samples of gum scrapings and tears should be tested on site by counterimmunoelectrophoresis and/or agar gel immunodiffusion. The remaining samples should be taken to the diagnostic laboratory on wet ice by courier.

Histopathology yields good supportive evidence if giant cells and inclusions are detected. Failure to demonstrate these changes does not, however, invalidate the provisional diagnosis of cattle plague. The preferred samples for histopathology are small pieces of affected mucosa and slices of lymph nodes. They should be forwarded to the laboratory in 10% formol-saline.

Differential diagnosis

Many febrile diseases have clinical manifestations suggestive of cattle plague. In cattle and buffaloes, the mucosal syndrome of bovine virus diarrhoea virus infection is clinically and pathologically indistinguishable. In addition, malignant catarrhal fever, infectious bovine rhinotracheitis, foot-and-mouth disease and Jembrana disease have all been confused with rinderpest. In sheep and goats, the greatest diagnostic confusion arises with goat plague. Clinical and pathological differentiation from bluetongue, Nairobi sheep disease and even sheep pox is often difficult.

Immunology

An attack of cattle plague confers a lifelong immunity in recovered animals. IgM-class antibodies emerge 5–7 days after the onset of illness and decline within a few weeks, being replaced by IgG-class antibodies. Peak antibody titres are attained about 4 weeks after the onset of illness and they persist for about 4 weeks. Thereafter, antibody titres fall to a persistent threshold level; on rare occasions, they fall below detectable levels. Re-exposure produces an anamnestic rise in antibody levels.

Control

National control strategies for cattle plague are pointless unless backed with legislative powers. Low-risk countries insure their freedom from cattle plague by prohibiting imports of domestic ruminants and pigs from areas where the disease is endemic. Today, if an outbreak occurs in a low-risk country, it is likely to be misdiagnosed at first by being mistaken for mucosal disease. Confirmed outbreaks in low-risk countries are eradicated by slaughtering the affected herds and placing the neighbouring herds under quarantine. Animals in the quarantine herds are clinically examined daily for 3 weeks.

High-risk countries are those linked geographically or commercially to countries where the disease is endemic. If there is a geographical boundary, high-risk countries protect their livestock by creating an immune barrier zone at least 20 km deep along the border. All even-toed ungulates within the barrier zone are vaccinated annually against cattle plague. The entry of live animal imports is restricted to specified ports of entry, where the animals are examined clinically and segregated if sick or vaccinated against cattle plague if healthy; a history of previous vaccination is ignored. High-risk countries should hold emergency stocks of potent cattle plague virus vaccine to enable outbreaks within the high-risk country to be sealed off by ring vaccination.

The control strategy in countries where the disease is prevalent is to lower the incidence. The initial step is to vaccinate all animals of all ages in the national herd. All vaccinated animals other than calves are permanently identified by ear-marks or fire-brands. Vaccination is repeated annually until serological surveys indicate that the immune status of the national herd exceeds 90%. Thereafter, calves are vaccinated annually and revaccinated the following year. Vaccination teams should now be supplemented by mobile surveillance and mobile containment teams. If over the next 5 years there have been no outbreaks of rinderpest, then serious consideration should be given to stopping vaccination and stepping up the activities of the surveillance teams.

Disease outbreaks in countries where the disease is endemic are contained by segregation of the affected animals and ring vaccination of the surrounding herds irrespective of whether or not they have been vaccinated before.

All of the vaccines in use today are lyophilized live attenuated virus vaccines. The most popular is still Edward's goat-adapted virus vaccine, but in Africa and the Middle East it has been supplanted by Plowright's tissue culture vaccine. Tissue culture derivatives of Nakamuru's lapinized cattle plague virus vaccine are used in the Far East and South East Asia.

Eradication

Cattle plague has been eradicated from three continents and most African and Asian countries. It is therefore likely that it will be the first animal plague to be eradicated worldwide.

Further reading

Scott, G.R., Taylor, W.P. and Rossiter, P.V. (1986). *Manual on the diagnosis of rinderpest*. Rome, F.A.O.

EPIVAG

Synonyms for epivag include infectious epididymitis and cervico-vaginitis of cattle. Epivag is a chronic venereal disease of cattle characterized by enlargement and induration of the epididymis in the bull and vaginitis, cervicitis and endometritis in the cow.

Aetiology

The causal agent is believed to be a virus belonging to the Beta-herpesvirinae subfamily of the Herpesviridae family of DNA viruses. In some accounts, the virus has been labelled bovine herpes virus-4. There is some doubt, however, as to whether this slow growing herpes virus is the cause, because Koch's postulates have yet to be fulfilled.

Occurrence

Epivag was so rampant in eastern and southern Africa in the 1930s that it was listed as a Notifiable Disease in South Africa and Zimbabwe and it led to the creation of the world's first national artificial insemination service to control the disease in Kenya. Today, the condition is rarely reported.

Species affected

Only cattle are affected. Indigenous African cattle possess a high innate resistance and clinical manifestations in them are rare. Imported exotic cattle and their crosses, on the other hand, have little resistance.

Transmission

Epivag is a venereal infection and is transmitted during coitus between infected and healthy animals. It may also be spread by the indiscriminate use of a contaminated speculum.

Clinical features

Affected bulls have enlarged and distorted testes. The lesions take 3–6 months to develop and sometimes longer. Enlargement and induration first involve the tail of the epididymis and later the head. Commonly, both epididymes are affected. Bulls are at first infertile and then became permanently sterile. The semen is affected before clinical signs are apparent; the volume is reduced, the appearance is watery and floccules of mucus are present. The fructose content falls or is absent. Buffer capacity is poor, the specific gravity is low and the pH high. Spermatozoa are few or absent and when present are abnormal in shape and motility.

The incubation period in cows lasts only a few days but the infection persists for months. The clinical response varies from slight hyperaemia of the vaginal mucosa with little or no discharge to severe vaginitis, cervicitis and metritis with a profuse thick yellow-white discharge. Most cows recover, but some become sterile from occlusion of the Fallopian tubes or from chronic fibrous peritonitis around the ovaries.

Pathology

The size and weight of the epididymes are increased. The cut surface is hard and the tubules are obliterated by dense fibrous tissue, although in early cases they are dilated by mucopurulent discharge. The colour of the cut surface varies from white to pale grey. Some testes have pin-head calcareous deposits. Bands and streaks of fibrous tissue may be evident.

Diagnosis

A presumptive diagnosis is based on the herd history, the clinical signs and semen examination. In contrast, lesions in the female are difficult to assess in the absence of disease in the male.

Differential diagnosis

Herds with affected bulls should be checked for brucellosis and, perhaps, tuberculosis. The clinical signs in the female are readily confused with those produced by infectious pustular vulvovaginitis. Lesions in epivag, however, persist for many weeks.

Immunology

In the absence of a precise aetiological identification, meaningful immunological data do not exist.

Control

All affected bulls should be slaughtered. Affected cows may be treated symptomatically and then later inseminated. The widespread use of artificial insemination using semen from clean bulls has brought the disease under control dramatically in eastern and southern Africa.

Further reading

Castrucci, G., Frigeria, F., Cilli, V., Donelli, G., Ferrari, M., Chicchini, U. and Bordoni, E. (1986). A study of a herpesvirus isolated from dairy cattle with a history of reproductive disorders. *Comparative Immunology, Microbiology and Infectious Diseases*, **9**, 13–21

EQUINE HERPES VIRUS ABORTION

In all countries with major horse-breeding programmes, equine herpes virus abortion is a significant cause of economic loss.

Aetiology

Three viruses are implicated in equine abortion. The most important is equine herpes virus-1 (EHV-1), the next is equine viral arteritis and the least important is equine herpes virus-4 (EHV-4). Until recently, EHV-1 and EHV-4 were thought to be the same virus, but hybridization trials have shown that they are distinct viruses with common antigens. Both cause rhinopneumonitis and abortion; the syndrome most often associated with EHV-1, however, is abortion, whereas the common syndrome following EHV-4 infections is rhinopneumonitis. Both are members of the Alpha-herpesvirinae subfamily of the Herpesviridae family of DNA viruses.

Occurrence

Equine herpes viruses have a worldwide distribution.

Transmission

Both viruses are shed principally in expired air but they may be shed also in uterine discharges following an abortion. Infectious aerosols deposit the virus on the epithelium of the nasal mucosa and conjunctiva initiating infection. Both viruses cross the placenta and congenital infection results.

Clinical features

The introduction of an infected excreter of EHV-1 into a stud may or may not be followed by a mild epidemic of an upper respiratory tract infection. One to four months later, abortions start, mares in the last term of pregnancy being the most susceptible.

Abortions occur without premonitory signs and there are usually no complications afterwards. The foetus is usually born dead. Foals close to term may be born alive but survive only for a few hours. Spread to in-contact foals may result in a fatal generalized disease manifested by respiratory distress. Encephalitis occasionally occurs in which the clinical signs range from slight inco-ordination to complete paralysis and death. Abortion storms may involve all the mares in the stud.

Unlike EHV-1 infections, abortions caused by EHV-4 virus are sporadic. Most EHV-4 infections occur in foals 2–12 months of age and are manifested by fever, anorexia and a profuse serous nasal discharge which later becomes mucopurulent. Most foals recover rapidly and completely.

Pathology

Gross lesions in EHV-1 aborted foetuses are most prominent in the liver, being manifested as numerous small necrotic foci. Microscopically, there is evidence of severe necrosis of the splenic white pulp and focal hepatic necrosis together with a marked inflammatory cell response. Typical intranuclear inclusion bodies are present in the lesions.

Diagnosis and differential diagnosis

A presumptive diagnosis of an EHV-1 abortion storm is based on an assessment of the history, clinical signs and *post mortem* lesions in aborted foals and confirmed by examination of frozen cryostat sections of liver by indirect immunofluorescence. Confirmation of suspected EHV-4 abortion or equine virus arteritis abortion is more difficult; techniques used include immunofluorescence of cryostat sections of foetal tissues, virus isolation in equine kidney cell cultures, and detection of antibodies.

Immunology

Horses infected with equine herpes viruses are infected for life and relapses and even reinfection is possible, despite the presence of circulating neutralizing antibody. Passive transfer of antibodies protects foals for several weeks.

Control

Sick horses with clinical signs of coughing, abortion or inco-ordination should be isolated immediately. Newly introduced animals should be kept completely separate from in-foal mares. Inactivated and live attenuated vaccines for EHV-1 virus are commercially available but their prophylactic value is doubtful.

Further reading

Campbell, T.M. and Studdert, M.J. (1983). Equine herpes virus type 1 (EHV-1). *Veterinary Bulletin*, **53**, 135–146.

EQUINE INFECTIOUS ANAEMIA

Also known as swamp fever, equine infectious anaemia (EIA) is a persisting viral infection of horses characterized by a variable clinical course that includes intermittent fever, depression, emaciation, oedema and death. The anaemia may be transient or progressive.

Aetiology

EIA virus is a member of the Lentivirinae subfamily of the Retroviridae family of single-stranded RNA viruses. Isolates vary in their antigenicity and virulence. It is readily inactivated by heat, lipid solvents and detergents.

Occurrence

EIA has been observed on all continents but its true homeland appears to be Central America and the north of South America. Important pockets elsewhere include Japan and tropical Australia. Even in its homeland its prevalence varies markedly, being greatest in valley bottoms and swampy areas and lowest in the mesa tablelands.

Species affected

The natural hosts are horses, mules and donkeys.

Transmission

The key mode of transmission involves bloodsucking tabanids which contaminate their mouthparts while feeding and transfer the virus to susceptible hosts when they feed again. It is a mechanical transmission and it is frequently mimicked by careless human beings using blood-tinged instruments on more than one animal. There is a tendency for a seasonal prevalence. A second important route of transmission is transplacental infection of the foetus. Infected mares which exhibit clinical signs during gestation invariably infect their foetus. Carrier mares, on the other hand, which remain healthy during their pregnancy, rarely infect their foetus.

Clinical features

Primary clinical reactions are usually manifested 1–3 weeks after exposure to infection. Sometimes, however, the primary reaction is inapparent and the first clinical episode occurs weeks or months after infection. Overt clinical signs in primary reactions are a sudden onset of fever – which usually persists for 3–4 days, but sometimes lasts for 1–3 weeks – together with the attendant signs of lacrimation, rhinorrhoea, sometimes epistaxis, and congested mucous membranes. Petechiae are commonly observed under the tongue. Anaemia is slight or absent unless the fever persists. There is, however, a marked initial leucopenia. Subcutaneous oedema commonly involves the ventral abdomen and legs. Most horses survive the primary reaction.

Multiple relapses occur at intervals varying from a few days to several weeks; sometimes there is apparent recovery for a year or more. The relapses are manifested as bouts of fever during which depression, anaemia and ventral oedema are evident. The relapse attacks usually last 3–5 days, but occasionally continue for up to 2 weeks. Emaciation and inco-ordination are progressive. Death supervenes during a febrile episode, the case mortality rate ranging from 30 to 70%.

Some animals survive despite being persistently infected. They are in good condition, non-febrile and not anaemic. Careful examination may reveal slight inco-ordination.

Clinical pathology

The anaemia is the result of an immunologically mediated destruction of erythrocytes coupled with bone marrow depression; consequently, there is an increased sedimentation rate and an increased plasma haemoglobin. Haemosiderocytes occur and there is a deposition of haemosiderin in liver, spleen and lymph nodes. Hypergammaglobulinaemia becomes evident if affected animals survive for 1–2 months. The marked leucopenia of the primary reaction is replaced by lymphocytosis and monocytosis in the relapse episodes.

Pathology

The outstanding features at autopsy in those few animals that die during the acute primary reaction are subcutaneous oedema, widespread serosal and mucosal haemorrhages, splenomegaly and hepatomegaly. The dominant findings in relapse deaths are splenomegaly, oedema of the dependent areas and emaciation.

The principle microscopic finding in early primary deaths is lymphoid necrosis manifested by empty germinal centres. The microscopic findings in relapse deaths are lymphoproliferative changes and anaemia.

Diagnosis

A provisional diagnosis is based on an assessment of the history, signs and lesions. Confirmation is readily achieved by Coggin's immunodiffusion test or an ELISA for the detection of antibodies; the presence of antibody indicates a presence of infectious virus. Commercial kits are available.

Confirmation of suspect primary clinical reactions depends on the detection of antigen in leucocytes by immunofluorescence tests.

Differential diagnosis

EIA shares clinical signs with several other diseases of horses. For example, subcutaneous oedema is also present in African horse sickness, dourine and equine arteritis. Anaemia is also a feature of babesiosis and dourine and progressive emaciation often occurs in equine surra caused by *Trypanosoma evansi*.

Immunology

Once infected, horses remain infected for life. Antibodies are produced within 4 weeks of infection, even though clinical signs are not seen until much later. They clear the virus from serum but not from leucocytes. The antibodies, however, do not confer protection. They can be detected by several *in vitro* tests but the most useful are the precipitating antibodies detectable by agar gel immunodiffusion.

Control

Treatment of infected horses is contraindicated because survivors are carriers. Infected horses should be isolated from susceptible horses. It is possible to eradicate equine infectious anaemia from a ranch or farm by regular screening for antibodies and slaughter of the reactors.

Horses should not be imported from known endemic areas but, if imported, they should be isolated until they have passed two clear tests. The control of insects is difficult but marshes should be drained, stables screened and, if necessary, insecticides should be used. Veterinarians and horse owners should take particular care to avoid using surgical instruments, particularly hypodermic needles, on more than one animal.

Further reading

Roberts, D.H. and Lucas, M.H. (1987). Equine infectious anaemia. *Veterinary Annual*, **27**, 147–150.

EQUINE VIRAL ARTERITIS

Equine viral arteritis (EVA) is a necrotizing pan-vasculitis of horses characterized by acute depression, fever, palpebral and limb oedema. Most pregnant mares abort while feverish.

Aetiology

The causal virus is the sole member of the *Arterivirus* genus of the Togaviridae family of RNA viruses. There is only one serotype. It is lipid sensitive.

Occurrence

Cases of EVA have been observed in North America, Europe, Africa and Asia. Serological surveys indicate that infection is widespread, although clinical outbreaks of the disease are rare.

Species affected

The horse is the only known natural host.

Transmission

Infected horses shed virus in all discharges and secretions. The major mode of transmission is by direct contact through the medium of infective droplets. Stallions may transmit the disease venereally for as long as 5 months. Transplacental transmission also occurs.

Clinical features

Incubation periods following contact transmission range from 1 to 4 weeks, whereas in venereal transmission they are as short as 3–4 days. Most infections are clinically inapparent, many are subacute and a few result in an acute systemic illness. Serious episodes occur sporadically in breeding studs in which the majority of the pregnant mares abort.

The clinical signs in subacute cases consist of a low-grade transient fever, transient anorexia, mild conjunctivitis, and a slight oedema of the legs and abdomen. In acute cases, the fever lasts up to 5 days and it is associated with deep depression, a stiff gait, limb oedema, peri-orbital oedema, conjunctivitis, lacrimation and rhinorrhoea. If the site of the lesions is the respiratory tract, nasal catarrh, coughing and dyspnoea are common. When the lesions affect the alimentary tract, colic and diarrhoea result. Abortion may occur at any stage of pregnancy, 20–60 days after exposure to the virus. Abortions may also occur when primary infections are clinically inapparent and frequently mares abort without showing premonitory signs.

Pathology

The basic lesion is a pan-vasculitis. The subcutaneous tissues, lymph nodes and visceral organs are congested, oedematous and haemorrhagic. Aborted foetuses are also oedematous.

Diagnosis

The variability of the clinical signs in cases of EVA renders a presumptive diagnosis difficult. Confirmation of the disease in adult horses requires isolation of the virus or the detection of antibodies. The specimens required for viral isolation are blood in anticoagulant and nasal swabs. Sera samples are examined for antibody either by complement fixation, ELISA or neutralization tests.

Antigen may be detected in cryostat sections of tissues from aborted foetuses.

Differential diagnosis

Most diagnostic confusion arises with abortion caused by equine herpes virus-1. Subacute and acute clinical cases in non-pregnant horses may be mistaken for equine influenza, equine infectious anaemia, and a mild form of African horse sickness.

Immunology

Horses recovering from post-natal infections are immune, whereas pre-natal infections may produce persistent lifelong carriers of the virus.

Control

Although live attenuated virus vaccines are commercially available, they only mask the clinical signs in infected horses and do not prevent virus replication and its shedding. Moreover, vaccination of mares in late pregnancy is not recommended because the vaccine virus may cross the placenta to infect the foal *in utero*. Control measures, therefore, are designed to limit the spread of EVA virus among breeding animals and are based on serological testing. Sero-positive animals are checked thereafter for virus shedding. Seropositive, virus-shedding stallions should only serve sero-positive mares. Sero-negative stallions should be tested annually for evidence of antibodies throughout the breeding season and should be used to serve sero-negative mares or previously vaccinated mares.

Further reading

Griffiths, C. (1987). Equine viral arteritis. *Journal of Equine Veterinary Science*, 7, 180–181.

EQUINE VIRAL ENCEPHALOMYELITIDES

The important neurotropic viral diseases of horses are accidental infections of mosquito-borne viral encephalomyelitides. Two sero-complexes of viruses are involved belonging to two families. The Togaviridae sero-complex includes the viruses that cause Eastern and Western encephalomyelitis (EEE/WEE) and Venezuelan encephalomyelitis (VEE) which occur in the Americas. The Flaviviridae sero-complex contains two viruses, one of which causes the disease known as Japanese equine encephalomyelitis in the Far East; the other is West Nile equine encephalomyelitis which causes disease in horses in the Camargue region of France and in Egypt. All the viruses implicated in equine encephalomyelitis induce disease in man.

Eastern and Western equine encephalomyelitides

The Eastern and Western equine encephalomyelitides are characterized by diphasic fevers, nervous signs and death.

Aetiology

The causal viruses are members of the *Alphavirus* genus of the Togaviridae family of RNA viruses. They cross-protect and are serologically related to the viruses causing VEE and Getah virus. They are not stable outside their mammalian hosts and vectors.

Occurrence

The diseases are endemic in the eastern and western states of Canada and the USA. They are an important cause of morbidity in both horses and man in the Americas; up to 4000 cases of equine encephalomyelitis occur annually in the USA, the majority being due to WEE. Both viruses also cycle in Central America, on the islands of the Caribbean and in the north of South America.

Species affected

The viruses cycle naturally and silently between wild birds and culicine mosquitoes belonging to the genus *Culiseta melanura*. In Jamaica, domestic fowls are major avian hosts of both viruses. In North America, the viruses overwinter in hibernating reptiles and amphibians. Minor natural hosts include wild rodents, skunks and foxes as well as domestic cats and dogs. Infections in donkeys, horses, mules and man are aberrant and accidental. Explosive epidemics of EEE virus regularly decimate hand-reared pheasants, a bird that is not indigenous to the USA.

Transmission

The vectors are culicine mosquitoes in which the virus multiplies. Outbreaks in exotic birds occur in the spring and are associated with the activity of *C. melanura*. Outbreaks in horses occur in late summer and a variety of mosquitoes are involved. Man, in addition, may contract infection, most commonly EEE, through handling infected horses and infected equine tissues; veterinarians and laboratory personnel in particular are at risk. Contact transmission of EEE virus between pheasants has also been reported.

Clinical features

Infections in horses are sporadic, clinically severe and often fatal; the case mortality rate with EEE approaches 90% and with WEE ranges between 20 and 40%. After an incubation period of 3–10 days, there is a sudden development of a high fever that is diphasic in character. The first febrile wave persists for 2–4 days and is often not observed. The second wave occurs 2–3 days later and is characterized by the onset of clinical signs of neuropathy. There is severe depression and affected horses adopt a characteristic straddled stance with the head lowered and ears drooping. Many horses are unable to swallow water and when they raise their head the water pours out of the mouth. Severe pruritus may lead to self-mutilation. A few animals are restless and hyperexcited. Some walk unsteadily in tightening circles and into obstacles. Many horses appear to be blind. Severely affected horses rapidly lose weight, become weak and eventually collapse. In panic attempts to rise they frequently injure themselves. Death supervenes within 5–10 days. Surviving animals rarely recover completely and usually exhibit some evidence of permanent neurological damage. In contrast, however, the clinical signs of some horses are subacute, being manifested by low-grade fever, anorexia and depression. There is rapid recovery in such cases. Moreover, serological surveys have indicated that inapparent infections occur.

Pathology

Gross changes are minimal. Microscopically, changes are restricted to the grey matter and are more extensive and severe in cases of EEE. There are no inclusion bodies.

Diagnosis

In the early stages, a diagnosis of colic or laminitis is common. Once neurological signs develop a presumptive diagnosis is readily made in endemic areas. The possibility of rabies, however, must always be considered. Confirmation of a suspect diagnosis should not be undertaken lightly. The specimens required are blood for serum and blood in heparin from live horses, and aliquots of the cerebral cortex, thalamus and hippocampus from dead horses. These should be forwarded to the laboratory fresh in containers on ice and in formol-saline. Rapid confirmation is most readily achieved by examining cryostat sections of the thalamus by an indirect fluorescent antibody test. Differentiation between the viruses of EEE and WEE requires isolation from blood collected early in the course of the disease. If horses survive, the convalescent serum sample should also be collected for comparison with the acute phase sample.

Differential diagnosis

One cannot differentiate between clinical cases of EEE, WEE and VEE. In areas where equine viral encephalomyelitides are endemic, differential confusion may arise from rabies and from the neuropathological syndrome associated with equine herpes-1 infections.

Immunology

Surviving animals possess a durable, probably lifelong, immunity to the homologous virus. Cross-protection between the alphavirus sero-complex is such that animals surviving VEE are also immune to EEE and WEE; animals surviving EEE are immune to WEE but not to VEE; and animals surviving WEE are susceptible to EEE and VEE.

Control

Horses at risk should be vaccinated annually with an inactivated cell culture vaccine. Monovalent and bivalent vaccines are available commercially and are usually given annually in the spring in two doses 4–6 weeks apart in previously unvaccinated horses. Thereafter, annual booster vaccinations should be carried out. On farms where a clinical case has occurred, steps should be taken to destroy the mosquito population using pesticides and drainage.

Further reading

Monath, T.V., McLean, R.G., Cropp, C.B., Parham, G.L., Lazuick, J.S. and Calisher, C.H. (1981). Diagnosis of eastern equine encephalomyelitis by immunofluorescent staining of brain tissue. *American Journal of Veterinary Research*, **42**, 1418–1421.

Venezuelan equine encephalomyelitis

Venezuelan equine encephalomyelitis (VEE) is an aberrant mosquito-borne viral infection of horses, donkeys and mules in Central America and tropical South America. The infections range in character from the subclinical to overt encephalomyelitis, the most common form being a fever associated with anorexia, depression and diarrhoea. The case mortality rate in horses developing encephalomyelitis is 40–80%.

Aetiology

The causal virus belongs to the *Alphavirus* genus of the Togaviridae family of single-stranded RNA viruses. There are four types and several subtypes, but only three subtypes of type I are pathogenic for horses. VEE virus also shares antigens with the viruses of EEE and WEE.

Occurrence

The virulent subtypes of VEE virus cycle silently in the tropical freshwater swamps of Central and South America. A second important ecological niche are meandering streams harbouring water lettuce. Periodically, the disease spreads north through Central America and once entered Texas. Non-virulent types and subtypes of the virus are widely distributed in the tropical Americas including the swamps of Florida.

Species affected

Endemic foci are maintained by silent cycles in swamp rodents and culicine mosquitoes which overspill into numerous other wild mammals including bats and monkeys. Birds are sometimes infected, but their role in the epidemiology of VEE is considered to be minor. Most, if not all, species of domestic animals are susceptible and usually undergo inapparent infection but, on occasion, overt disease and death have been observed in dogs, goats and sheep. The important aberrant hosts are horses, mules and donkeys, and man.

Transmission

All the types and subtypes of VEE virus are mosquito-borne and transovarial transmission in mosquitoes occurs. Mosquitoes infect horses, donkeys and mules but, in addition, contact transmission through aerosols may occur between sick and healthy animals. Experimentally, transplacental transmission has been demonstrated in horses. VEE viraemias in horses are high and infected horses act as amplifier hosts allowing a variety of bloodsucking insects to transfer infection mechanically. Man is infected from mosquito bites, from handling human patients and clinically infected animals and their tissues.

Clinical features

The incubation period is remarkably short, ranging from 12 to 36 hours after infection. The clinical responses of horses may be peracute, acute or subacute. Peracute reactions are characterized by diphasic fevers and encephalomyelitis, affected horses being anorexic and depressed. Diarrhoea is common and weight loss is rapid. Leucopenia and viraemia are evident during the first febrile wave. Clinical signs of encephalomyelitis occur during the second febrile wave which begins three or more days after the start of the short prodromal fever; the signs range from drowsiness to hyperexcitability, but there is not the intense pruritus seen in EEE infections. As the disease progresses, convulsions become increasingly frequent and are followed by collapse, prostration and death. Death may occur within 24 hours of the onset of neurological disorder, but it usually supervenes within 5 days.

About half of the horses affected with VEE virus do not develop encephalomyelitis. Nevertheless, many of these horses are acutely ill and some die. They exhibit high fevers which persist until death or for 2–4 days in animals that survive. Attendant signs include anorexia, depression, tachycardia, leucopenia, abdominal pain and diarrhoea. The weight loss is rapid.

Subacute reactions are manifested as short low-grade fevers and affected animals usually survive.

Pathology

The carcase is dehydrated. The predominant gross lesions are haemorrhages on the costal pleura and parietal peritoneum. The liver and kidneys are pale and friable. The lymph nodes are oedematous, translucent and often haemorrhagic. The gross appearance of the brain varies from no visible lesions to extensive necrosis and haemorrhage; the most consistent lesion is hyperaemia. Cerebral meninges tend to be oedematous. The spinal cord is grossly normal. Many of the lesions are immunologically mediated.

Diagnosis

Many equine diseases share clinical signs with VEE and a presumptive diagnosis is therefore not easy unless frank encephalomyelitis is present. Confirmation requires laboratory facilities. The specimens required are heparinized blood and serum from febrile cases, and portions of spleen and brain from dead animals. They should be forwarded to the laboratory on ice. Slices of brain and card should also be forwarded in formol-saline for histopathology. Recovered cases should be bled again for convalescent serum.

Differential diagnosis

Horses dying from VEE virus infection present more haemorrhagic lesions than horses dying from EEE or WEE. Nevertheless, it is often impossible to differentiate the three infections from clinical signs and *post mortem* lesions. In addition, rabies occurs in the endemic areas and should be considered.

Immunology

Recovery from infection with a non-virulent or virulent type or subtype confers a lifelong resistance which is associated with the presence of humoral neutralizing antibodies. This acquired resistance also protects horses from infection by EEE and WEE viruses.

Control

Horses at risk should be protected by vaccination; a live attenuated virus vaccine, designated TC-83 vaccine, was used to contain the epidemic wave that threatened the USA. The mass vaccination was supplemented by mosquito abatement through aerial spraying and by applying movement restrictions on all horses, mules and donkeys. Inactivated virus vaccines are now available commercially, and include a trivalent vaccine containing inactivated EEE, WEE and VEE viruses.

Further reading

Warton, T.E. (1981). Venezuelan, eastern and western encephalomyelitis. In *Virus diseases of food animals* (E.P.J. Gibbs, ed.), Vol. 2, pp. 587–625. London, Academic Press.

Japanese equine encephalomyelitis

Also known as Japanese B encephalitis, Japanese equine encephalomyelitis (JEE) is an accidental, mosquito-borne viral infection of man and horses, characterized by fever and encephalitis. Newborn piglets act as amplifier hosts of the virus and undergo inapparent infections. There is transplacental transmission of the virus in infected pregnant pigs causing teratogenic defects in the foetuses and abortion.

Aetiology

The causal virus is a member of the *Flavivirus* genus of the Flaviviridae family of RNA viruses. It is related to three other members of the genus, namely, St. Louis encephalitis virus, Murray Valley encephalitis virus and West Nile virus. All four viruses cause disease in man, but only JEE and West Nile virus cause disease in horses. There are at least two serotypes of JEE virus.

Occurrence

JEE is widely distributed in Asia over an area that stretches from the Indian subcontinent through to the Far East and the Pacific islands. It is found mainly in rural areas.

Species affected

The virus cycles naturally and silently between night herons and culicine mosquitoes. In the late spring and early summer, newborn piglets act as amplifier hosts increasing enormously the number of infected mosquitoes. Aberrant infections in a wide range of animals follow thereafter. The principal aberrant hosts that react clinically when infected are man and horses.

Transmission

JEE virus is transmitted by mosquitoes that breed in freshwater fish ponds and rice paddies. In temperate areas of Asia, the vector is *Culex tritaeniorhyncus* and in tropical Asia *C. gelidus*. The role of transovarial transmission in mosquitoes is in dispute. Although epidemiological studies suggest that air-borne transmission of JEE virus is rare, experimental studies have shown that aerosol transmission between sick and healthy animals and man is possible.

Clinical features

Infected horses develop fevers after incubation periods of 1–2 weeks duration. The clinical reactions may be peracute, acute or subacute. The overall case mortality rate is around 5%, but may be as high as 30–40% in acute and hyperacute cases.

Peracute reactions are characterized by their short course and the development of encephalitic signs from the onset of fever. The fever is high and infected horses sweat profusely, wander aimlessly, are demented and photophobic. Self-inflicted abrasions are common. Muscular tremors worsen, inco-ordination increases and posterior ataxia develops. Affected horses collapse and die within 4 days of the onset of clinical signs.

Most horses survive acute reactions, which are manifested by a high fluctuating fever of 4–12 days duration and low-grade encephalitic signs. Affected horses are drowsy, anorexic, swallow with great difficulty, stagger and may fall. Transient neck rigidity and radial paralysis have been observed. Mucous membranes are injected, sometimes jaundiced and often contain petechiae. Rhinorrhoea is common, the discharges being serous to greenish mucoid in character. Recovery appears to be complete.

Subacute reactions are characterized by transient low-grade fevers, partial anorexia and congestion of mucous membranes. Recovery is uneventful.

Infections in adult non-pregnant pigs are clinically inapparent. Infected pregnant sows, however, abort, produce mummified foetuses or give birth to stillborn, congenitally abnormal piglets. Newborn piglets infected after birth rarely show clinical changes, but if they do they are low-grade encephalitic signs.

Pathology

The spectacular gross lesions are small haemorrhages on all serous surfaces, congested lungs, congested cerebral blood vessels and numerous petechiae on the meninges. Microscopically, the dominant lesion is a diffuse non-suppurative encephalomyelitis with perivascular cuffing. There are no inclusion bodies.

Diagnosis

Early cases are often diagnosed as colic, but when other signs evolve it is relatively easy to arrive at a presumptive diagnosis based on the history and the clinical signs. In some countries, the possibility of rabies must be considered. Confirmation requires the detection of antigen by immunofluorescence in cryostat sections of brain tissues or by isolation and identification of the virus. The specimens required are blood for serum and blood in heparin from early cases and aliquots of brain tissue from horses that have been dead less than 12 hours. Slices of tissue should also be forwarded to the laboratory in formol-saline for histopathology.

Differential diagnosis

Differential diagnostic problems may arise in cases of tetanus and rabies.

Immunology

Recovered animals and man develop a durable immunity which is lifelong. The progeny of immune mares are passively protected for a few weeks.

Control

Prophylactic vaccination of horses at risk is the most practical and efficient control measure available; in Japan, for example, annual vaccination is essential. Inactivated virus vaccines are readily available commercially to protect horses and they have been used in sows to protect against stillbirths. Attenuated vaccines are administered to piglets to stop the amplification of the field virus. Nationwide vaccination in Japan of human beings with inactivated and attenuated vaccines have almost eradicated the disease from man and cases today are usually only seen in unimmunized foreigners or people over 35 years of age. Nevertheless, the Japanese operate an early warning system whereby newborn piglets are bled for evidence of IgM antibodies and, if the incidence rate of IgM antibodies increases rapidly, vaccination of the human population is undertaken.

Further reading

Takashima, J., Watanabe, T., Ouchi, N. and Hashimoto, N. (1988). Ecological studies of Japanese encephalitis virus in Hokkaido: Interepidemic outbreaks of swine abortion and evidence for the icnes to overwinter locally. *American Journal of Tropical Medicine and Hygiene*, **38**, 420–427.

West Nile encephalomyelitis

West Nile encephalomyelitis (WNE) is an aberrant mosquito-borne viral infection of man and horses characterized by low-grade fever and encephalomyelitis. Total or partial blindness is a common sequel in affected horses.

Aetiology

The causal virus is a member of the *Flavivirus* genus of the Flaviviridae family of RNA viruses and is therefore related to Japanese encephalitis, Murray Valley encephalitis and St. Louis encephalitis viruses.

Occurrence

WNE virus is widely distributed in Africa, western Asia and southern Europe. Clinical disease in horses has only been observed in Egypt and southern France.

Species affected

WNE virus cycles silently and naturally in wild birds and culicine mosquitoes. Antibodies have also been detected in the sera of dogs, bats, monkeys and rodents. Man and horses sometimes react clinically when infected, but morbidity rates are much lower than infection rates.

Transmission

WNE virus is mosquito-borne and therefore has a seasonal preference. In Africa, the main vector is *Culex univittatus*, in Asia it is *Culex vishnui*, and in France *Culex modestus*. The virus has also been isolated from soft ticks, particularly *Ornithodoros moubata*, but the epidemiological significance of soft-tick infections is not clear.

Clinical features

The duration of the natural incubation period is not known. The onset of illness is not dramatic, being manifested by low-grade fever and inco-ordination, which progressively worsen to ataxia in 2–4 days. Many affected animals are jaundiced but other systemic signs are minimal. Some cases are hyperexcitable. Within a further 6 days, horses either recover or become prostrate, paralysed and die. Few recover completely and most show evidence of neurological damage; in particular, blindness which may be total or partial. Up to 30% of clinical cases terminate in death, but many more horses succumb later from their disabilities.

Pathology

Lesions observed *post mortem* in Egypt were congestion and petechiation of the mucous membrane of the urinary bladder, congestion of alimentary tract mucosa and severe congestion of the cerebral surface. In contrast, in France, gross changes were conspicuous by their absence. Histopathological examination revealed a non-suppurative encephalomyelitis.

Diagnosis and differential diagnosis

As with the other equine viral encephalomyelitides, the early clinical signs in West Nile infections are often mistakenly attributed to colic. As the disease progresses, a presumptive field diagnosis becomes easier. The possibility of rabies, however, must always be considered. Confirmation requires the demonstration of antigen in cryostat sections of the brain by immunofluorescence or isolation of virus from nervous tissues. Histopathological examination of a portion of brain is a useful supplementary diagnostic aid.

Immunology

Surviving horses develop a lifelong resistance which is manifested by the presence of humoral antibodies.

Control

The morbidity of WNE has not warranted the development and use of vaccines. Affected cases should be treated symptomatically. Wild white horses of the Camargue that are blinded by the disease are shot on humane grounds.

Further reading

Joubert, L., Oudar, J., Hannoun, C., Beytout, D., Corniou, B., Guillon, J.C. and Panthier, R. (1970). Épidémiologie du virus West Nile; étude d'un foyer en Camargue. IV. La méningo-encéphalomyélite du cheval. *Annals de l'Institut Pasteur*, **118**, 239–247.

FOOT-AND-MOUTH DISEASE

Synonyms for foot-and-mouth disease (FMD) include aftosa and aphthous fever. FMD is a highly infectious viral disease of all domesticated and wild even-toed ungulates. It is characterized by fever and the appearance of vesicles in and around the mouth and muzzle, on the feet and on the teats and udder. Death is rare except in very young animals. Man is susceptible.

FMD is a disease of major economic significance because of the speed with which it spreads through animal populations if left uncontrolled, causing very heavy losses in production, particularly milk production.

Aetiology

FMD virus is a member of the *Aphthovirus* genus of the Picornaviridae family. There are seven immunologically designated serotypes, viz., O, A, C, SAT 1, SAT 2, SAT 3 and Asia 1. In the past, cross-complement fixation tests were used to divide each serotype into many subtypes. Today, differences within serotypes are determined by genomic analysis.

FMD viruses are acid and alkali labile and heat-sensitive.

Occurrence

Only a handful of countries have never been infected with FMD, viz., New Zealand, Japan, and the Central American countries lying between Mexico to the north and Colombia in the south. It has been eradicated from Australia, Canada and the USA. Most countries in Europe are now free of the disease, but the infection is endemic in most of Asia, many parts of Africa and most South American countries.

The O, A and C serotypes are prevalent in Africa, Asia, Europe and South America.

The SAT 1 serotype occurs in Africa and Asia. The SAT 2 and SAT 3 serotypes are limited to Africa and Asia 1 occurs only in Asia.

Species affected

Probably all cloven-hoofed animals are susceptible to FMD virus. Clinical cases are most frequently seen in cattle, pigs and sheep. The true natural host of the SAT serotypes is probably the wild African buffalo. FMD has also been reported in elephants. Clinical disease in man is rare, but people handling infected animals may harbour the virus in their nasopharynx for more than 24 hours.

Transmission

In addition to being disseminated directly and indirectly, FMD virus is capable of being wind-borne. Aerosols of infective droplets generated by cattle and pigs survive for many hours under suitable environmental conditions, particularly if the relative humidity is greater than 70% and the temperature is low. Plumes of infected aerosols may spread the virus downwind over a distance of 250 km. In the tropics, however, the most important method of spread is by direct contact between animals. Young calves are infected indirectly by being fed infected milk. Similarly, infected swill fed to pigs frequently initiates new foci of the disease. Veterinarians handling infected animals risk spreading the disease to other animals if they handle them within 24 hours.

FMD virus persists in the pharyngeal tissues of many animals after recovery. In convalescent cattle, for example, the virus has been recovered intermittently for up to 2 years. The carrier state in sheep and pigs, however, is measured in weeks. With the exception of the wild African buffalo, recovered carriers are not infectious.

Clinical features

Cattle. The first signs of illness in cattle following an incubation period of 3–8 days are dullness, depressed appetite, mild fever, and a marked fall in milk production. Profuse salivation is stimulated by the development of blanched vesicles on the dorsal surface of the tongue, the dental pad and the inner lips, producing strings of saliva that hang from the mouth. Movement of the lips gives rise to a characteristic smacking sound. Vesicles 1–10 cm in diameter are also found on the nostrils and muzzle. The lesions readily rupture and the necrotic epithelium sloughs off, leaving large raw ulcers which frequently become super-infected. Resolution occurs within 2–3 weeks.

Vesicles also develop on the coronary bands of the foot, the bulbs of the heel and the interdigital clefts. The resulting swelling and pain leads to marked lameness and affected animals are often seen shaking their feet. Rupture of the lesions brings relief but the exposed ulcers are liable to secondary infections. Lactating cows often develop vesicles on the teats and udder and they are therefore predisposed to mastitis. Abortion frequently occurs in pregnant animals. Mortality in adult cattle is rare.

Pigs. The incubation period of FMD in pigs is longer by a few days than that in cattle. Affected pigs are recognized by the presence of froth and salivation around the mouth. Vesicles are commonly found on the snout and they rupture easily, leaving shallow clean ulcers. Foot lesions are more easily detected because the vesicles become confluent, circling the coronary band and extending over the heels into the interdigital spaces. The pain leads to lameness and it may be so marked that the pigs walk on the tips of their toes. The hooves often slough. Vesicles similarly encircle the accessory digits.

Sheep. The incubation period in sheep may be as long as 13 days and the clinical signs are more muted than in other species. Vesicles on the tongue are transitory and are difficult to detect. Foot lesions lead to lameness, but differentiation from footrot is difficult.

Neonates. Mortality in sucking neonates may be high. Vesicles are not prominent and death is due to acute myocardial necrosis. In particular, FMD must be suspected in all sudden death cases in newborn piglets. Some survivors of neonatal FMD may exhibit severe dyspnoea when exercised and they are colloquially known as "panters".

Pathology

In addition to the lesions observed in the live animal, vesicles and ulcers may be seen on the pillars of the rumen. The acute myocardial necrosis seen in neonates is manifested by the appearance of small greyish foci in the myocardium, giving it a striped appearance – the so-called "tiger" heart. Similar necrotic foci may also occur in skeletal muscles.

Diagnosis

The clinical signs, particularly salivation and lameness occurring simultaneously with vesicles, should be regarded as FMD until proven otherwise. In countries where control vaccination is practised, confirmation and identification of the serotype of virus involved is essential. The samples required are fresh vesicle fluid and epithelial fragments from ruptured and unruptured vesicles. A sample should be forwarded to the laboratory in glycerol-saline in a thermos flask containing cold chill-packs but not wet ice. When samples from early lesions are received in the laboratory, a result can be obtained within 3 hours. In the past, the detection of antigen by complement fixation was the common method, but it is being supplanted by enzyme-linked immunosorbent assays (ELISA). Biochemical techniques are thereafter used to identify the genomic characteristics of the isolate to ensure that the most suitable vaccine is selected to control the epidemic within a few days.

Differential diagnosis

In the Americas, vesicular stomatitis is readily mistaken for FMD. In Europe and Asia, the major differential confusion is swine vesicular disease, a benign enterovirus infection of pigs and man. Many viral diseases, however, produce lesions on the mucosal surfaces that may be confused with FMD. Similarly, teat lesions may be confused with orthopox and parapox infections and bovine herpes mammillitis.

Immunology

The early antibodies in recovered animals are IgM immunoglobulins and will neutralize both homologous and heterologous serotypes. The later developing IgG antibodies are serotype-specific and to a varying degree isolate-specific. The duration of immunity following natural infection is limited. Antibodies passed in the colostrum will protect the sucking young for up to 5 months. Recovered animals may be infected immediately afterwards with one of the other serotypes and develop clinical disease.

Control

Low-risk countries ensure their freedom from FMD by controlling the importation of live animals and prohibiting the importation of animal meat products. Imported live animals are quarantined on arrival and while in quarantine are tested for the presence of virus in the pharyngeal tissues and for the presence of antibodies. Outbreaks in low-risk countries are controlled by applying a "stamping out" policy.

In high-risk and endemic areas, control of FMD is based on the strategic use of inactivated vaccines. Mono-, bi-, and trivalent vaccines containing one, two or three serotypes respectively are commercially available. In the past, the inactivating agent was usually formalin, but better results have followed the use of beta-propiolactone (BPL) or acetylethyleneimine (AEI). Modern vaccines contain adjuvants such as aluminium hydroxide, saponin or purified mineral oil.

Antibodies appear 4 days after vaccination and reach a peak 3 weeks later. The duration of immunity in cattle following a single dose of inactivated vaccine lasts 3–4 months and is extended to about 1 year if the cattle are revaccinated. Vaccination of pigs is difficult and only minimal protection is afforded except with oil adjuvanted vaccines which provide protection for a few months.

Further reading

Kitching, R.P. (1989). Development of foot and mouth virus strain characteristics – a review. *Tropical Animal Health and Production*, **21**, 153–166

GOAT PLAGUE

Synonyms for goat plague include peste des petits ruminants, PPR, kata, erosive stomatitis and enteritis of goats, goat catarrhal fever and stomatitis-pneumoenteritis complex. Goat plague is a viral contagion of goats and, less commonly, sheep, characterized by fever, erosive stomatitis, enteritis, pneumonia and death. Therefore, it mimics cattle plague.

Aetiology

Goat plague virus is a member of the *Morbillivirus* genus of the Paramyxoviridae family and shares antigens with other members of the genus. In particular, goat plague and cattle plague viruses partially cross-protect. They are distinguished by serum neutralization tests.

Occurrence

Goat plague is endemic in the nomadic herds and flocks that graze the sahel area of Africa. Transhumance introduces the virus into the herds and flocks in the south precipitating disastrous epidemics. Large importations of goats and sheep from Africa have introduced goat plague to several countries in the Middle East. More recently the disease has been recognized in India.

Species affected

The natural hosts are goats and sheep. In addition, captive wild ruminants have reacted severely and died in a zoological garden in the Middle East. Natural infections in cattle have not been authenticated but, experimentally, cattle may be infected; the reactions are symptomless and the virus is not shed. Similarly, pigs are susceptible to experimental infection and, like cattle, they are dead-end hosts.

As nomadic goats and sheep have a high innate resistance to goat plague virus, they undergo subacute reactions. In contrast, goats and sheep belonging to settled farmers south of the sahel have a low innate resistance and the disease in goats, in particular, is fulminating and usually fatal. The indigenous goats and sheep in the Middle East also possess a low innate resistance and when infected react severely.

Transmission

Infective aerosols are generated from virus shed by sick goats in all secretions and excretions and they initiate new infections when inhaled by susceptible in-contact goats or sheep, the virus entering the new host through the cells of the upper respiratory tract and the conjunctiva.

Clinical features

The clinical course of goat plague mimics that of cattle plague. A short prodromal fever follows an incubation period of 2–6 days and is accompanied by a serous nasal discharge that rapidly becomes profuse and catarrhal stimulating sneezing. Mucosal erosions appear shortly after the onset of fever and diarrhoea develops 2–3 days later. Ocular and nasal discharges now become mucopurulent, dry and encrust the nares and mat the eye-lids. The breath is fetid. Depression is intense and often the terminal stages are complicated by bronchial pneumonia. The mortality rate in goats other than the nomadic sahel goat ranges from 77 to 90%, and death usually occurs within a week of the onset of illness.

Subacute reactions are more common in sheep and are manifested by nasal catarrh, low-grade fever, recurring crops of mucosal erosions and intermittent diarrhoea. Most recover after a course of 10–14 days.

The most common activated complication is pasteurella pneumonia, but other latent enteric and haemoparasites may be exacerbated. Labial orf lesions, for example, commonly develop in surviving goats.

Clinical pathology

The acute disease is characterized by a severe leucopenia associated with destruction of lymphocytes.

Pathology

The carcase is dehydrated and soiled with fluid fetid faeces. Mucopurulent discharges encrust the peri-orbital and peri-nasal areas. The necrotic stomatitis is extensive, the abomasum and ileo-caecal valve are engorged and along the length of the colon rather inconspicuous "zebra" stripes occur. Lymph nodes are enlarged. A prominent *post mortem* finding is a purulent bronchopneumonia which masks an underlying primary viral pneumonia manifested as areas of level red consolidation.

The spectacular microscopic changes are associated with the mucosal erosions, depressed lymphoid tissues and consolidated lung lobules. Multinucleated giant cells containing intranuclear and intracytoplasmic inclusions are found in pneumonocytes and epithelial cells.

Diagnosis

Cases in goats and sheep possessing a low innate resistance are readily recognized from the clinical signs and *post mortem* findings. Confirmation is best achieved by the detection of specific antigens in lymph nodes and tonsils from animals killed early in the course of the disease. Unlike cattle plague, cases of goat plague usually contain high levels of antigen at death. Antigen can be sought on the spot in the field by counter-immune electrophoresis or by agar gel immunodiffusion.

It is always desirable to attempt to identify the causative virus by cross-neutralization tests, so that it can be checked to show that it is goat plague virus and not rinderpest virus. To this end, blood in EDTA together with samples of lymph nodes and tonsils are sent to the laboratory to be inoculated on to primary lamb kidney cells.

Differential diagnosis

Goat plague and cattle plague in goats are indistinguishable, clinically or pathologically. When goat plague was first observed in West Africa, it was misdiagnosed as bluetongue. Diagnostic confusion can also occur with heartwater, caprine pleuropneumonia and Nairobi sheep disease.

Immunology

Surviving goats and sheep develop a lifelong active immunity associated with the presence of humoral neutralizing antibodies. Specific antibody may also be detected in the sera of survivors by complement fixation and measles haemagglutination-inhibition tests.

Control

Scant attention has been paid to the control of goat plague in the endemically infected flocks and herds in the sahel. Settled herds and flocks at risk through contact with transhumant herds and flocks should be vaccinated with tissue culture-adapted cattle plague virus vaccine. An attenuated goat plague virus vaccine has been developed, but it is not widely available. Control is enhanced if live animals are not purchased in markets and introduced into settled village flocks. A particular danger is the goat or sheep sent for sale to a market and brought back home unsold.

In epidemics, sick animals should be segregated immediately and be given hyperimmune antiserum. Contact animals should be vaccinated and observed daily for clinical signs of disease. If they sicken, they should be transferred to the segregated sick flock.

Further reading

Taylor, W.P. (1984). The distribution and epidemiology of peste des petits ruminants. *Preventive Veterinary Medicine*, 2, 157–166.

HOG CHOLERA

Synonyms for hog cholera include swine fever and classical swine fever. Hog cholera, a serious virus disease of pigs, has two distinct syndromes, viz., a chronic persistent infection acquired pre-natally and a post-natal acute contagion characterized by fever, widespread haemorrhages, ataxia and death that is indistinguishable from African swine fever (ASF).

Aetiology

Hog cholera virus is a member of the *Pestivirus* genus of the Flaviviridae family of RNA viruses. It is related to the viruses of bovine virus diarrhoea and Border disease of sheep. The pestiviruses differ from all other Flaviviridae viruses by being non-arthropod-borne. They are related serologically. Only one type of HC virus is known, although strains vary widely in virulence. The virus is relatively stable and will survive in frozen carcases for years and in cured or salted pig-meat products for months.

Occurrence

Hog cholera emerged in the USA about 1830 after settlers imported European breeds of pigs. Since then, the disease has spread to every country with a major pig industry. Today, it is widely distributed in Central and South America, Asia and parts of Europe.

Species affected

The true natural hosts are domestic and wild pigs.

Transmission

The progeny of persistently infected carrier sows are infected when the virus crosses the placenta. Post-natal infection occurs either directly through close contact between sick and healthy pigs, the infection being acquired by inhalation, or indirectly through ingestion of feed contaminated by fresh infected secretions or excretions. A common source of new outbreaks is the feeding of infected pig-meat scraps. Once the disease is established within a herd, its spread is hastened by mosquitoes and tabanids.

Clinical features

Many congenitally infected piglets die *in utero* and are aborted. Others are born alive but are weak, deformed or trembling. Some are born apparently healthy but are persistently viraemic, become carrier sows and so maintain the cycle.

Post-natal infections may be acute, chronic or mild following an incubation period of 3–10 days. The acute disease is manifested by an abrupt loss of appetite, a sudden high fever and thirst. Affected pigs huddle and bury themselves under their bedding. Depression is marked and they are reluctant to move. Early constipation is followed by diarrhoea and vomiting. As the disease progresses, skin discolouration of the abdomen and necrosis of the ear tips and tail become evident. Conjunctivitis is usually severe and the eye-lids are often stuck together by dry exudate. Respiratory distress is sometimes evident. Inco-ordination, circling and trembling precede posterior paraplegia and convulsions. Females may abort. The case mortality rate may reach 90%.

The chronic form may occur in pigs that survive the acute form or may be seen in pigs that never show any signs of primary infection. Affected pigs have bouts of fever, depression and inappetence. Encrusted skin lesions are common and death supervenes in about 30 days and is associated with secondary bacterial infection.

In the subacute form, the clinical signs are very variable and are frequently missed. Affected pigs fail to thrive and pregnant sows may abort.

Pathology

The gross changes are predominantly haemorrhagic; submucosal and subserosal petechiae are widespread and larger haemorrhages affect the intestinal mucosa, lungs, spleen, lymph nodes and kidneys. In chronic cases, there is often evidence of a fibrinous pneumonia and button ulcers may be found in the intestinal mucosa in the region of the ileo-caecal valve.

Microscopically, the prominent lesions involve the small blood vessels and capillaries. Significant lesions in the central nervous system are perivascular cuffing and gliosis. There are no inclusion bodies.

The pathology of hog cholera cases is indistinguishable from that of ASF.

Diagnosis

The severity of the signs and lesions caused by hog cholera virus vary enormously. A presumptive diagnosis, therefore, must be confirmed by the detection of antigen. The samples required are tonsil, kidneys, spleen, ileum, submandibular and mesenteric lymph nodes, and brain together with blood in anticoagulant for virus isolation. Half of the organ samples should be sent in containers on water-ice and half in formol-saline. In countries where ASF also occurs, any presumptive diagnosis of hog cholera should also be screened for the presence of ASF.

Differential diagnosis

Both clinically and pathologically, hog cholera resembles ASF and differentiation requires laboratory facilities. Misdiagnoses also occur with acute septicaemias, pseudo-rabies, thrombocytopenic purpura and warfarin poisoning.

Immunology

Many pre-natally infected piglets do not develop antibodies and remain antibody-free throughout their life. Post-natally infected pigs that recover are immune for life and develop high titres of neutralizing antibody which are transferred to the piglets in the colostrum protecting them for up to 4 months.

Control

Low-risk areas maintain their freedom from hog cholera by a total ban on the importation of live pigs or pig-meat products. In addition, the feeding of uncooked swill is forbidden. Outbreaks of hog cholera in low-risk countries are controlled by the total slaughter and destruction of infected herds and the tracing of all movements into and out of herds. In countries where hog cholera is endemic, losses are kept under control by vaccination of the pig herds; in most countries, the vaccine used is a live virus vaccine. Hog cholera has been eradicated from many countries and this is, perhaps, a disease that is a candidate for total global eradication.

Further reading

Harkness, J.W. (1985). Classical swine fever and its diagnosis: A current view. *Veterinary Record*, **116**, 288–293.

IBARAKI DISEASE

Also known as Kaeshi disease, Ibaraki disease is an acute arthropod-borne disease of cattle characterized by fever, ulcerative stomatitis and dysphagia that leads to dehydration and emaciation.

Aetiology

The causal virus of Ibaraki disease is a member of the *Orbivirus* genus of the Reoviridae family of double-stranded RNA viruses. It is very closely related to the virus causing epizootic haemorrhagic disease of deer and less closely to bluetongue virus. In the presence of proteins, Ibaraki virus is remarkably stable.

Occurrence

Ibaraki virus is widely distributed in the Far East and South East Asia and the adjacent archipelagos. Clinical episodes are more frequently recorded in the late summer and autumn in Japan and Korea.

Species affected

The disease has only been observed in cattle. Attempts to infect sheep experimentally have failed.

Transmission

Like other orbiviruses, Ibaraki virus is arthropod-borne, but data as to the species of arthropods involved are meagre; however, *Culicoides* are suspected. Transplacental transmission occurs in pregnant cattle.

Clinical features

The natural incubation period is not known. The onset of illness is abrupt, being manifested by fever and its attendant signs of depression, anorexia, lacrimation, conjunctivitis and rhinorrhoea. Visible mucous membranes are congested and eroded and salivation is profuse. Erosions also appear on the muzzle and around the external nares and become encrusted. In a few cases, similar encrusted erosions affect the coronets causing lameness. Lesions have also been observed on the udder. Many animals develop painful swelling of the leg joints.

The fever usually lasts 2–3 days, but sometimes it persists for 7 days. The most distinctive sign is dysphagia, i.e. difficulty in swallowing, which occurs in 25% of the affected animals when the fever and other initial symptoms have subsided. The difficulty in swallowing leads to dehydration and emaciation and occasionally to aspiration pneumonia which is the major cause of death in affected animals. The overall case mortality rate is about 10%, but in animals with dysphagia 35% are expected to die or are slaughtered.

Pathology

In addition to the erosions and ulcers observed in life, erosions and ulcers affect the oesophagus, larynx, pharynx and the abomasum. Carcases are dehydrated and the contents of the rumen, reticulum and abomasum are dry. Aspiration pneumonia is a common finding.

The significant microscopic lesion is degeneration, necrosis and haemorrhage of the striated muscles of the oesophagus, larynx, pharynx and abomasum. Neutrophil infiltration is prominent around the degenerated muscle fibres.

Diagnosis

An assessment of the history of an outbreak with particular emphasis on the seasonal incidence and geographical prevalence together with the clinical signs and *post mortem* lesions form the basis of a presumptive field diagnosis. Confirmation depends upon isolation of the virus in cell cultures or embryonated chicken embryos and its serological identification.

Differential diagnosis

Ibaraki disease in cattle mimics bluetongue in sheep. On rare occasions, cattle infected with bluetongue develop similar clinical signs. Differential confusion may also arise with rinderpest, the mucosal syndrome of bovine virus diarrhoea virus infection, malignant catarrhal fever and even foot-and-mouth disease.

Immunology

Complement-fixing and neutralizing antibodies occur in the sera of recovered animals, but the dynamics of the serological responses are not known.

Control

Affected animals should be nursed symptomatically and particular attention should be paid to counteracting the dehydration because of the depressed water intake. An attenuated live virus vaccine is used to immunize cattle at risk in Japan and protection of up to 3 years is claimed.

Further reading

Ung-Bok Bak, Chang-Kook Cheong, Hee-In Choi, Chang-Woo Lee, Hyo-Sung Oh, Young-Ok Rhee, Myung-Rae Cho and Young-Il Lim (1983). An outbreak of Ibaraki disease in Korea. *Korean Journal of Veterinary Research*, **23**, 81–88.

INFECTIOUS BOVINE RHINOTRACHEITIS

Synonyms for infectious bovine rhinotracheitis (IBR) include bovid herpes virus-1 disease and red nose. IBR is a persistent viral infection of cattle characterized by fever, rhinitis with rhinorrhoea and tracheitis. In recent years, abortogenic variants have emerged.

Aetiology

IBR virus is a member of the Alpha-herpesvirinae subfamily of the Herpesviridae family of double-stranded DNA viruses. It is serologically identical to infectious bovine pustular vulvovaginitis virus, but their DNA restriction-endonuclease digestion patterns differ. Although IBR virus is relatively stable, a temperature-sensitive mutant has been developed, which is in use as a live attenuated virus vaccine.

Occurrence

IBR has a worldwide prevalence. The abortogenic variants first emerged in the USA, but have since spread to other countries.

Species affected

Antibodies avidly reactive with IBR virus are prevalent in many species of wild and domesticated ruminants, but clinical disease seems to be limited to cattle and domestic buffaloes. Most epidemics in cattle occur in animals over 6 months of age, because younger calves are seldom at risk.

Transmission

Overt clinical cases shed large quantities of virus in their breath and in respiratory and ocular discharges producing aerosols that infect susceptible in-contact animals.

Pre-natally, there is transplacental transfer of abortogenic variants from the cow to the foetus. Abortion usually follows.

Clinical features

Most clinical reactions are subacute, but some are acute. The incubation period ranges from 2 to 6 days. Animals affected subacutely develop low-grade fevers, mild rhinitis and conjunctivitis. The milk yield in lactating animals is depressed. Recovery is rapid, occurring 3–5 days after the onset of fever.

Acute cases have higher fevers and more profuse nasal and ocular discharges which become mucopurulent causing respiratory distress. The appetite is lost. Depression is obvious and coughing indicates bronchopneumonia. Coalescing pustules cause necrotic plaques in the upper respiratory tract mucosae. Super-infection with opportunist bacterial pathogens is common and may have serious effects.

Abortogenic variants of IBR virus are alleged to cause 25% of pregnant cattle to abort and the interval between exposure and abortion ranges from 8 days to several months. Aborted foetuses have usually been dead for several days before expulsion and, consequently, are autolysed, have brownish friable tissues and are often decomposed. Calves infected *in utero* in the last stages of pregnant may be born alive only to succumb from an acute febrile form of IBR, manifested by respiratory distress and diarrhoea.

Most uncomplicated cases of IBR recover. The virus lies latent in cranial ganglia and may be activated by stress. Relapses are never as severe clinically as the primary infections.

Pathology

Death, except in newborn calves, is usually associated with secondary bacterial infections. Pathological examination of neonatal deaths reveals white necrotic lesions on the mucosae of the mouth, tongue, oesophagus and the stomachs. Diffuse peritonitis may also be present.

In animals slaughtered early in the course of the disease, histopathological examination will reveal acidophilic intranuclear inclusions in epithelial cells.

Diagnosis

Presumptive diagnoses based on the clinical signs and history are readily confirmed by detecting virus antigen in the nuclei of cells collected on nasal swabs. Cryostat sections of liver and spleen from non-autolysed aborted foetuses will also reveal the presence of the virus in the nuclei of the cells.

The detection of antibodies in mature, non-vaccinated animals has diagnostic significance, indicating the presence of the virus.

Differential diagnosis

Differential diagnostic problems include foot-and-mouth disease, rinderpest, mucosal disease and malignant catarrhal fever.

Immunology

The development of neutralizing antibodies 1–2 weeks after the onset of infection does not affect the persistence of the virus in recovered animals. Recovery is attributed to cell-mediated immune mechanisms. Antibodies transferred in the colostrum will protect calves for 1–6 months.

Control

The prevalence of IBR is very high. Nevertheless, isolation of newly purchased animals is a wise precaution and vaccination of breeding stock is recommended to mitigate losses from abortion. Live attenuated vaccines may be administered intramuscularly or, preferably, by the intranasal route. Intranasal vaccination has also been recommended in the face of an acute outbreak in the hope that it will reduce the severity and duration of the disease.

Further reading

Nettleton, P.F. (1986). The diagnosis of infectious bovine rhinotracheitis. *Veterinary Annual*, **26**, 90–99.

INFECTIOUS PUSTULAR VULVOVAGINITIS

Synonyms for infectious pustular vulvovaginitis (IPV) include coital exanthema, infectious pustular vaginitis, infectious pustular balanoposthitis, and genital syndrome of bovid herpes virus-1. IPV is a persistent viral infection of cattle transmitted by coitus or by artificial insemination, and characterized by fever, vulvovaginitis and leucorrhoea in heifers and cows and by balanoposthitis in bulls.

Aetiology

IPV virus is a member of the Alpha-herpesvirinae subfamily of the Herpesviridae family of DNA viruses. It is serologically identical to infectious bovine rhinotracheitis virus but differs in its DNA restriction-endonuclease digestion pattern.

Occurrence

IPV has a worldwide distribution. In the past, it was widely distributed in Europe through the practice of using "travelling" bulls.

Species affected

Antibodies avidly reacting with the viruses of IBR and IPV are prevalent in many wild and domesticated ruminants. Clinical disease, however, seems to be limited to cattle and domesticated buffaloes.

Transmission

IPV virus is usually transmitted by coitus. Semen from infected bulls may be contaminated with the virus and transmission may follow artificial insemination.

Clinical features

IPV virus attacks the epithelium of the urogenital tract of both sexes, giving rise to multiple focal pustular lesions. Affected animals develop fever, depression and inappetence. In cows, oedema of the vulvar labia is marked and the vagina inflamed. Pustules tend to coalesce, forming false pseudomembranes and produce a thick yellowish discharge. Vaginal irritation is intense, stimulating frequent micturation. Affected bulls are reluctant to serve and adhesions associated with the balanoposthitis may lead to permanent inability to serve.

Infertility is transient. IPV virus, unlike IBR virus, is not associated with abortion.

The acute disease in both sexes lasts only a few days and complete resolution occurs within 2 weeks. Recovered animals, however, are carriers, and relapses occur following stress or the use of corticosteroids.

Pathology

IPV is benign. The examination of biopsies of affected mucosa collected early in the course of the disease will reveal the presence of typical herpes intranuclear inclusion bodies.

Diagnosis

A presumptive diagnosis based on the clinical signs and history is readily confirmed by detecting virus antigen in the nuclei of cells collected on swabs of an infected urogenital tract. The detection of antibodies in non-vaccinated animals has diagnostic significance by indicating the presence of the virus.

Differential diagnosis

Although IPV has been confused with foot-and-mouth disease, rinderpest and mucosal disease, a careful clinical examination will indicate the restricted nature of the lesions.

Immunology

Neutralizing antibodies appear 1–2 weeks after the onset of the clinical signs. However, the virus is cell-associated and the presence of antibody does not prevent relapses. Antibodies transferred in the colostrum, however, will protect calves for several months.

Control

Affected animals should be treated symptomatically and temporary cessation of the breeding programme is recommended. Partial prophylaxis may be achieved by using IBR vaccines because of the close serological relationship between the two viruses. The vaccine does not prevent infection but limits the severity of the clinical signs.

Further reading

Straub,O.C. (1983). The IBR-IPV disease complex. *Veterinary Medical Review*, **2**, 119–131.

INFLUENZA

Influenza is an acute respiratory disease characterized by epidemic episodes. The causal viruses have been isolated from many species of animals as varied as man, birds and whales. Three types of the virus are known, but only influenza virus A is implicated in epidemics in domesticated animals. Subtypes of influenza A tend to be species-specific.

Equine influenza

Aetiology

Equine influenza is caused by influenza virus A, a species of the *Influenzavirus* genus of the Orthomyxoviridae family of RNA viruses. The subtypes affecting horses are known as equine 1 and equine 2. They are differentiated by their haemagglutinin and neuramidase antigens; equine 1 is an H7N7 virus and equine 2 an H3N8 virus. Both viruses are antigenically stable, but there is recent evidence of antigenic drift occurring in equine 2 virus.

Occurrence

Epidemics of equine influenza have occurred on all continents except Australasia. They tend to spread rapidly and involve horses in many countries because of the frequent all-year-round transport of horses for racing and breeding.

Species affected

The equine 1 and 2 subtypes of influenza A virus only affect horses.

Transmission

The transmission of influenza virus is epitomized by the couplet "Coughs and sneezes cause diseases". Close aerosol contact is necessary for the spread of the virus. Infected horses shed virus for up to 10 days in the nasal secretions and expired air. Virus in inhaled droplets settles on the epithelium of the upper respiratory tract where it multiples.

Clinical features

A high fever is evident after an incubation period of 1–3 days. The fever persists for 1–2 days and is associated with a dry hacking cough. The submandibular and pharyngeal lymph nodes are enlarged. Affected horses are depressed and lose their appetite. A nasal discharge, which is at first serous, becomes mucopurulent. Recovery begins 1–2 weeks later, provided the horses are nursed and rested. Failure to do so may result in them developing secondary bacterial bronchitis or catarrhal bronchial pneumonia. Deaths are rare except in foals deprived of colostrum.

Pathology

There are no specific lesions. The mucous membranes of the upper respiratory tract are hyperaemic or inflamed. In fatal cases, bronchial pneumonia or lobular pneumonia is present.

Diagnosis

A presumptive diagnosis of an epidemic of acute cases of equine influenza is relatively easy but in partially immune animals is much more difficult. Confirmation is most readily achieved by inoculating nasal washings from febrile horses into the amniotic and allantoic sacs of 9-to 11-day-old embryonated chicken eggs. Isolated virus is identified by haemagglutination and haemagglutination-inhibition tests.

Differential diagnosis

Many viruses attack the upper respiratory tract of horses and their differentiation requires laboratory facilities.

Immunology

Recovered horses develop an immunity associated with the production of neutralizing antibody. It is transient and lasts for only a few months. Partially immune horses allow the virus to cycle silently and may initiate fresh epidemics when such horses are moved into a susceptible stud.

Control

Premises on which equine influenza epidemics occur should be placed in quarantine for at least 4 weeks and the same restrictions should apply to the stablemen handling the diseased horses. Thereafter, the premises should be cleaned and disinfected together with the equipment and horse boxes.

The major control technique is regular and frequent vaccination using a bivalent inactivated vaccine. The primary vaccination should be boosted by a second dose 8–12 weeks later. Thereafter, horses are revaccinated every 3–6 months.

Further reading

Tumova, B. (1980). Equine influenza – a segment in influenza virus ecology. *Comparative Immunity and Microbiology of Infectious Diseases*, 3, 45–59.

Swine influenza

Aetiology

Several subtypes of influenza type A virus affect swine including some derived from man. The current common subtype affecting pigs is H1N1.

Occurrence

Swine influenza has a worldwide distribution.

Species affected

The swine subtypes of influenza A virus have been known to spread to man and to domesticated birds.

Transmission

Transmission of swine influenza virus requires close aerosol contact.

Clinical features

Although the virus is prevalent in all pig populations, disease is relatively rare. Clinical signs appear after an incubation period of 1–3 days and are manifested by a reluctance to move, huddling in corners and a high fever. Rhinitis and conjunctivitis develop. Affected pigs sneeze and cough, and their respirations are laboured and abdominal in character. Depression, anorexia and prostration are common. Most pigs recover quickly within a week, but if secondary bacterial infections supervene the mortality rate may be 5–10%.

Pathology

There are no specific lesions. Deaths are associated with the lesions of secondary bacterial pneumonias.

Diagnosis

Most swine influenza infections in pigs are not diagnosed. Suspicions, however, are aroused when there are acute epidemics. Confirmation requires the isolation of the virus from nasal washings in embryonated chicken eggs and thereafter its identification.

Differential diagnosis

Diagnostic problems have arisen in the past with outbreaks of enzootic pneumonia, haemophilosis, pasteurellosis, chlamydiosis and pseudorabies.

Immunology

Recovered pigs develop a transient immunity associated with neutralizing antibodies.

Control

The best control measure is to keep a closed herd because most outbreaks occur after the introduction of a new pig into a susceptible herd. Attenuated live and inactivated vaccines have been developed, but they have had little success in controlling the disease.

Further reading

Sanford, S.E., Josephson, G.K.A. and Key, D.W. (1983). An epizootic of swine influenza in Ontario. *Canadian Veterinary Journal*, **24**, 167–171.

LUMPY SKIN DISEASE

Synonyms for lumpy skin disease (LSD) include Ngamiland disease and pseudourticaria. LSD is a malignant pox of cattle characterized by fever, cutaneous nodules, mucosal ulcers and generalized lymphadenitis.

Aetiology

LSD virus is a member of the *Capripoxvirus* genus of the Poxviridae family of double-stranded DNA viruses. It is closely related to the capripoxvirus that produces sheep and goat pox. Like many pox viruses, LSD virus is relatively heat stable, but it is inactivated by exposure to chloroform and ether.

Occurrence

The original homeland of LSD was Zimbabwe, but today the disease is endemic throughout Africa south of the Sahara and in Malagasy. Recent epidemics have occurred in Egypt and Israel.

Species affected

LSD has only been observed in cattle, but antibodies have been detected in the sera of African buffaloes. Fatal infections have been induced in giraffe and impala experimentally. Despite the cross-protection between LSD and sheep pox viruses, natural transmission has not been recorded between cattle and sheep or between sheep and cattle.

Transmission

LSD virus is arthropod-borne, several genera of bloodsucking insects being involved. The major vector, however, is still unknown. Outbreaks are seasonal, occurring at the onset of the rainy season. Point epidemics are sporadic and occur in years with above average rainfall. The virus may cross the placenta.

Clinical features

The natural incubation period ranges from 2 to 4 weeks, but the incubation period following experimental infection is around 1 week. Clinical reactions may be peracute, acute, subacute or inapparent.

Peracute reactions are characterized by the generalization of the nodules to the tissues of the upper respiratory tract causing respiratory distress and death within 10 days.

Acute reactions are characterized by a sudden onset of fever with the attendant signs of staring coat, depression, rhinitis and conjunctivitis. The fever is usually biphasic, the second febrile peak being associated with the sudden appearance of cutaneous nodules. These are intradermal, firm, raised, round and circumscribed, varying in diameter from 0.5 to 5.0 cm. They appear in many different sites simultaneously, but others appear over the succeeding 2–4 days. The predilection sites are the head and neck, limbs, perineum, genitalia and udder. Sometimes the whole body is covered with nodules. Lymphadenitis follows the appearance of the nodules and persistent painful oedema develops in one or more limbs, lower abdomen and/or brisket. The overlying skin sometimes necroses and sloughs, to leave a large open suppurating wound. Pox in the mucosa of the oral pharynx are at first nodular but quickly erode to leave deep ulcers. Their presence gives rise to noisy respirations and profuse salivation.

The skin nodules occupy the full thickness of the skin and sometimes penetrate into the subcutaneous tissue and underlying muscle. Some nodules are slowly resorbed, others become indurated and persist for years, but most develop into sit-fasts. In the later stages of the disease, all three types of nodular reaction are present. Sit-fast formation begins when the skin around the nodule becomes necrotic and a central cylindrical core of tissue begins to separate from the surrounding healthy skin. The central core necroses and in a period of 5–7 weeks the necrotic core is sloughed, leaving a granulating floor which heals as a disfiguring pock that damages the hide.

Subacute reactions are manifested by the evolution of a few nodules without a systemic disturbance.

Morbidity is extremely variable. A notorious virgin soil epidemic in South Africa in 1944 involved 8 million cattle and several affected farms reported mortality rates greater than 50%. Elsewhere in Africa, morbidity is about 0.5% and the case mortality rate about 2%. Surviving animals in the South African epidemic were severely debilitated and convalescence was prolonged, but elsewhere in Africa a marked loss of condition is not a common feature. Pregnant cows may abort and a foetus with skin lesions has been observed.

Pathology

The cut surface of the nodules is dull and pinkish-grey and the subcutis is often infiltrated by red serous fluid. Sit-fasts are usually raised above the level of the surrounding healthy skin. Microscopically, the nodules are variolous in morphology.

In animals that die, nodules are found in visceral organs, particularly the lungs and the tissues of the upper respiratory and digestive tracts, as well as cutaneously. Nodules in the parenchyma of the tissues are intact, but those in the upper respiratory and digestive tracts are quickly eroded into ulcers. All lymph nodes are enlarged.

Diagnosis

Typical cases are easily recognized clinically during point epidemics but difficulties arise during interepidemic periods. Confirmation is best sought by examining a biopsy sample from an early skin nodule by electron microscopy. Supportive diagnostic aids include virus isolation on the chorio-allantoic membrane of embryonated hen eggs or in tissue cultures, and histopathology. Excised early nodules are the preferred specimens and should be forwarded to the laboratory, half in 10% formol-saline and half-frozen.

Differential diagnosis

Lumps on cattle are common in Africa. The most difficult to differentiate from LSD in the early stages are the nodules of the Allerton type of pseudo-lumpy skin disease; later stages are readily distinguished. Other conditions known to cause confusion include the lesions of demodicosis, onchocercosis, globidiosis, ringworm, skin tuberculosis, photo-sensitization and urticaria. Difficulties often arise from streptothricosis, which may co-exist with LSD, and from tick and insect bites.

Immunology

Recovered animals will react to challenge 3–4 months later. The challenge lesions are localized and the typical accelerated immune reactions contain infectious virus.

Humoral antibodies play little role in the defence of the animal to reinfection and cell-mediated immune mechanisms are probably more important.

Control

Quarantine measures do not prevent the spread of LSD. Prophylactic vaccination is therefore widely used. In East Africa, the vaccine is a sheep and goat pox virus propagated in cell culture. In South Africa, a bovine isolate of LSD virus has been attenuated by serial passage in cell cultures and in embryonated eggs. Antibodies persist for 3 years in cattle after vaccination.

If the disease occurs, affected animals should be segregated in insect-proof buildings and in-contact animals should be vaccinated.

Further reading

Woods, J.A. (1988). Lumpy skin disease – a review. *Tropical Animal Health and Production*, **20**, 11–17.

MAEDI-VISNA

Synonyms for maedi-visna include chronic progressive pneumonia (CPP), atypical pneumonia, lung sickness and Laikipia lung disease. Maedi and visna are non-febrile, slow progressive diseases of sheep and goats and are different clinical manifestations of the same viral infection. The maedi syndrome is a slowly progressive interstitial pneumonia, whereas the visna syndrome is a slow, progressive demyelination. A mixed syndrome has recently been observed. All syndromes invariably terminate fatally.

Aetiology

The causal virus is a *Lentivirus* of the Retroviridae family of RNA viruses. It is closely related to a *Lentivirus* of goats that causes arthritis and/or encephalomyelitis.

Occurrence

Maedi-visna is present in all continents of the world except Australasia. Both syndromes may occur in one flock, but the maedi syndrome is much more common than the visna syndrome.

Specific affected

Disease is only seen in adult sheep and goats. Breed differences in susceptibility are suspected but not proven, whereas there is clear evidence that there are breed differences in regard to the severity of the lesions.

Transmission

The major mode of transmission is excretion of the virus in colostrum or milk and its ingestion by lambs and kids. Less commonly, transmission may occur between closely confined individuals when infected droplets in aerosols generated by splashing milk are inhaled. The virus does not cross the placenta and has not been isolated from semen.

Clinical features

The incubation period in maedi exceeds 2 years and may take 8 years. The onset of clinical signs is insidious; affected animals fail to thrive despite having a good appetite. They tend to lag behind the flock and gradually show signs of respiratory distress which progressively worsens over many months. Dyspnoea may be induced if affected sheep are forcibly exercised. Death is often precipitated by secondary bacterial pneumonia.

The incubation period in the visna syndrome is shorter and signs may occur in sheep as young as 2 years old. The onset is insidious, the early sign being slight inco-ordination. Affected animals lag behind the flock, stumble and fall without reason, and progressively lose condition. Lip and facial muscles tremble and the ataxia progressively worsens. Paresis follows and leads to paraplegia. Affected animals stay alert. The overt clinical course may last for 1 year or longer, with periods of remission. Death is inevitable.

Pathology

The spectacular gross lesions in cases of maedi are the enlarged heavy lungs which are sponge-rubber in consistency, pale grey or greyish brown in colour, and fail to collapse when the thorax is open. Frothy fluid is not present in the bronchi or trachea. Microscopically, there is a chronic, diffuse interstitial pneumonia. The alveolar septa are thickened and infiltrated by mononuclear cells.

There are no gross lesions in visna. Microscopic examination reveals demyelination and a diffuse encephalomyelitis.

Diagnosis

The clinical signs and *post mortem* lesions lead to a presumptive diagnosis which may be confirmed histopathologically. Mononuclear cells in smears of affected lungs of cases of maedi often contain intracytoplasmic inclusions that stain greyish blue with Giemsa.

Differential diagnosis

Maedi must be differentiated from ovine pulmonary adenomatosis and visna from scrapie.

Immunology

In the early stages of infection there is a short viraemia which disseminates the virus to the tissues throughout the body. This stimulates an immune response manifested by the appearance of humoral antibodies and the development of a cell-mediated immunity. A variety of serological tests are available to detect antibodies, such as serum neutralization, complement fixation, agar gel immunodiffusion and ELISA.

Control

Serological surveys have revealed that the prevalence of infection far exceeds the prevalence of clinical morbidity. The ability of the virus to persist in the presence of antibody nullifies the possibility of a vaccine. Disease-free flocks can be maintained by only purchasing animals that have passed two serological tests. The incidence of disease in endemically infected flocks may be depressed by regular 6-monthly serological tests, removing all positive reactors. In small flocks, it may be possible to break the cycle of infection by removing the lambs at birth before they have received colostrum and rearing them by hand in isolation.

Further reading

Dawson, M. (1987). Pathogenesis of maedi-visna. *Veterinary Record*, 120, 451–454.

MALIGNANT CATARRHAL FEVER

Synonyms for malignant catarrhal fever (MCF) include bovine malignant catarrh (BMC), bovine herpesvirus-3 infection and alcephaline herpesvirus-1 infection. MCF is a febrile, frequently fatal, necrotic catarrh of large domesticated ruminants and deer acquired through association with wildebeest and/or sheep.

Aetiology

Two pathogenic agents are involved. One, ACV-1, is a herpesvirus of wildebeest that is a member of the Gamma-herpesvirinae subfamily of the Herpesviridae family of double-stranded DNA viruses, and the other is an as yet unidentified agent (SAA) harboured by sheep. The diseases induced by both agents are clinically identical.

Occurrence

MCF has a worldwide distribution. The wildebeest-associated agent, ACV-1, occurs in Africa and in zoological gardens worldwide. The SAA is found wherever sheep and cattle are husbanded together.

Species affected

ACV-1 virus cycles silently in wildebeest, other alcephalines and oryx. The SAA affects sheep, goats, mouflons and musk-oxen.

The aberrant dead-end hosts of ACV-1 are cattle, deer and elk, and of SAA cattle, banteng and domesticated buffaloes.

Transmission

In wildebeest and alcephalines, the ACV-1 virus passes through the placenta into the foetus. Cell-free virus is shed in the nasal and lacrimal secretions of wildebeest calves undergoing primary infections shortly after birth. Aberrant hosts inhale infected aerosol droplets generated by young wildebeest calves directly or by sniffing contaminated pastures.

The mode of transmission of SAA is unknown. Infections in dead-end hosts, however, are associated with parturition in sheep.

Infected cattle are *not* infectious to other in-contact cattle. Transplacental transmission, however, has been recorded on a few occasions in cattle.

Clinical features

The incubation period in aberrant hosts is approximately 3 weeks, although it is sometimes longer. Outbreaks are seasonal, being linked to the natural parturition seasons of wildebeest and sheep. Nasal and ocular sero-mucoid discharges precede the sudden onset of high fever that persists throughout the course of the disease. Depression is severe and anorexia is total. Hyperplasia of the superficial lymph glands of the head and neck is obvious.

The nasal and oral mucosae are at first deeply congested. Thereafter, petechiae, erosions and diptheresis rapidly develop. The nasal discharges become mucopurulent and fetid and form long tenacious strings. Saliva drools from the mouth. The muzzle becomes dry, cracked and encrusted with exudate and the nostrils become blocked with debris causing respiratory distress. Photophobia causing persistent blinking of the eyes and excessive weeping occurs early in the course of the disease. Both corneas are infiltrated from the periphery by lymphocytes and gradually become opaque. In addition, encephalomyelitis is often manifested by muscular tremors, inco-ordination, torticollis and aggressive behaviour.

Diarrhoea and dysentery occur only occasionally in ACV-1 infections, whereas it is relatively common in SAA infections. Similarly, dermatitis and laminitis are more frequently observed in cases where sheep are incriminated. Areas of hairless skin become red or even purple, exude and become encrusted.

Clinically affected cattle die 4–13 days after the onset of illness. A rare chronic form of the disease may linger on for several weeks. Few clinical cases survive.

Pathology

The carcase is emaciated, soiled and fetid. The spectacular gross lesions are hyperplasia of the cranial and cervical lymph nodes, necrosis of the upper respiratory tract down as far as the bronchi, necrotic stomatitis, pseudo-infarcts in the kidneys, ecchymosis of the urinary bladder mucosa and bilateral corneal opacities. Congestion and haemorrhagic striping of the gastrointestinal tract is commonly noted in SAA infections, but is less common in ACV-1 infections.

The striking histopathological feature is the infiltration of many tissues by large lymphoblastoid cells together with a destruction of smaller lymphocytes. Diffuse areas of necrosis appear in many tissues. A focal fibrinoid necrotizing vasculitis, involving both arteries and veins, is a conspicuous feature and, in the past, was considered diagnostic. Prominent perivascular cuffing together with diffuse encephalitis is usually present.

Diagnosis

A presumptive diagnosis is based on the history, clinical signs and *post mortem* lesions; of particular importance is a history of contact with parturient wildebeest or sheep. Confirmation is most commonly sought by histopathology, for which infected tissues are forwarded in 10% formol-saline. The detection of rising antibody titres to ACV-1 virus has been advocated as a diagnostic tool. ACV-1 virus may be isolated in bovine thyroid or bovine testes cells if they are seeded with whole cells from fresh samples from suspected cases.

Differential diagnosis

A differential diagnosis should include rinderpest, the vesicular diseases, bovine virus diarrhoea and ingestion of caustic substances.

Immunology

Infected animals remain infected for life. ACV-1 virus-induced antibodies in surviving animals are detectable by several serological techniques, such as immunoperoxidase, indirect immunofluorescence, complement fixation and neutralization tests. These humoral antibodies appear in the circulation 8 days before the onset of fever.

Using ACV-1 virus in serological tests, it has been possible to demonstrate the presence of antibodies reactive to ACV-1 virus in sheep from many countries. In addition, in the course of SAA infections in cattle in Europe, North America and Australia, rising titres of antibodies specific for ACV-1 virus develop. Therefore, the evidence strongly supports the hypothesis that SAA is an herpesvirus.

Control

Contact between potential aberrant hosts and natural hosts should be avoided, particularly when parturient and in the weeks thereafter. A successful vaccine has yet to be developed.

Further reading

Plowright, W. (1986). Malignant catarrhal fever. *Revue Scientique et Technique de le l'Office International des Epizooties*, **5**, 897–918.

MOKOLA RABIES

Mokola rabies is a recently recognized neuropathy of cats and dogs caused by Mokola virus, a rabies serotype. The significance of the disease is that cats and dogs vaccinated against classical rabies virus are not protected against infection with Mokola virus.

Aetiology

Mokola virus is a serotype of rabies virus and belongs to the *Lyssavirus* genus of the Rhabdoviridae family of RNA viruses.

Occurrence

Mokola virus was isolated originally from a shrew (*Crocidura* sp.) trapped in the Mokola district of Ibadan in Nigeria. The first isolations of the virus outside West Africa occurred in Zimbabwe.

Species affected

Data are scanty. The natural host in West Africa appears to be the shrew. The virus has also been isolated from the brain of a harsh-furred mouse (*Lophuromys sikapusi*) caught in the Central African Republic. Two human cases have been reported from Nigeria. The first known cases in domesticated animals occurred in cats and dogs in Zimbabwe in the early 1980s. Experimental attempts to infect cats, however, failed, whereas a jackal and a mongoose also experimentally exposed were infected.

Transmission

The saliva of an infected shrew is infectious and the major mode of transmission is through biting. Experimentally the virus has been shown to replicate in *Aedes* mosquitoes, and transovarial transmission has been observed.

Clinical features

The clinical signs of Mokola virus infections in cats and dogs mimic those caused by classical rabies virus. Although the disease evolves through prodromal, excitative and paralytic phases, the dominant sign presented to the clinician is that of "dumb" rabies. Case mortality rates are unknown.

Pathology

Significant gross lesions have not been reported. Microscopic examination revealed extensive meningo-encephalitis with neuronal degeneration and necrosis, gliosis and marked perivascular and meningeal lymphocytic infiltrations. Occasional intracytoplasmic inclusions were present in neurons, but they did not have the inner structure characteristic of classic Negri bodies.

Diagnosis

In the original outbreak in Zimbabwe, fluorescent antibody tests for rabies antigens failed, but subsequent examination revealed very weak fluorescence. White mice inoculated intracerebrally died within 9 days, and their brains showed the same weak fluorescence. A locally prepared conjugate made from serum of guinea-pigs hyperimmunized with Mokola isolates gave strong fluorescence with smears from Mokola virus-infected brains, but it gave poor fluorescence when the smears were prepared from brains infected with classic rabies virus.

Differential diagnosis

Differentiation of Mokola viral infections from classic rabies necessitates isolation of the virus and its identification by cross-neutralization tests in weaned mice.

Immunology

Infected animals that survive develop antibodies that are strongly reactive to Mokola virus and weakly reactive to classic rabies virus. Cats and dogs immunized with live rabies vaccine are not protected against infection with Mokola virus. Trials in experimentally infected mice confirmed the absence of any cross-protection between Mokola and classic rabies viruses.

Control

The current rabies vaccines used to protect domesticated animals will not give protection against Mokola virus infection. All suspect cases of rabies in Africa in previously vaccinated animals should be checked also for the presence of Mokola virus.

Further reading

Foggin, C.M. (1983). Mokola virus infection in cats and dogs in Zimbabwe. *Veterinary Record*, **113**, 115

NAIROBI SHEEP DISEASE

Also known as Kisanyi goat disease, Nairobi sheep disease (NSD) is a tick-borne viral infection of sheep and goats characterized by a febrile, haemorrhagic gastroenteritis in naive animals exposed for the first time to infected rhipicephalic ticks. It is the most pathogenic virus infection of sheep and goats in eastern Africa, with mortality rates in naive sheep of up to 90%.

Aetiology

NSD virus is a member of the *Nairovirus* genus of the Bunyaviridae family of RNA viruses. It is heat labile and closely related to two other tick-borne virus infections, namely, Ganjam virus which provokes a similar disease in sheep and goats in India, and Dugbe virus which infects cattle in West Africa but without inducing clinical reactions. All three viruses cause a mild febrile illness in man characterized by generalized abdominal pain, headache and backache.

Occurrence

The distribution of NSD virus follows the distribution of the principal tick vector, *Rhipicephalus appendiculatus*, and the virus is known to have survived in areas where the disease has occurred but has not been recognized subsequently for many years. Overt disease has been reported form East Africa, Ethiopia, Somalia and Zaire. Serological surveys, however, have revealed a much wider distribution in Africa.

Species affected

NSD virus cycles silently between indigenous sheep and goats and rhipicephalic ticks. Clinical disease occurs when sheep and goats reared in tick-free areas are moved into tick-infested areas or where sheep and goats from tick-infested areas enter tick-free areas while still harbouring infected ticks which in turn feed on and infect naive sheep and goats. Inapparent natural infections also occur in antelopes, and there is some evidence that the common peri-domestic rat of East Africa, *Arvicanthis abyssinicus*, is also naturally infected. Strangely cattle are alleged to be refractory.

The antibody prevalence in man is high in eastern and southern Africa. On rare occasions, naturally acquired infections in man are clinically apparent, but most clinical cases in man are laboratory-acquired infections.

Transmission

The common vector of NSD virus is the brown tick, *R. appendiculatus*, but other species of *Rhipicephalus* and *Amblyomma* ticks occasionally act as vectors. Both trans-stadial and transovarian transmission in the tick occur, but the latter appears to be dependent upon an infective feed at the adult stage. The virus survives for at least 18 months in unfed ticks.

NSD virus has been isolated from a pool of *Culicoides* in East Africa, but the epidemiological significance of the isolation has not been assessed.

Clinical features

The incubation period ranges from 4 to 15 days. Clinical signs in animals reared in areas infested with infected ticks are usually not observed. In contrast, the clinical response of naive adult sheep is peracute, being manifested by the sudden onset of a high fever with marked attendant signs of depression, anorexia, mucopurulent nasal and ocular discharges, dyspnoea and fetid dysentery. Some affected animals die within 3 days, but in others the course of the disease is prolonged for 5–9 days. Surviving pregnant animals abort. The actions in young lambs and kids are not as severe as in adults. Case mortality rates may approach 90%.

Pathology

The striking gross lesions at *post-mortem* are the severe haemorrhagic gastroenteritis and the hyperplasia of all lymphoid tissues. In addition, petechiae often stud the epicardium and ecchymoses involve the endocardium. Dermal haemorrhages have been observed in foetuses of pregnant ewes that die. Microscopic examination reveals a glomerulo-tubular nephritis, myocardial necrosis and coagulative necrosis of the gall bladder.

Diagnosis

If there is a history of recent movement of naive animals into a tick-infested area, the clinical signs and *post mortem* lesions will give rise to a presumptive diagnosis of NSD. In contrast, a presumptive diagnosis of NSD is not readily considered when the outbreak occurs in a tick-free area. Confirmation requires isolation of the causal virus, either in BHK 21 cells or in infant mice, and its identification by immunofluorescence or immunoperoxidase staining. The specimens required are blood in anticoagulant collected from febrile cases and pieces of spleen and mesenteric lymph node from dead animals, and they should be forwarded to the laboratory in fresh wet ice.

Differential diagnosis

The differentiation of haemorrhagic gastroenteropathies in tropical sheep and goats is difficult. In some areas, the possibility of goat plague and rinderpest must be considered. Diagnostic confusion also arises with coccidiosis, parasitic gastroenteritis and salmonellosis.

Immunology

A natural attack confers in survivors a lifelong immunity associated with the production of humoral antibodies. A cryptic record dating back to the 1930s hints that persistence or latency of the virus may occur; the report has yet to be confirmed or refuted.

Control

Infections of NSD virus are silent in endemic areas and the infection does not warrant the application of control measures there. Sheep and goats imported into tick-infested areas, however, should be vaccinated prophylactically before movement or as soon as possible after they arrive. Attenuated and inactivated methanol-precipitated vaccines are available, the latter being the more efficient.

Further reading

Davies, F.G. and Mwakima, F. (1982). Qualitative studies of the transmission of Nairobi sheep disease virus by *Rhipicephalus appendiculatus (Ixiododia ixodidae)*. *Journal of Comparative Pathology*, **92**, 15–20.

ORF

Synonyms for orf include contagious pustular dermatitis, contagious ecthyma and soremouth. Orf is a benign zoonotic pox of sheep and goats characterized by the development of eroded granulomas on mucosal sites and encrusted granulomas on dermal sites.

Aetiology

Orf virus is a member of the *Parapoxvirus* genus of the Poxviridae family of DNA viruses. In moist conditions the virus is relatively heat labile, but when desiccated the virus will survive for years at room temperature. It resembles and is related to the other members of the *Parapoxvirus* genus.

Occurrence

Orf is distributed worldwide and is probably the most common viral disease of sheep. The prevalence of epidemics tends to be biannual, the first peak being associated with the disease in sucking lambs and a later second peak when the disease attacks naive stock lambs. Sporadic clinical cases, however, may be observed at any time.

Species affected

Orf is a disease of domesticated and wild sheep and goats. Man and dogs are also susceptible.

Transmission

The source of new outbreaks in sucking lambs is believed to be a flare up of a persistent infection in a stressed ewe following parturition. The virus thereafter spreads rapidly to the other lambs in the flock, both directly and indirectly. Morbidity approaches 100% in lambs reared indoors and ranges from 30 to 60% on the range. An essential precursor for infection, however, is the necessity for a break in the integument of the skin or lips. Ewes nursing affected lambs often develop crops of transient lesions on their teats which sometimes lead to mastitis. Susceptible weaned lambs acquire infection when sold through markets as store animals.

Man is frequently infected through handling infected animals, but man-to-man infection appears to be rare. Dogs and hounds become infected when fed affected carcases.

Clinical features

Orf is regarded as a benign non-febrile affliction, but nevertheless, it has been known on rare occasions to kill. In some countries, deaths from secondary myiasis are not uncommon.

The basic lesion is a papule that enlarges to become a granuloma, which is seen in its purest form when the peri-odontal gums of sucking lambs are attacked. It is seen in its grossest form as a giant granuloma super-infected with many fungi and *Dermatophilus congolensis*, a lesion commonly described in many textbooks as strawberry foot-rot. Mucosal granulomas become eroded and ulcerated. On dermal sites, orf granulomas are encrusted. The lesions in sucking lambs tend to be peri-orbital and peri-labial, whereas those in store lambs are usually found on the legs and in the interdigital clefts. Any wound, however, may become infected, e.g. ear notches, castration wounds and tail amputation sites. In ewes, the teats become encrusted with multiple lesions.

Persistent orf infections have been identified in hornless rams, the site of the virus being the keratinized knobs on the crown of the head associated with the trauma of butting. The site of persistent infections in ewes has yet to be discovered. The course of the primary infection is 4–6 weeks. Giant orf granulomas, however, take up to 6 months to resolve.

Pathology

Orf granulomas are found only on the skin and on the mucous membranes of the upper alimentary tract and the lower urogenital tract. The histopathology of the lesions is characterized by hyperplasia of the dermal papillae, ballooning degeneration of epithelial cells and intracytoplasmic inclusion bodies early in the course of the infection.

Diagnosis

Although a clinical diagnosis is easy, misdiagnoses are common when the granulomas appear on sites other than the head, legs and teats. The scabs covering dermal sites are firmly adherent and if removed forcibly reveal a forest of swollen dermal papillae which quickly flood with blood. The under-surface of the scab is a cast of the swollen dermal papillae and is pitted with holes.

The samples required for the confirmation of a provisional diagnosis are scrapings of the surface of the granuloma or the scab from early lesions.

Differential diagnosis

Sheep pox and orf are frequently confused. Similarly, bluetongue was mistaken for orf for many years in Texas. Eroded granulomas on the surface of the tongue have been diagnosed as foot-and-mouth disease.

Treatment

The resolution of the lesions is significantly enhanced by intermittent injections of low immunosuppressive doses of levamisole hydrochloride. Frequent applications of ointment formulations of antiviral drugs such as idoxuridine and acyclovir have been claimed to speed resolution.

Immunology

Humoral antibodies play a minor role in the host defence and antibodies transferred in the colostrum do not protect sucking lambs. Cellular immunity is probably the major clearance mechanism. Reinfections are manifested in 95% of previously infected animals by accelerated immune reactions characterized by the development of transient orf granulomas, the course of the lesion being limited to 1–2 weeks.

Control

In the absence of endemic orf, vaccination is contraindicated. Live vaccines, however, do have a role to play in deliberately infecting in-contact animals in the face of an outbreak. The technique ensures that the outbreak will be contained within 6–10 weeks, instead of grumbling on for 3–4 months. Vaccines should also be used to protect fattening lambs and cast ewes moved from disease-free farms to endemic farms, the animals being vaccinated as soon as possible after arrival.

Further reading

Robinson, A.J. and Balassu, T.C. (1981). Contagious pustular dermatitis (orf). *Veterinary Bulletin*, **51**, 771–782.

OVINE PULMONARY ADENOMATOSIS

Synonyms for ovine pulmonary adenomatosis (OPA) include jaagsiekte and driving sickness. OPA is a contagious slow progressive lung tumour of sheep characterized by a production of a copious secretion into the respiratory tract leading to dyspnoea, wasting and death.

Aetiology

The causal agent has not been unequivocably identified, but a prime suspect is a lentivirus of the Retroviridae family of RNA viruses.

Occurrence

OPA is widespread throughout the world except Australasia.

Species affected

The major victims are sheep, but occasionally goats are affected. Diseased animals are not usually detected before they are 2–3 years old. On rare occasions, however, OPA has been diagnosed in lambs as young as 5 months.

Transmission

OPA is a contagious disease transmitted in aerosols when there is close direct contact between healthy and affected sheep. Transplacental transmission does not occur.

Clinical features

Morbidity in flocks endemically infected is low. In contrast, morbidity is high with losses of up to 60% when a previously disease-free flock becomes infected. The incubation period extends over several months and even years and the onset of illness is insidious, progressing slowly into a non-febrile chronic pneumonia. Affected sheep breathe sharper and deeper and lag behind the rest of the flock when they are moved.

They remain bright and alert at first and do not lose their appetite. The respiratory distress becomes progressively worse and their breathing becomes noisy due to air bubbling through the copious fluids secreted into the respiratory tract. Simultaneously, there is progressive emaciation. Death is the inevitable sequel after a prolonged clinical course of several months. It is sometimes precipitated by a secondary pasteurella pneumonia.

Pathology

The tumours involve only the lungs and the pulmonary lymph nodes. The lungs do not collapse when the thorax is opened and the tumour lesions are readily recognized as sharply demarcated fawn-grey areas which when cut have a granular surface and ooze a frothy fluid. A frothy fluid also fills the trachea and bronchial passages. The microscopic lesion is an alveolar adenomata.

Diagnosis

The so-called wheelbarrow test aids a presumptive diagnosis in the field; when the hind legs of an affected sheep are raised so that the head is lower than the thorax, a frothy sero-mucoid fluid flows from the nostrils. The volume of the fluid ranges from 25–500 ml/day. Histopathology will confirm a presumptive diagnosis.

Differential diagnosis

The principal diagnostic confusion occurs with cases of maedi. Histopathology differentiates between these diseases.

Immunology

In the absence of conclusive evidence as to the nature of the causal agent, the immune response of affected sheep is unknown.

Control

Specific tests to pick out affected sheep in the early stages of the disease are not available. If sheep are detected or suspected, they should be culled and they should be separated from healthy sheep. If possible, newly purchased sheep should be segregated from the rest of the flock for several years. It has been suggested that it should be possible to establish an OPA-free flock by removing lambs at birth, segregating them and feeding them with colostrum from OPA-free ewes.

Further reading

Sharp, J.M. (1981). Slow virus infections of the respiratory tract of sheep. *Veterinary Record*, **108**, 391–393.

PIG POX

Pig pox or swine pox is a benign pox exclusive to pigs, characterized by the appearance of numerous encrusted pustular weals in the skin of the abdomen and groin and, less commonly, the back. Mortality is rare except in neonates.

Aetiology

Pig pox virus is the only member of the *Suipoxvirus* genus of the Poxviridae family of DNA viruses.

Occurrence

Pig pox has a worldwide distribution.

Species affected

Pig pox virus affects only pigs and experimentally it can only be grown in cells derived from pigs. Naive pigs of all ages are affected when exposed to the virus. Most epidemics, however, occur in sucking and newly weaned pigs.

Transmission

The common mode of transmission is through the activities of the sucking pig louse (*Haematopinus suis*) and stable flies (*Stomoxys calcitrans*). Louse-associated lesions are found on the abdomen and groin, whereas stable fly-associated lesions appear along the back. In addition to arthropod-vector transmission, there is strong evidence of vertical transmission *in utero*; for example, pig pox virus has been recovered from generalized cutaneous lesions observed on stillborn piglets.

Clinical features

The incubation period ranges from 4 to 14 days and the course of the disease lasts 5–6 weeks. At the onset of the macular rash the pigs are quiet, eat less and have a slight transient fever. The macules quickly become papules, which in turn become pustular and umbilicated exuding serum which encrusts in the centre. Although the encrustations are at first red-brown, they rapidly blacken. The pocks are circular, 1–2 cm in diameter and have a peripheral hyperaemic ring conspicuous in light skin pigs. Lesions on the lips and tongues of sucking pigs commonly spread to the teats of the nursing sows. Encrustation is complete 10 days after the onset of the macular rash, and the scabs drop off 3–4 weeks later. The healed skin is not scarred.

Most outbreaks of pig pox are uncomplicated, but occasionally cutaneous streptococcal abscesses have been observed concurrently.

Pathology

Pocks occur only on the skin and on the mucous membrane of the oral cavity. Lymph nodes draining affected skin show slight lymphadenitis. Microscopic examination reveals changes typical of pox infections, including ballooning degeneration and eosinophilic intracytoplasmic inclusion bodies. Pig pox infections, however, may be distinguished from vaccinia infections of pigs by the presence of intranuclear vacuoles.

Diagnosis

A provisional diagnosis is based upon the history, particularly the history of the presence of lice and/or stable flies, and the clinical appearance of the lesions. Specimens required for confirmation of a provisional diagnosis are scraping of the lesions and scabs from early lesions.

Differential diagnosis

In the past, the most common confusion arose with vaccinia infections spread from recently vaccinated human beings. Today, confusion is most likely to arise from an exudative epidermatitis, often seen in sucking pigs, the aetiology of which is unknown. The restricted distribution of the vesicles of foot-and-mouth disease differentiate it from pig pox.

Immunology

Pigs that have recovered from pig pox are alleged to be totally refractory to reinfection. Recovery is associated with the production of antibodies, detectable by agar gel precipitation tests and by counter-immunoelectrophoresis.

Control

The age-related prevalence of pig pox indicates that the infection is more widespread than commonly accepted, but there is no demand for a vaccine to control the disease. Essential preventive measures are the control of lice and insects.

Further reading

Olufemi, B.E., Ayoade, G.O., Ikede, B.O. and Akpevie, S.O. (1981). Swine pox in Nigeria. *Veterinary Record*, **109**, 278–280.

PSEUDOLUMPY SKIN DISEASE/BOVINE MAMMILLITIS

Synonyms include bovid herpesvirus-2 infection, Allerton virus disease, bovine herpes mammillitis, bovine ulcerative mammillitis and dermopathic herpes.

Pseudolumpy skin disease and bovine mammillitis are different clinical manifestations of the same herpesvirus infection. Pseudolumpy skin disease is characterized by a low-grade transient fever and by exudative cutaneous plaques. Bovine mammillitis is non-febrile and the plaques are localized to the skin of the teats and udder. Trauma at milking quickly converts the plaques into ulcers which become encrusted.

Aetiology

Bovid herpesvirus-2, the causative agent, is a rapidly growing member of the Alpha-herpesvirinae subfamily of the Herpesviridae family of DNA viruses.

Occurrence

The pseudolumpy skin disease syndrome is endemic in eastern and southern Africa and the USA. The bovine mammillitis syndrome occurs in Australia, Europe and the USA.

Species affected

The syndromes of pseudolumpy skin disease and bovine mammillitis have only been observed in cattle. However, the virus has also been isolated from ulcers in the upper alimentary tract of dead debilitated African buffaloes. Although no disease has been observed, antibodies have been detected in the sera of bushbuck, eland, giraffe, hippopotamus, impala, oryx and waterbuck.

Transmission

Both syndromes have a seasonal prevalence and biting insects are believed to initiate infection. Traumatized skin appears to be the favoured site for virus multiplication.

Clinical features

Pseudolumpy skin disease syndrome. The disease is first manifested after an incubation period of 5–9 days by the development of a moderate fever and mild lymphadenitis. Within a few days, numerous cutaneous plaques emerge. They are circular or oval with a diameter of 1 cm, are hard and firm and have a red periphery. Over the next 3 days, the plaques enlarge to a diameter of 3–5 cm. Their centres are depressed, exude, and form a thin brown crust. The skin beneath the crust dies and peals off 2 weeks later, leaving a bald patch of new skin covered with fine grey scales. New hair covers the site within 2 months. The number of plaques ranges from 1 to 2 to many, and they may be found at any cutaneous site, the most common being the face, neck, back and perineum.

Mammillitis syndrome. Lesions of bovine mammillitis are most commonly seen in first calving heifers, 2–3 days after parturition. The lesions develop more frequently on the teats than on the udders. The disease is first manifested by the appearance of painful plaques. They are round in shape and have a diameter of between 1 and 3 cm, and the skin covering them has a reddish-blue colour. They quickly ulcerate. In mild cases, the ulceration is superficial and pain is absent or limited, but in more severe cases the ulcers become confluent and may involve two-thirds of the circumference of the teat. They exude profusely and become encrusted. The resulting scabs are removed in the process of milking, leaving extensive painful lesions. Some ulcers on the teats spread to involve the skin of the udders. Acute mastitis is a common sequel and it arises as a result of the sensitivity of the teats which prevents the animals being milked normally. Calves sucking affected cows become infected after an incubation period of about 10 days and they develop ulcerative lesions on the muzzle, buccal mucosa and tongue, together with fever and loss of condition.

The course of the disease varies with the number and severity of the lesions, ranging from 2 to 6 weeks in mild cases, to 2–3 months in those with extensive ulceration. Some severely affected animals have to be slaughtered.

Pathology

Pathological changes are limited to the sites of the lesions. Histopathological examination of biopsies reveals numerous syncytia with intranuclear inclusions in fresh samples. Samples taken a few hours later show evidence of severe necrosis of epidermal cells with heavy infiltration with polymorphonuclear cells.

Diagnosis

Pseudolumpy skin disease syndrome. The benign nature of pseudolumpy skin disease is such that many clinical cases are missed. A presumptive diagnosis is readily confirmed histopathologically by electron microscopic examination of a biopsy sample of an early lesion or by isolation of the virus in bovine testes or bovine kidney cells.

Mammillitis syndrome. A presumptive diagnosis of bovine mammillitis is based upon the history and the clinical signs. Specific confirmation is readily achieved by histopathological or electron microscopic examination of biopsies and by virus isolation.

Differential diagnosis

Pseudolumpy skin disease is not important, but in Africa it confuses the diagnosis of the much more serious lumpy skin disease. Histopathological examinations of biopsy will readily distinguish the two virus infections. Bovine mammillitis tends to be more severe than other teat conditions of cattle, such as pseudocowpox, cow pox, foot-and-mouth disease and vesicular stomatitis. Nevertheless, it may be necessary to isolate the virus or demonstrate its presence by electron microscopy.

Treatment

Treatment of cases of pseudolumpy skin disease is not warranted. Treatment of bovine mammillitis, however, should be attempted by using bland emolients. Ointment formulations of anti-DNA viral preparations will probably speed healing, but their use is contraindicated in milking cattle where the milk is intended for human consumption.

Vaccines are not available commercially, although experimental vaccines have shown some promise. Wild virus, injected intramuscularly, provides protection.

Immunology

Latency in recovered animals has been suspected, but attempts to prove it have failed. Antibodies in recovered animals allegedly render them immune for at least 4 years. They are readily detected by ELISA.

Further reading

Connor, R.J. and Mukangi, D.J.A. (1986). Concurrent outbreak of pseudo-lumpy skin disease and acute *Trypanosoma vivax* infection in cattle. *Tropical Animal Health and Production*, **18**, 127–132.
Scott, F.M.M. and Holliman, A (1986). Outbreak of bovine herpes mammillitis in Cumbria. *Veterinary Record*, **118**, 81–82.

RABIES

Synonyms for rabies include hydrophobia, lyssa and classic rabies. Rabies is a viral infection of mammals, transmitted in the saliva of a rabid animal and usually, but not always, manifested by a fatal encephalomyelitis.

Aetiology

Rabies virus is a member of the *Lyssavirus* genus of the Rhabdoviridae family of RNA viruses. The *Lyssavirus* genus contains six official serotypes, namely, rabies, Lagos bat, Mokola, Duvenhaag, Obodhiang and Kotonkan. There are, however, several other ill-defined agents which may well be serotypes of rabies. A report in late 1989 raised the number of rabies serotypes to 25 but the authenticity of many of these has yet to be confirmed.

The most important serotype is rabies virus; however, in addition, two other serotypes are known to be fatal for man, namely Duvenhaag and Mokola virus. Mokola virus has recently caused an epidemic of a rabies-like disease of cats and dogs in Zimbabwe.

Occurrence

Rabies virus occurs worldwide, except in Antarctica and Australasia. Several countries which are islands or have short land boundaries are also free of the disease.

Species affected

All mammals are susceptible, but the most important hosts are bats and carnivores. Rabies is not a major disease of food animals, except in cattle in Latin America.

Ecologically, rabies virus occupies two distinct niches – a sylvatic and an urban niche. The sylvatic niche is widespread and the maintenance hosts of the virus in the sylvatic niche vary with the geographical location. In South and Central America, the maintenance host is the vampire bat, in Europe and North America the fox, in Africa and Asia the jackal, in the Middle East and Eastern Europe wolves, in North America skunks – and, recently, the raccoon – and in India and South Africa the mongoose. Cattle are the common aberrant hosts involved in sylvatic rabies.

The maintenance host in the urban niche is the dog, particularly the stray dog. Urban rabies is a major public health problem in affected countries and poses a major hazard to veterinarians working in those countries.

Transmission

Rabid animals usually excrete virus in their saliva 2 days before they show clinical signs and throughout the course of the disease which normally lasts less than 10 days. In addition, dogs in Africa and Asia have on occasion been known to survive rabies and excrete the virus in their saliva for months. Similarly, vampire bats will excrete rabies virus for several months. Transmission usually occurs when infected saliva is deposited in a bite wound. Less common routes of transmission include the following: transplacental infection in the skunk; aerosol infection in bat caves; and ingestion of an infected carrier. Iatrogenic transmission has occurred in man following transplants of corneas taken from an infected patient.

Two of the official rabies serotypes, Obodhiang and Kotonkan, are arthropod-borne; the remainder are transmitted by biting animals.

Rabies virus deposited in a bite wound penetrates striated muscle cells where either it multiplies or becomes sequestered as a sub-viral particle. Within a few hours, newly formed virus particles enter the peripheral nervous system through the neuromuscular spindles and move passively through the axoplasm to the spinal ganglia and hence into the cord and brain to multiply in neurons. Thereafter, the virus spreads from the central nervous system passively in the axoplasm of peripheral nerves; in particular, it moves down the lingual nerve to the salivary glands where it multiplies in acinar cells. Infection of other non-neural cells also occurs, e.g. in the cells of the cornea and hair follicles.

The mechanism whereby the virus that is sequestered in the muscle cells at the site of the wound is triggered to initiate rabies replication in the nervous system is not known. Sequestration of the virus, however, is believed to be responsible for the occasional very prolonged incubation period that has been recorded.

Clinical features

In most clinical cases of rabies, the incubation period is 3–8 weeks, but authenticated reports double this and there are documented incubation periods of up to 1 year.

The course of the clinical disease ranges from 2 to 10 days. There are three clinical phases: prodromal, excitative and paralytic. If the excitative phase dominates, the clinician refers to "furious" rabies, but if the paralytic phase dominates, then the clinical description is "dumb" rabies.

The prodromal phase is manifested by a change in the normal behaviour of the animal, e.g. friendly dogs become irritable and fierce dogs become affectionate. Affected cattle stray away from the herd and affected dairy cows stop milking. The prodromal period in dogs lasts 2–3 days, in cats about 1 day and in cattle it is measured in a few hours.

In the excitative phase, affected animals are hypersensitive, very restless and will attack and bite without warning. There is usually a voice change; dogs, for example, develop a characteristic low-pitched hoarse howling, cats mew continuously, cattle grind their teeth and bellow constantly in a low-pitched voice, sheep bleat incessantly and horses frequently grind their teeth and whinny and may be diagnosed as having acute colic. All species are sexually stimulated. Dogs develop a depraved appetite. The furious phase lasts 1–4 days.

The paralytic phase is a progressive motor paralysis which begins posteriorly, and which is followed by flaccid paralysis and death. Affected animals are quiet and not irritable and only bite when provoked. They cannot eat or drink and drool saliva.

Pathology

Gross lesions are conspicuous by their absence. The presence of foreign bodies, such as sticks, stones and pieces of metal, in a dog's stomach is indicative of the depraved appetite of the dog.

Characteristic microscopic lesions are found in the central nervous system. A non-suppurative encephalomyelitis is manifested by perivascular cuffing and gliosis. In addition, there is neuronal degeneration and the presence of inclusions known as Negri bodies in the cytoplasm of affected neurons is diagnostic. They range in size from 2 to 8 μm and may be round or oval and contain an inner matrix or basophilic granules. Negri bodies are most readily detected in the neurons of the hippocampus of affective carnivores and in the Purkinje cells of herbivores.

Diagnosis

The provisional diagnosis is based upon the history and the clinical signs. Suspect cases should be isolated in secure premises and held for 10 days. Death, however, is not an inevitable sequel.

Confirmation of rabies in a live animal is achieved either by examining impression smears of the eyeball or cryostat sections of a biopsy of an outer edge of a tactile hair follicle using direct immunofluorescence.

When an animal dies, the head should be removed and forwarded on ice to the diagnostic laboratory. Do not attempt to remove the brain or brain stem in the absence of a suitable vice. The cranium is opened, the brain removed and Ammon's horn is exposed. Impression smears of the cut surface of Ammon's horn and squash smears of pieces of tissue from Ammon's horn are prepared. While wet, some preparations are dipped into Seller's stain. The others are air-dried, fixed in acetone and coated with antibody conjugated with fluorescein isothiocyanate. If inclusion bodies or specific antigen are not detected, then suspensions of brain tissue are prepared and inoculated intracerebrally into mice. The mice are examined daily for 21 days and any that die are examined for specific immunofluorescence.

Differential diagnosis

All cases of encephalomyelitis in animals in countries where rabies is endemic should be handled as if they were rabies until proven otherwise. If rabid signs develop in vaccinated animals in Africa, infection with the Mokola serotype of rabies should be considered.

Treatment

Vigorous symptomatic treatment of human patients with clinical signs of rabies have been known to save lives. The technique is not recommended for animals.

In man, personal prophylaxis following a bite from a suspect animal is important. The wound should be thoroughly irrigated and scrubbed with plenty of water and soap to remove the contaminating saliva and to abrade the affected tissues. Medical advice should be sought thereafter.

Veterinarians and other high-risk personnel should be vaccinated before exposure to rabies. Booster doses of vaccines should be administered as soon as possible after exposure.

Immunology

Both non-specific and specific immunological responses protect the host against rabies. Both live attenuated and adjuvanted inactivated vaccines are used to protect animals. They are prepared either from embryonated eggs or cell cultures. A few countries still use inactivated vaccines prepared from infected brain tissues. However, these are not recommended as they are not efficient.

Control

Rabies-free countries apply the most stringent regulations in respect of the importation of animals from rabies-infected areas. All imports are quarantined for several months, and in many countries the animals are vaccinated with an inactivated vaccine immediately upon entering the country.

Urban dog rabies is best controlled by destroying stray dogs and licensing and vaccinating all other dogs. Legislative powers and penalties are essential.

Tremendous strides have been made in the past decade to limit the spread of sylvatic rabies. In particular, the control of rabies in foxes by the systematic distribution of baits laced with vaccine has yielded spectacular results. The control of vampire bat rabies in Latin America depends primarily on vaccination of the bovine hosts, supplemented by the injection of anticoagulants into cattle which, while harmless to the cattle, kill bats. The control of other forms of sylvatic rabies is fragmentary and relies on public awareness of the risks.

Further reading

Kuwert, E.M., Merieux, C., Koprowski, H. and Bogel, K. (eds) (1985). *Rabies in the tropics*. Berlin; Springer-Verlag.

RIFT VALLEY FEVER

Synonyms for Rift Valley fever (RVF) include infectious enzootic hepatitis of sheep and cattle, and Zinga virus disease. RVF is a mosquito-borne infection of domesticated ruminants, camels and man, characterized by acute fever, hepatitis and death in young animals and by abortion in pregnant animals. Human infections in the past were not considered to be serious, being manifested as an influenza-like illness; however, in recent years, a fatal haemorrhagic form of RVF has emerged and it is classified now as one of the most dangerous pathogens of man.

Aetiology

RVF virus is a member of the *Phlebovirus* genus of the Bunyaviridae family of single-stranded RNA viruses. It is stable outside the host, retaining its infectivity under adverse environmental conditions.

Occurrence

RVF virus is widely distributed in Africa, but major epidemic episodes in animals and humans are relatively rare, occurring in 5-to 20-year cycles. The virus survives in the interepidemic periods in mosquito eggs, laid on vegetation in dambos which are shallow depressions in the forest edges. Dambos are only flooded in years when the rainfall is so excessive that it raises the water-table. The eggs then hatch and a new population of infected mosquitoes emerges. RVF may have been introduced into Egypt and Mauritania with cattle carrying infected *Myalommia* ticks.

Species affected

Clinical disease has only been observed in sheep, goats, cattle, camels, domesticated buffaloes and man. Antibodies, however, have been detected in a wide variety of hosts, but there is doubt as to how specific these are because the 30 members of the *Phlebovirus* genus cross-react. There is a remarkable age-related innate resistance to RVF virus; the case mortality rate in lambs less than 1 week old exceeds 90% whereas the rate in lambs over 1 week old drops to 20%. Apart from abortion, infection in adult animals is subacute. Modern isolates of the virus, however, are highly virulent for man.

Transmission

Epidemics in domesticated animals are initiated by the bites of infected mosquitoes. Thereafter, infected aerosols generated by virus-infected aborted fluids spread the disease rapidly through the flock or herd. Man is usually infected by the aerosol route through handling infected animals or tissues in the laboratory. Many species of *Culex* and *Aedes* mosquitoes are implicated in the transmission of RVF during epidemics, but the mosquito that lays infected drought-resistant eggs is *Aedes meintoshi*.

Clinical features

The incubation period may be as short as 12 hours or as long as 96 hours. Most, if not all, infected pregnant sheep, cattle and camels abort affected foetuses. Peracute reactions occur in newborn lambs which die within hours of infection. Acute reactions occur in older lambs and calves and very occasionally in adult sheep. Affected animals have a high fever, vomit and stagger, collapsing and dying when the fever regresses

24–48 hours later. Other prominent signs are a profuse purulent nasal discharge and sometimes a haemorrhagic diarrhoea.

Subacute reactions occur in adult sheep, cattle and camels. There is a low-grade fever, partial inappetence and general weakness. Jaundice is prominent. Lactation stops temporarily. Mortality is low in adult animals and many undergo inapparent infections.

Uncomplicated RVF in man runs a course of 4–7 days. The clinical signs mimic acute influenza and consist of a transient fever, severe muscle pain, headache, photobia and anorexia. Full recovery occurs. RVF encephalitis in man is characterized by a biphasic febrile episode, with the central nervous system signs developing during the second febrile wave. These consist of irritation, confusion, stupor and sometimes coma. Other patients show hypersalivation, teeth grinding, visual hallucination and vertigo. Partial or full recovery occurs after 50 days. RVF retinitis is evident 1–3 weeks after the primary febrile illness and is associated with the development of retinal lesions, which are usually bilateral. Half the patients have a permanent loss of central vision. Haemorrhagic RVF is a new disease, first observed in South Africa in 1975. It is characterized by a very acute febrile illness, accompanied with jaundice. Widespread haemorrhages develop in 2–4 days, and death usually occurs within another 3–6 days. A few patients recover after a long slow convalescence.

Pathology

The basic lesion is a focal necrosis of the liver, but in young animals the foci coalesce to form a diffuse necrotic lesion; the liver is bright yellow and studded with subcapsular haemorrhages. It is not enlarged. In slaughtered affected adult sheep or cattle, the focal necrosis of the liver is discrete. In addition to the hepatitis, there are haemorrhages in most other organs and tissues. Microscopic examination of the liver reveals well-defined primary foci of severe coagulative necrosis, which are predominantly centrilobular. Hyaline intracytoplasmic inclusions occur and, occasionally, eosinophilic intranuclear inclusions may be detected.

Diagnosis

Index cases are usually misdiagnosed, but once an epidemic is underway the field diagnosis is relatively easy. Rapid confirmation may be achieved by examining cryostat sections of the liver for antigen by immunofluorescence. If necessary, virus can be isolated from the liver, spleen or serum from affected animals by the inoculation of mice or cell cultures. Retrospective serological diagnosis is useful to measure the extent of an epidemic, but it is essential to use neutralization tests and not haemagglutination-inhibition tests.

Differential diagnosis

Wesselsbron disease mimics RVF clinically and differentiation requires laboratory facilities. The prominent hepatic lesion in aborted foetuses and dead neonates helps to distinguish RVF from other causes of abortion in cattle and sheep.

Immunology

The active resistance engendered by a natural attack is lifelong. Passive protection is conferred on the sucking young through the ingestion of colostrum which will protect for about 5 months.

Control

Because of the long gaps between epidemics, routine annual vaccination is rarely attempted. In East Africa, an early warning system has been established with the meteorological department, which alerts the veterinary authorities when there is a high risk of the water-table being raised. Vaccination of the animals at risk can then be initiated before the epidemic starts. Both inactivated and attenuated virus vaccines are used, the former being considered to be more appropriate for pregnant animals. Veterinarians and laboratory personnel at risk should be immunized. An experimental formalin-inactivated virus vaccine grown in diploid foetal-raised, lung cells is available from the Salk Institute, PO Box 25, Swiftwater, Pennsylvania, USA.

Further reading

Shimshony, B. and Barzilai, R. (1983). Rift Valley fever. *Advances in Veterinary Science and Comparative Medicine*, **27**, 347–425.

ROTAVIRUS DIARRHOEA

Rotaviruses are one of the major causes of diarrhoea in neonatal animals.

Aetiology

The causal viruses belong to the *Rotavirus* genus of the Reoviridae family of double-stranded RNA viruses. There are many serotypes, most of which are host-specific. They are stable over a wide pH range and resist lipid solvents. The only active disinfectants are iodophors and phenol compounds. Proteolytic enzymes in the small intestine of most animals enhance infectivity. Rotaviruses are particularly prevalent on premises where animals are reared intensively.

Species affected

Rotaviruses cause diarrhoea in calves, foals, lambs and piglets. Some types infect and produce disease in babies. Clinical disease is age-related, seldom occurring in animals less then 1 week old or over 2 months old. Infections in adult animals are clinically inapparent.

Transmission

Rotaviruses are shed in the faeces of infected animals and survive at ambient temperatures in faeces for several months. Faecal contamination of water supplies also leads to spread of infection.

Clinical features

The incubation period is less than 24 hours. Columnar epithelial cells of the duodenum and ileum are destroyed by rotaviruses and are replaced by cuboidal cells without a brush border. Maladsorption and diarrhoea follow. Death is attributable to dehydration and/or secondary bacterial infection, but most animals recover within 3–4 days. The absorptive function of the gut, however, is impaired for several weeks. The severity of the enteritis ranges from the production of soft faeces to profuse watery diarrhoea with yellow-coloured faeces. The fluid loss causes severe dehydration.

Pathology

Young animals dying from severe rotavirus infection have sunken eyes and are severely dehydrated, soiled and fetid. The spectacular gross lesion is distension of the intestine with fluid consisting of unadsorbed milk and water. Lung changes, if present, are associated with secondary bacterial infection.

Diagnosis

The clinical signs and *post mortem* lesions together with the age-related incidence are not pathognomonic. Diagnosis requires the detection of the virus in the faeces, the most rapid method being polyacrylamide gel electrophoresis, which separates the RNA genomic segments for comparison with control rotavirus segments. Commercial kits are available which employ ELISA antigen-capture techniques. If an electron microscope is available, virus particles in the faeces may be detected after negative staining and identified by immuno-aggregation by specific antiserum. Serological testing for antibodies will identify endemically infected herds.

Differential diagnosis

In addition to dietary-induced gastroenteritis, numerous other pathogens cause diarrhoea in newborn animals. They include salmonella, enteropathogenic strains of *Escherichia coli* and chlamydia. Cryptosporidia protozoa are also frequently incriminated. In addition, coronavirus diarrhoea may cause diagnostic confusion.

Immunology

Rotaviruses are widely distributed, and most adult domesticated animals have antibodies. Antibodies passively transferred in the colostrum give some protection to neonates.

Control

At the onset of diarrhoea, affected animals should be taken off milk and fed water and electrolyte solutions containing glucose for 30 hours. Antibiotics have a role to play in combating secondary bacterial infection.

The significant prophylactic measures are (1) a reduction in the stocking density, (2) prevention of a build-up of faecal contamination in rearing houses by regular cleansing, and (3) vaccination of the dam to boost the antibody level in the colostrum and milk over a longer period. Inactivated vaccines are now commercially available.

Further reading

Snodgrass, D.R., Terzolo, H.R., Sherwood, D., Campbell. I., Lees, J.E. and Synge, B.A. (1986). Aetiology of diarrhoea in young calves. *Veterinary Record*, **119**, 31–34.

SCRAPIE

Scrapie is an infectious and progressively degenerative fatal encephalopathy of goats and sheep.

Aetiology

The nature of the infectious agent of scrapie has yet to be confirmed. The most likely candidate is a tiny genome of single-stranded DNA protected by protein and wrapped around fibrils of host protein. It resists destruction by chemical and physical treatments which inactivate bacteria and conventional viruses. It is not unique, being a member of a group of several unconventional degenerative diseases of the nervous system, such as Creutzfeldt-Jakob disease and Kuru in man, chronic wasting disease in North American deer, transmissible mink encephalopathy and, probably, to the recently discovered bovine spongeiform encephalopathy.

Occurrence

Scrapie has spread to North America, Africa and Asia with the export of sheep from Europe.

Species affected

Natural infections of scrapie are most common in sheep, but they also occur in goats. A recently identified host gene controls the rate of the agent's replication and hence the length of the incubation period. Transmissible mink encephalopathy was induced in mink fed scrapie-infected sheep carcases. The source of bovine spongiform encephalopathy is believed to have a similar source.

Transmission

The major mode of transmission of the scrapie agent is by the vertical route. Some lambs are probably infected pre-natally, but the majority are affected in the early post-natal period. Foetal membranes from infected ewes are infectious and horizontal spread of the agent occurs when they are eaten by a susceptible sheep. Because of the hardiness of the scrapie agent, susceptible sheep grazing contaminated pastures are at risk.

Clinical features

The incubation period is long; typically, sheep infected as neonates exhibit the first clinical signs a few weeks after they have given birth for the second time, i.e. when they are at least 3 years old. The disease is non-febrile and the onset insidious. Experienced shepherds note a change in the animals' behaviour and they test their suspicions by kneading a fold of the skin over the spine which stimulates a severe twitching of the lips in infected animals. The behavioural changes progress to overt neurological signs, in particular, pruritis, and local motor inco-ordination. Affected sheep continually nibble parts of the skin and rub or scrape against objects constantly. The appetite is not impaired and the affected ewes continue to nurse their lambs. The course of the overt disease lasts 1–2 months, a rapid weight loss occurring just before death. A few sheep die suddenly and unexpectedly, but others linger on for 6 months.

Pathology

There are no gross lesions other than self-inflicted wounds and broken fleeces. The prominent microscopic lesion is vacuolation of the grey matter of the brain without any signs of demyelination or inflammation. Ultra-structural studies of negatively stained detergent extracts of affected brain have revealed the presence of fibrils. These scrapie-associated fibrils or SAFs are not the scrapie agent, being derived from infected host cells. They have diagnostic significance. Another specific scrapie lesion is the production of cerebral amyloid.

Diagnosis

The presumptive diagnosis of scrapie is based upon the clinical signs and is relatively easy in countries where the disease is endemic. The diagnosis is confirmed by the histopathological demonstration of vacuolated neurons and the ultra-structural demonstration of SAFs.

Differential diagnosis

The early clinical signs of scrapie are readily confused with external parasitism from lice and mange mites. The neurological signs may be confused with visna, tick-borne encephalitides, pseudorabies and focal symmetrical encephalomalacia.

Immunology

Failure to identify the exact nature of the scrapie agent nullifies attempts to detect an host immune response despite early replication of the agent in the lymphoreticular system before infecting the brain and despite the fact that the disease only develops in immuno-competent animals.

Control

In endemic areas of Europe many commercial flocks are either apparently free of clinical scrapie or the prevalence is so low as to be of no economic significance. In other flocks 10-15 per cent of a flock may die from scrapie before the normal culling age is reached. Control of the disease, where necessary, may be achieved by slaughtering out whole maternal blood lines coupled with breeding flock replacements from aged ewes. Recently the use of thoroughly washed embryo-transplants has been advocated to break the cycle of infection.

Further reading

Kimberlin, R.H. (1981). Scrapie. *British Veterinary Journal*, **137**, 105–112.

SHEEP AND GOAT POX

Synonyms for sheep and goat pox include capripox, sheep pox, goat dermatitis and stone pox. Sheep and goat pox is a malignant pox of sheep and goats characterized by fever, cutaneous nodular pocks and visceral pocks. It has the reputation of being the most virulent pox disease of livestock, and epidemics in previously disease-free countries kill most affected animals.

Aetiology

Sheep and goat pox are caused by a single virus that is a member of the *Capripoxvirus* genus of the Poxviridae family, along with bovine lumpy skin disease virus. It is ether-sensitive and acid-labile. On the other hand, it is relatively heat-stable even at 37°C.

Isolates of sheep and goat pox virus vary widely in their host specificities; some readily infect sheep and goats, whereas others infect only sheep or only goats.

Occurrence

Sheep and goat pox is endemic in southern Europe, Africa north of the equator, in the Middle East, the Asian subcontinent and China. An ill-defined benign goat pox has been reported from Norway and California, but the clinical descriptions of this disease more closely resemble orf than sheep and goat pox.

Species affected

Natural infections of sheep and goat pox are restricted to sheep and goats, despite the fact that the virus is closely related to the virus of lumpy skin disease of cattle. Man is not susceptible.

Transmission

The various modes of transmission of sheep and goat pox virus are ill-defined. Although both direct and indirect contact occur, the virus is not highly infectious. The high prevalence of lung lesions in infected animals suggests the possibility of aerosol transmission. On the other hand, intradermal inoculation of the virus is the most effective way to infect sheep, suggesting that biting arthopods play a role in transmission. The virus will also enter through abraded skin, and sheep and goats may acquire infection by rubbing themselves against objects contaminated with saliva or lesion exudate deposited by infected sheep and goats. The practice of night-herding sheep and goats in stockades for their protection encourages transmission by any of the above routes.

A carrier state has yet to be confirmed. The hair and wool of recovered sheep and goats, however, is usually contaminated with the virus, and this contamination persists for many months.

Clinical features

The incubation period is 7 days or less. Clinical reactions may be peracute, acute, subacute or inapparent and mortality may vary from 5 to 80%. Lesions, as well as mortality, tend to be more severe in lambs than in adult sheep.

Peracute infections occur in indigenous lambs and in exotic sheep imported into an endemic area or affected in a wave of a virgin-soil epidemic. They are characterized by generalized haemorrhages, widespread cutaneous ulceration and death. The course is usually too short for pocks to develop.

The onset of acute reactions is sudden and manifested by a high fever, nasal and ocular discharges and salivation. Animals lose their appetite. Papules appear 24 hours later on mucous membranes and thin-skinned areas of the body. At first they are circumscribed, oedematous and hyperaemic. The number varies widely, but if the lesions are numerous they tend to become confluent. The appearance of the skin lesion varies; in some outbreaks they are vesicular, and in others they are nodular. The pocks in the upper respiratory and upper alimentary tracts erode and ulcerate. Within a week the high fever regresses and the papules exude and encrust. In the days that follow, the crust becomes a scab that gradually darkens. Irritation is intense and self-mutilation is common. Death may occur at any stage after the appearance of the pocks. Nodular lesions may be resorbed, indurate or heal by sit-fast formation within 5–6 weeks, leaving a permanent depressed scar. Naive pregnant sheep and goats abort.

Subacute reactions are often missed. The fevers are muted and transient and the lesions are often restricted to particular sites like the head and under the tail.

Clinical pathology

Studies on the clinical pathology of sheep and goat pox infection are conspicuous by their absence. An early leucocytosis is dramatically enhanced when the lesions necrose.

Pathology

The carcase is often emaciated and fetid. Pocks in the form of white nodules occur in many viscera as well as cutaneously. Mucosal lesions are ulcerated. The histological changes are typical and the detection of Borrel cells is regarded as being pathognomonic; they are found around blood vessels and between collagen bundles and are characterized by swollen cytoplasms with large vacuoles and large oval nuclei with enlarged nucleoli. Many of the Borrel cells and many epithelial cells contain eosinophilic intracytoplasmic inclusion bodies.

Diagnosis

A provisional diagnosis is based on the history of the outbreak, clinical signs and *post mortem* lesions, and confirmation is seldom sought in animals that die. In animals that survive, confirmation is essential to differentiate sheep and goat pox from orf. The preferred samples are early pocks.

Differential diagnosis

Other skin infections rarely exhibit the explosive character of virgin epidemics of sheep and goat pox, but in endemic areas orf, mange, streptothricosis and bluetongue often create difficulties in differential diagnosis. Electron microscopy is particularly valuable for differentiating sheep and goat pox virus from orf virus.

Immunology

Recovery from infection is associated with the production of antibodies. The antibodies, however, are not neutralizing antibodies, and passive protection is not conferred to the lamb in the colostrum. Resistance to the full effects of reinfection is attributed to cell-mediated immune mechanisms.

Control

Low-risk areas ensure their freedom from sheep and goat pox by prohibiting the importation of sheep and goats from endemic areas. In high-risk areas, control is difficult if herds and flocks are herded communally or are owned by nomads; infected animals should be destroyed and in-contact animals should be vaccinated. In countries where sheep and goat pox are endemic, prophylactic vaccination is recommended.

Many live and killed vaccines have been developed and used to control sheep and goat pox. Some are derived from strains of the virus that infect goats and sheep equally, some have been developed from sheep-specific strains and others from goat-specific strains. The best appear to be live attenuated vaccines that induce a good take in the vaccinated animal. Intradermal challenge of properly vaccinated animals results in accelerated immune reactions at the sites of challenge. The accelerated immune reactions are not associated with fever and do not cause abortion. Susceptible control animals challenged intradermally, develop febrile systemic reactions, generalized pocks and many die.

Further reading

Kitching, P. (1983). Progress towards sheep and goat pox vaccines. *Vaccine*, **21**, 4–9.

VESICULAR STOMATITIS

Vesicular stomatitis attacks horses, cattle and pigs in North, Central and South America, producing vesicles in the oral mucosa, in the skin over the coronary band and in the interdigital skin of the foot. It is a major cause of economic loss in dairy cattle. In addition, it is readily confused with foot-and-mouth disease in cattle and pigs.

Aetiology

The causal virus is a member of the *Vesiculovirus* genus and is the type virus of the Rhabdoviridae family of single-stranded RNA viruses. It is readily inactivated by temperatures above 60°C and by low and high hydrogen-ion concentrations. Common disinfectants are effective in destroying it. There are six distinct serotypes, two of which cycle in domestic animals, namely the New Jersey and Indiana serotypes.

Occurrence

The disease is endemic in the tropics and subtropics of the western hemisphere. Periodically, the disease extends northwards and southwards with dramatic results.

Species affected

The common natural domesticated hosts are horses, cattle and pigs. Sheep and goats are also susceptible, but they rarely contract the disease. Man is readily infected when handling affected animals or diagnostic specimens in the laboratory. The virus cycles in a wide variety of forest mammals, overspilling into domesticated animals seasonally at the time of maximal arthropod activity.

Transmission

The major mode of transmission of the Indiana serotype is through the bite of phlebotomine sand flies in which there is transovarial transmission. The New Jersey serotype is also believed to be transmitted by arthropods, but the specific species is unknown. Both serotypes are readily transmitted through skin abrasions, such as those caused by ill-fitting milking machine parts. Infective aerosols are responsible for most human infections.

Clinical features

Fever develops after an incubation period of 2–3 days. Simultaneously, circumscribed thin-walled vesicles erupt on the tongue, oral mucosa, along the coronary bands or in the interdigital skin. In lactating cows, the teats are a primary site of infection. In a given outbreak in a herd, the site of vesiculation is often a single location in all affected animals. Vesicles frequently coalesce and rupture leaving very shallow erosions which heal quickly. There is hypersalivation, anorexia, lameness and loss of condition. The occurrence of teat lesions is often followed by severe mastitis. The course of the uncomplicated disease is around 7–10 days. Death is not a sequel.

Vesicular stomatitis infections in man resemble influenza and usually resolve without complications. Encephalitis, however, has been reported.

Diagnosis and differential diagnosis

In countries free of foot-and-mouth disease, a presumptive diagnosis of vesicular stomatitis is readily made from the history and clinical signs. In countries at risk from foot-and-mouth disease, confirmation is essential to differentiate between it and vesicular stomatitis, bearing in mind that both conditions have occurred simultaneously in a herd. Specimens required are either the vesicular fluid or tissue scrapings from the area around the lesion. The examination of serum for antibodies is a useful supplementary aid for confirming a diagnosis.

Immunology

Recovery is associated with the appearance of humoral antibodies, but these do not prevent reinfection through skin abrasions. There is no cross-immunity between the two serotypes.

Control

Explosive outbreaks north and south of the endemic area are difficult to control. Affected animals should be nursed and rested and lesions soothed with emollients.

Prophylactic vaccination is used in dairy herds to prevent interruption of milk production. The vaccines are live attenuated viruses and are administered intramuscularly. Pigs are protected with inactivated vaccines.

Further reading

Knight, A.P. and Messar, N.T. (1983). Vesicular stomatitis. *Compendium on Continuing Education for the Practicing Veterinarian*, 5, S517–S522.

WESSELSBRON DISEASE

Wesselsbron disease is a mosquito-borne virus infection of sheep, cattle and man. The causal virus is widely distributed in southern Africa. On rare occasions, abortion storms in ewes and fatal febrile hepatitis in newborn lambs have been observed that mimic the clinical signs of Rift Valley fever.

Aetiology

Wesselsbron virus is a member of the *Flavivirus* genus of the Flaviviridae family of the single-stranded RNA viruses. It is not resistant to environmental stresses.

Occurrence

Serological surveys have shown that Wesseslbron virus is active throughout Africa south of the Sahara. Disease outbreaks, however, have only been observed in sheep, cattle and man in southern Africa.

Species affected

The natural hosts appear to be domestic and wild ruminants, wild ground-living birds, camels and man. The virus has also been isolated from the brain of a dog which was suspected to have had rabies. Horses, pigs and monkeys have been infected experimentally.

Transmission

The principal vectors are species of *Aedes* mosquitoes. Transplacental transmission is common in pregnant ruminants and lambs and calves have been with born antibodies, having recovered from an *in utero* infection. Stockmen, veterinarians and laboratory personnel are exposed to risk when they handle infected tissues, generating infective aerosols.

Clinical features

The vast majority of infections of ruminants with Wesselsbron virus are subclinical. A few adult sheep undergo subacute infections manifested by a transient low-grade fever, depression and anorexia. In contrast, infections in newborn lambs are much more severe. After an incubation period of less than 2 days, there is a sudden surge of fever which abates within 24 hours. Two days later, a second febrile wave occurs that persists for 2–3 days. Affected lambs are listless, weak, have staring coats, sunken flanks and respiratory distress, their respirations being abdominal in character. Occasionally, there is overt encephalitis. The mortality rate in newborn lambs approaches 30%.

Wesselsbron virus is both teratogenic and abortogenic. Infected ewes may abort, give birth to stillborn lambs or expel congenitally abnormal lambs. Lambs born alive from infected ewes may themselves be ill or have apparently recovered; the latter possess precolostral antibodies.

Most human infections are clinically inapparent, but laboratory-acquired infections tend to be overt. The illness consists of fever, headache, backache, and aching bones and joints. The convalescence is prolonged and there may be a residual disturbance of vision.

Pathology

The gross lesions in dead newborn lambs range from a mild to severe icterus and a slight to moderate hepatomegaly, the liver being yellow to orange-brown in colour with congested areas distributed throughout. In addition, there is a generalized lymphadenopathy and the mucosa of the abomasum contains petechiae and ecchymoses. Microscopic examination of the liver reveals the presence of intracytoplasmic and intranuclear inclusions in many necrotic hepatocytes.

Diagnosis and differential diagnosis

The clinical signs of Wesselsbron virus infections in newborn lambs and pregnant ewes resemble Rift Valley fever so closely that differentiation in the field is impossible. Confirmation requires the isolation and serological identification of the virus, the tissues required being brain and liver.

Immunology

Recovered animals are immune for life. Workers in West Africa have suggested that the absence of reported clinical cases there may be due to the presence of other flavivirus antibodies in the sera of domestic animals.

Control

Clinical episodes are so rare that control measures are seldom undertaken. An attenuated virus vaccine is available commercially in South Africa, and it may be used alone or in combination with Rift Valley fever vaccine. It should not be administered to pregnant animals.

Further reading

Barnard, B.J.H. and Voges, S.F. (1986). Flaviviruses in South Africa. *Onderstepoort Journal of Veterinary Research*, 53, 235–238.

Other diseases

A.N. Morrow and M.M.H. Sewell

EQUINE ANHIDROSIS

Inability to sweat even after severe exercise (anhidrosis), which occurs in some horses in the humid tropics.

Aetiology

This breakdown in acclimatization to a hot humid climate is thought to be multi-factorial in origin, probably involving physiological inhibition or malfunction of the sweat glands due to prolonged stimulation or overstimulation with secondary endocrine or electrolyte derangement.

Occurrence

Anhidrosis has been encountered in all types of riding horses in areas where a warm climate is accompanied by long periods of high atmospheric humidity, including parts of India, the Far East and the Caribbean. When there are marked annual variations in temperature and humidity, the disease tends to be seasonal, being most common during hot weather and in the wetter months. Cases may be encountered throughout the year in countries where the temperature and humidity are consistently high.

Species affected

The condition is more commonly encountered in horses imported from temperate countries,though it has been reported in horses bred in hot humid climates. Arab horses may be less susceptible.

Clinical features

The first sign is usually tachypnoea after exercise and there may be excessive sweating at this stage. However, the areas in which sweating occurs become restricted over a few weeks or months and are eventually limited to a few places such as the brisket, under the saddle, the perineum and the crest of the neck. Partial anhidrosis may occur.

The body temperature is raised even at rest and after severe exercise may reach 40.5°C. The coat develops a harsh, dry appearance and in severe cases loss of hair may occur, especially on the face, sides and neck. Affected horses become progressively more unfit for fast work and may show signs of distress after only moderate exercise. The appetite may become capricious and polyuria may be noticed. Sudden death may occur during or immediately after severe exertion.

Pathology

There are no characteristic lesions and the sweat glands are histologically normal.

Diagnosis

The disease can be recognized from the history and clinical signs. The injection of 0.5 ml of 1:1000 epinephrine fails to elicit the normal localized patch of sweating.

Treatment

Affected animals should be exercised only moderately and in the cooler part of the day. Steps should be taken to reduce the heat load by providing well-ventilated or air-conditioned housing, hosing the animal with water and feeding a light diet made up largely of green fodder, bran and chaff. Transferring affected animals to a cooler environment usually leads to a considerable improvement.

There is no consistently effective chemotherapy, although oral administration of a commercial electrolyte mixture has been reported to lead to some improvement in about half the cases treated.

M.M.H.S.

EPIZOOTIC LYMPHANGITIS

Epizootic lymphangitis is an infectious equine disease which, in its classical form, is characterized by nodules and chronic suppurating ulcers on the skin with inflammation of the associated lymphatic vessels and nodes.

Aetiology

It is caused by the yeast-like tissue form of the dimorphic fungus, *Histoplasma farciminosum*. The organism forms mycelia in the external environment and is relatively resistant to ambient conditions.

Occurrence

The disease prevails in an endemic form in some countries of West, North and North-East Africa and the Middle East. It is also reported from the Indian subcontinent and the Far East.

Species affected

The infection is restricted to horses, mules and rarely donkeys.

Transmission

The incidence is high only when large numbers of animals are collected together, as transmission usually involves infection of wounds by flies contaminated by feeding on open lesions on infected animals. Contaminated grooming kits and saddlery can also be responsible. When animals are individually owned and stabled, the disease remains sporadic.

Clinical features

Lesions consist of nodules and abscesses on the skin and mucous membranes and are most commonly found on the head, neck, shoulders and limbs. The chronic nature of individual lesions is one of the most striking features of the disease.

The first sign of infection consists of a small, painless swelling. The subcutaneous tissue around the nodule becomes oedematous, raising the nodule above the surface of the skin. The nodule gradually enlarges, softens and finally bursts, discharging a thick oily yellow pus. The local superficial lymphatic vessels draining the area become enlarged and prominent, and small swellings appear on the enlarged vessels. The new nodules eventually rupture and the disease continues to spread along the lymphatics.

Individual lesions become larger, the flow of pus increases, and a chronic granulating ulcer develops at the point of rupture over a period of 10 days, after which the discharge thickens and eventually hardens into a scab. A few days later the scab is sloughed off and another flow of pus occurs. The process is repeated several times with the ulcer becoming slightly larger on each occasion until after 6–8 weeks when the granulating surface may be over 1 inch in diameter. The lesions heal slowly. Scab formation and sloughing continue, but each time the ulcerated surface is a little smaller until finally only a scar remains. The development and regression of a lesion may take up to 3 months.

More serious lesions occur when large lymph nodes are involved. Small abscesses are formed within the nodes and these eventually coalesce to form huge subcutaneous swellings, often projecting several inches from the surface of the body. The swellings, which are extremely painful, eventually rupture through the skin, discharging large quantities of thick bloodstained yellow pus. A granulating fistula persists for some time, continually discharging pus. Healing finally occurs after many weeks. The general health of the animal is usually otherwise unaltered.

Pathology

The lesions, as described, are usually confined to the skin and subcutaneous tissue. The lymphatic ducts are greatly enlarged and often surrounded by thick layers of fibrous tissue. The enlarged ducts are filled with thick yellow pus. Primary infection of the lungs, the nasal mucosa and the conjunctiva has been recorded. Histological examination shows the presence of the tissue phase of the organism, especially in the cytoplasm of macrophages.

Diagnosis

An advanced typical case showing "cording" of the lymphatics and progressive ulceration is highly suggestive of the disease in areas of endemic infection, but confirmation of the diagnosis requires microscopic demonstration of the lemon-shaped, yeast-like cells in pus, preferably from an unopened abscess. These may be seen in wet preparations but are best stained with Claudius, Gram or Giemsa. The organism may be grown in culture on Sabouraud's dextrose agar containing 2.5% glycerol, Brain Heart Infusion agar with horse blood added, or on dextrose, glycerol PPLO medium. Growth is slow, with colonies of the organism, in its mycelial form, appearing after 4–8 weeks when cultured at 25°C. Conversion to the yeast form occurs if subcultured four or five times at 8-day intervals on BHI agar containing 5% blood at 35–37°C.

In areas where the disease is endemic, chronic nasal discharge and conjunctivitis should be regarded with suspicion and smears prepared from the discharges. A post-mortem examination may be necessary to give a definitive diagnosis of lung involvement. Cording is seen only a considerable time after infection and routine examination of wounds in areas of endemic disease will frequently reveal infection. Many of these recover spontaneously without showing any of the classical signs.

Skin tests and various serological tests including complement fixation tests, agglutination tests, immunodiffusion, ELISA and indirect immunofluorescence have been described as an aid to diagnosis.

The disease can be confused with cutaneous glanders (farcy), but a mallein test will differentiate, and with ulcerative lymphangitis, which is more acute and is caused by *Corynebacterium pseudotuberculosis*.

Treatment

Treatment of clinical cases is often unsuccessful. In endemic areas where slaughter is not always possible sodium iodide intravenously, excision of the lesions where feasible, administration of antifungal drugs or a combination of these methods may be attempted, but recurrences up to a year later are common.

Clotrimazole inhibits growth of the organism in culture.

Immunology

Most infected animals show well-marked allergic reactions to the injection of culture filtrates of the fungus. Spontaneous recovery sometimes occurs and complete immunity results. An experimental heat attenuated vaccine is claimed to give a degree of protection.

Control

The disease can be eradicated by isolation and slaughter, but in most areas where it is endemic this is not possible. Nevertheless, destruction should be advocated in advanced cases. Control measures should include early effective isolation or disposal of infected horses, protection of wounds from flies, cleaning and disinfection of infected stalls and equipment and control of fly breeding. Steps should be taken to avoid tick sores, saddle galls and other injuries and materials used for dressing wounds must be destroyed immediately.

A.N.M.

HORN CANCER

Horn cancer is a carcinomatous condition, which affects the horn base of zebu cattle. It usually manifests itself as highly vascular excrescences of squamous epithelial tissue.

Aetiology

The precise cause is unknown, but an associated impairment in cell-mediated immunity has been shown to be caused by a humoral factor which affects the T-lymphocytes. Most cases have a history of previous mechanical injury to the horn. Chronic irritation from the use of "head-ropes" for securing the long-horned animals or from practices such as paring or polishing the external layers of the horn may be predisposing factors. The high prevalence in adult castrates suggests that a hormonal mechanism may be involved.

Occurrence

The condition is largely confined to India, but cases have been reported in Zebu cattle in Indonesia, Iraq and South America. Similar but probably unrelated conditions have been described in sheep, goats and rhinoceroses and also in cattle in the Sudan.

Species affected

In India, horn cancer affects about 1–2% of 5-to 10-year-old bullocks with prominent horns. It is less common in cows and buffaloes, rare in bulls and not seen in young cattle. It affects all breeds, but the prevalence is relatively high in the Hariana cattle breed.

Clinical features

The earliest sign is a slight drooping of the horn at its base. This deformity increases until the horn bends downwards and becomes loose. It then becomes detached from the skin at its base, exposing the horn core. This usually presents as highly vascular greyish or yellowish nodular excrescences which are covered with foul-smelling mucoid or bloodstained exudate. If the neoplasm has invaded the frontal sinus, there is an intermittent purulent rhinorrhoea. Ophthalmia and opacity of the cornea are infrequent concommitant features.

Constitutional disturbances are generally absent, but as the condition advances the animal shows uneasiness and becomes emaciated. In neglected cases death may occur due to toxaemia, maggot infestation and secondary bacterial infection.

Pathology

There is a squamous-cell carcinoma of the horn epithelium with characteristic keratinized "cell nests". Metastatic spread to the regional lymph nodes is common and further spread to organs such as the lungs and liver may occur, particularly in longstanding cases.

Diagnosis

Diagnosis is fairly easy in characteristic cases in which the cauliflower-like growths at the horn base and the other clinical features occur. The similar condition in Sudanese cattle is restricted to the interior of the horn core but may be suspected if the animal shakes or tilts its head or persistently rubs its horns on fixed objects. Confirmatory diagnosis is by histological examination of biopsy tissue.

Treatment

Early cases may respond to surgical excision provided there has been no invasion of the internal organs. Irrigation of the frontal sinus with acid-pepsin solution may be advantageous. A combination of surgery and immunotherapy with a saline-phenol allogeneic extract may be successful in more advanced cases.

Control

Dehorning young long-horned animals, particularly those with a familial history of horn cancer, is probably the most reliable measure.

Further reading

Chauhan, H.V.S., Kalva, D.S. and Mahajan, S.K. (1980). Studies on horn cancer preliminary trials of immunotherapy. *Australian Veterinary Journal*, **56**, 509–510.

Naik, S.N., Balakrishnan, C.R. and Randelia, H.P. (1969). Epidemiology of horn cancer in Indian Zebu cattle. *British Veterinary Journal*, **125**, 222–230.

M.M.H.S.

Index